| DATE DUE | | | |
|---|---|---|---|
| | | | |
| | | | |
| | | | |
| | | | |
| | | | |
| | | | |
| | | | |
| | | | |
| | | | |
| | | | |
| | | | |
| | | | |
| | | | |
| | | | |

# Cellular Controls
# in Differentiation

*Based on the Unilever Jubilee
Symposium held in Vlaardingen,
Holland during December 1980*

# Cellular Controls
# in Differentiation

Edited by
Clive W Lloyd
David A Rees
*Unilever Research, Colworth Laboratory,
Sharnbrook, Bedford, England*

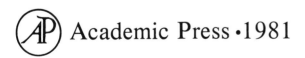 Academic Press •1981

*A Subsidiary of Harcourt Brace Jovanovich, Publishers*
London  New York  Toronto  Sydney  San Francisco

ACADEMIC PRESS INC. (LONDON) LTD
24/28 Oval Road
London NW1


*United States Edition published by*
ACADEMIC PRESS INC
111 Fifth Avenue
New York, New York 10003

*574.87*
*C33*
*12 6738*
*nov.1983*

*British Library Cataloguing in Publication Data*
Cellular controls in differentiation.
1. Cell differentiation - Congresses.
I. Lloyd, C.W. II. Rees, D.A.
574.1'7      QH607
ISBN 0-12-453580-1

LCCCN 81-67883

Designed by Ken Allan and Claire Jones
Unilever Research, Colworth Laboratory, Bedford

Printed in Great Britain

# Contributors

**Sydney Brenner** MRC Laboratory of Molecular Biology, University Medical School, Hills Road, Cambridge CB2 2QH

**Klaus Weber and Mary Osborn** Max Planck Institute for Biophysical Chemistry, D-3400 Goettingen, FRG

**Antti Vaheri and Kari Alitalo** Department of Virology, University of Helsinki, Haartmaninkatu 3, SF-00290 Helsinki 29, Finland

**Mark C Willingham and Ira H Pastan** Laboratory of Molecular Biology, National Cancer Institute, Bethesda, Maryland 20205, USA

**Philip Cohen** Department of Biochemistry, University of Dundee, Dundee DD1 4HN, Scotland

**Philip Coffino** Department of Medicine and Microbiology, S-412, University of California, San Francisco, California 94143, USA

**Donald Metcalf** Cancer Research Unit, Walter and Eliza Institute for Medical Research, Royal Melbourne Hospital, PO 3050, Victoria, Australia

**Natalie M Teich and Janice Rowe** Imperial Cancer Research Fund, Lincoln's Inn Fields, London WC2A 3PX

**Nydia G Testa and T Michael Dexter** Peterson Laboratories, Manchester M20 9BX, England

**Arthur H Pardee and Ruth Sager** Sidney Farber Cancer Institute and Harvard Medical School, Departments of Pharmacology and Microbiology, 44 Binney Street, Boston, Massachusetts 02115, USA

**Bohdan Wasylyk, Claude Kedinger, Jeff Corden, Paulo Sassone-Corsi and Pierre Chambon** Laboratoire de Genetique Moleculaire des Eucaryotes du CNRS, Unite 184 de Biologie Moleculaire et de Genie Genetique de l'INSERM, Institut de Chimie Biologique, Faculté de Médicine, 11 Rue Humann, 67085 Strasbourg, France

**Piet Borst** Section for Medical Enzymology and Molecular Biology, Laboratory of Biochemistry, University of Amsterdam, Jan Swannerdam Institute, Box 60,000,1005 GA Amsterdam, The Netherlands

**Richard L Gardner** Sir William Dunn School of Pathology, South Parks Road, Oxford OX1 3RE, England

**Harvey Eisen, R Gjersen and S Hasthorpe** Unité d'Immunoparasitologie, Institut Pasteur, Paris, France

**Antonio Garcia-Bellido** Centro de Biologia Molecular, (Consejo Superior de Investigaciones Cientificas), Universidad Autónoma de Madrid, Spain

# Preface

This volume is based on the proceedings of a Symposium organised by Unilever to mark its Jubilee Year - the fiftieth anniversary of our formation by the merger of two groups of Companies, one Dutch and the other British, in 1930. We chose the subject 'Cellular Controls in Differentiation' because biological issues have always been prominent in our own Research and Development, and because this particular topic holds great intellectual challenge - promising even more excitement as our understanding of cellular mechanisms continues to unfold. We were very pleased that a wide range of distinguished speakers and guests were able to join us at our Vlaardingen Laboratory in the Netherlands, December 14-18 1980, to take stock of present understanding.

In addition to the conceptual advances, we can - in due course - expect practical implications to emerge from this area of research, for society and for Unilever. However we did not feel it appropriate for this Symposium to dwell upon possible industrial application - instead we have concentrated on the underlying scientific principles. In so doing, we would like to acknowledge the contribution that has been made to the success of Unilever over its first fifty years by advances in fundamental science, and show our belief in the importance of a lively scientific community for the future of our own and other industries. With this in mind, it is hoped that by meeting the costs of the Symposium and subsidising the volume, the proceedings will reach a wider readership than would otherwise be possible.

Differentiation - the process whereby cells act out just part of their gene-encoded repertoire according to spatial and temporal cues - is undoubtedly complex. Because of this, as Sydney Brenner points out in his Keynote Address, its complete understanding will probably first require the solution to many subsidiary problems of cellular behaviour. In this Symposium we have attempted to sample just such a broad range of disciplines: from molecular to development biology.

Topics were selected which are showing particular progress and which -

because of the increased understanding they offer - are producing echoes in previously distant fields. It is hoped that some of this interdisciplinary excitement will emerge both from the juxtaposition of papers and from question periods.

Undoubtedly, there are so many strands yet to be discovered that we cannot hope to draw any more than a patchy picture of tissue differentiation from selected fragments of current science. But our grasp of cell structure and function has improved so very quickly, and on such a broad front over the last decade that it is tempting to feel that we are at the edge of a new era of intellectual synthesis. It is for this reason that we feel it appropriate to take stock of some of the areas from which are likely to emerge the elements of a total understanding of cellular differentiation.

August 1981                                                    C. W. Lloyd
                                                               D. A. Rees

# Contents

# 1
# Keynote Address

# Genes and Development

*Sydney Brenner*

Mr Chairman, Minister, Ladies and Gentlemen. Our meeting today celebrates the fiftieth anniversary of Unilever, and it gives me great pleasure to open the proceedings. I am older than Unilever and I assume they are expecting wise advice; however, since I am only a little older I will not be able to tell you much you do not already know. During the past fifty years biological science has undergone a number of revolutionary changes and the pace of change increases every day. Not only have our powers of analysis increased by the acquisition of a vast array of new techniques, but with the discovery of a range of cloning methods, both cellular and molecular, it is said that biology has entered a new, synthetic phase: that of the construction of organisms. Genetic and cellular engineering and their possible benefits for us are widely discussed both in the technical and lay press and there are now many efforts to exploit and apply the new molecular biology to medicine, agriculture and industry.

So much has been written about genetic engineering and changing organisms in a directed way that many people may think that there is now nothing further to do. On the contrary, the subject is still in its infancy and, in fact, I claim that in one particular sense it does not yet exist. The essence of engineering is *design* and it is the implementation of a *plan* that distinguishes the engineer from the tinkerer and separates intentional human activity from the chance events of nature. Today, no-one can order a new organism like a unicorn, or a dragon, or a centaur, because nobody knows how to design one, let alone build it. Consider the centaur. It is a very old mythical beast and the man who first drew one simply cut off the torso of a man and stuck it onto the bottom of a decapitated horse. This is not genetic engineering but hopeful transplantation surgery, and you could not make real centaurs that way. In addition, it only takes a little reflection about the internal anatomy of this animal to realise that there are intractable problems about connecting two pairs of lungs and two cardiovascular systems, two digestive systems and two spinal cords with two sets of forelimbs. Even if we resolved such physiological and anatomical contradictions the real question is not that of making it by grafting but whether anybody could actually write down the specifications in a genetic form from which centaurs could be made. It is not possible to do this for real organisms above a certain level of complexity let alone for fantastic beasts and it is clear the central problems of mythical biology are the same as those of real biology.

The remarkable paradox is that we know that the total explanation of all organisms already resides within them. Biological systems are elaborate systems of a very particular kind containing within themselves an internal representation in the form of their genetic material. I do not wish to call this a *program*. We tend to talk loosely about genetic programs and we should be careful about the implications of this language even when used metaphorically. In most present-day computing systems programs are encoded in the imperative. They say *Do, Add, Read, Write*. The human programmer delivers instructions to the machine and it is a very particular machine, acting sequentially in time, largely doing one thing at any one moment. Do genes encode the imperative? Is there anything in our genomes that could be the Make-a-Hand program? Or even *called* this? The genome could be more like a *menu* than a *program* and, moreover, it could be like a Chinese menu in which the courses could be eaten in any order or even together, rather than like a French menu which carries with it a strict temporal order. This is just another way of saying that perhaps a better computer metaphor to think about in connection with biological systems is that of an information retrieval system rather than one which performs calculations and perhaps the elementary activity of biological systems is more like function evaluation rather than instruction.

The difficulties we have in talking about biological systems at this level can be more easily seen by the following consideration. We could say 'It's perfectly simple; all we have to do is to work out the entire DNA sequence of any organism and there is the total explanation'. We may imagine someone standing up at some future conference to declare 'I will now tell you everything about *Drosophila*' and then proceeding to intone 'A G G C T T A' and so on for $10^8$ or so bases. For small viruses or for mitochondria, this would make sense but for organisms of the complexity of *Drosophila* the sequence would be largely meaningless. The syntax would be there but the semantics would be absent. And here is the heart of the matter; we will only understand the internal representation when we discover how it maps onto the structure and function of organisms and only when this is known will we be able to begin to think of designing and building new organisms.

Is there a general answer to this question of mapping genetic space onto organismic space? It would be very important and interesting if there were some set of rules which we could use to analyse the problem. It has often been said that we might be able to decompose it into two: one concerning a *logical* relationship between genome and organism, and another, more mechanistic, connection which will involve the details of gene structure and expression and the functions of gene products. The first, it has been suggested, might be revealed by careful genetic experiments interpreted by clever geneticists. However, for a successful interpretation we need to know whether organisms have a general organisational structure in the logical sense and we should realise that this may not necessarily be connected with their morphology. Perhaps this rather opaque statement can best be illustrated by examples taken from simple systems. Let us consider *Escherichia coli* growing on a simple medium. Every 30 minutes each bacterium must take another one, synthesising a large number of complicated molecules from simple components, copying a DNA accurately and then partitioning everything into two cells. This is accomplished by a few thousand different chemical reactions, all carried out simultaneously and mixed up in a very small space. At first sight, this seems a totally intractable problem. Thus, not so long ago, it was argued that the enzymes composing a sequential biosynthetic pathway would need to be assembled into one structure so that each enzyme could hand over its product to the next one to ensure efficiency. For electron transfer this still seems to be true but such an 'assembly line' model is no longer tenable for most small molecule pathways. How is it then accomplished? The answer is that in the small volume of a bacterium diffusion is fast enough to put most small molecules everywhere; the transit time for a molecule of molecular weight 500 is about 1 msec. The elementary event in the system is a molecular collision and even though most of these for a given substrate involve the wrong enzyme or even the wrong place on the right one, the number of random collisions is nevertheless so large that a substrate will hit a binding site with reasonable frequency. The binding site is the *heart of the matter*, unlike a computer where a signal is sent from one part to another by a wire connecting the two, the bacterium does not have physical addresses and uses a *broadcast* system instead with *logical* addresses; each enzyme simply ignores the irrelevant messages and only those fitting its binding site are retained and acted upon. It is this special hardware that enables the bacterium to be an effective multiple parallel system without paying an enormous tax in elaborate wiring diagrams. Similar arguments apply to the control systems, and it is easy to show that regulation works on the basis of locally controlled anarchic demons bound together only by a global property of resource partitioning in which greed is punished by death. There is no master control, a single supervisor or monitor, as some might once have assumed, based on intuitive experience of man-made systems.

The same applies to a problem like bacteriophage morphogenesis. We now know that the shape and structure of something like phage T4 is not explicitly and uniquely represented in its genome; and there are no guiding jigs or hands which build the structure in the cell and which need to be separately specified. The key process is *self-assembly* which depends on the *bonding properties* of many different protein molecules so that the representation of the structure is *distributed* over many genes in the DNA. Thus, until we discovered the construction paradigm of viruses no sense could be made of the genetic specification of virus structure.

If we now return to more elaborate organisms, those which contain many different cells all generated from one egg, to search for a general organisational principle, we should be careful not to rely too much on intuition or experience with man-made systems. The rules we think inevitable for systems of some complexity may not be universal principles but simply reflect the limitations of our own minds. We tend to be more at home with hierarchical structures and sequential processes and it is common to find these in many models of development and its genetic control. The following should serve to show the difficulties faced by general arguments about complex systems. It has been supposed that the organism must be partitioned in some way to give it a modular structure. The basis of this could in principle be anything - anatomical parts, or physiological systems, or developmental pathways. It is these modules that would be the logical basis for the internal genetic representation. Indeed the explicit basis could be provided by the mechanism of a 'master control gene', one governing each module. Such hypotheses are very familiar. Modular representation is not only appealing for control purposes but there are also advantages for a complex system undergoing evolutionary change. Large computer programs are always organised on a modular basis in order to localise stringently the effects of any changes. If this were not so, a change would have ramifying unpredictable effects and the debugging process would be impossible. Thus by analogy it is argued that the genes are also arranged in closed logical packets allowing changes to take place in one subsystem without affecting the others. Notice such systems minimise the complexity of control information at the expense of the duplication of low level actions: if the latter are cheap, this is a good way to do it. You may recall that the existence of isozymes has been thought to reflect this modular organisation. However, there is a different general argument equally plausible on general principles, which gives a different answer.

Suppose there are no completely disjoint sets of genes but that most genes participate in all, or many, developmental processes. These, we assume, are structured in two layers: one set of *kernel* processes which are inaccurate and another set of *refinement* processes which can reduce and compensate for the unreliability of the first. It can be argued that at a given level of complexity biological processes must be intrinsically noisy. Thus it is not possible with the existing molecular hardware for a cell reproducibly to synthesise a set of exact numbers of molecules of one protein. This has to be approximated by adding a feedback control mechanism which can set different levels but with a statistical variance. Crystallographers are familiar with this in their work where, because of intrinsic errors in methods, they aim first at a messy 'ballpark' answer and then progressively improve this by a series of refinements. What is important is that refinement can be done by a linear optimisation process which makes small random changes in any component followed by the measurement of a global value such as an energy minimum. If the *sign* of the change is positive the state is retained, else it is rejected. Such systems can find an optimum but do not need to take particular account of any intricate internal structure in achieving this end; they have distinct advantages for evolution. Thus, one begins with a messy, inaccurate 'sort of fly' which is then progressively refined into a fly. Of course, in this process many changes will have 'unpredictable' consequences, but, unlike computer programming, natural selection is cheap and has plenty of time to work.

These examples should serve to illustrate the difficulty of general arguments for complex biological systems, but this does not mean that they are futile. Thus, in each of the cases discussed above there will be different consequences for mutations of various genes. I doubt whether there is enough evidence to decide between them but it is worthwhile emphasising that a large number of mutations produced experimentally in higher organisms yield animals with variable phenotype: many mutants of *Drosophila* are referred to as having poor penetrance or low expressivity. And of course we should remember that when there are two models to distinguish, the possibility that both are wrong should also be considered.

From these considerations and others based on our own experimental work, I am drawn inexorably to the conclusion that it is unlikely that we will easily find general principles of wide application to the developmental and other problems of higher organisms. It seems that answers to questions about the relation between genomes and complex organisms will come from detailed knowledge of the structure and expression of individual genes and from an insight of how their products participate in the biochemical and cellular processes underlying development. The advent of gene cloning as an analytical tool, coupled with the application of powerful biochemical methods to good experimental systems now makes it feasible to tackle a large number of questions in higher organisms and pursue them to some depth. This may sound like a typically conservative - some might even say reactionary - molecular biological approach but I venture to predict that not only can it be done this way but that it will be done this way. If science is the art of the soluble, molecular biology is the art of the inevitable.

# 2
# Cell Morphology

That interaction between cells and their surrounding matrix is important for the maintenance of tissues has been known for a long time to embryologists but now appears to be moving rapidly towards a molecular explanation.

For instance, it is now established that many of the social properties of cells (their morphology, contact and growth behaviour) can be attributed to some interaction between fibrillar extracellular proteins and proteins which are organised into skeletal assemblies in the cytoplasm.

In this first section Drs Weber & Osborn and Vaheri & Alitalo present different sides of the cytoskeleton/pericellular matrix interaction which is beginning to provide a deeper understanding of key properties of metazoan development.

# Aspects of the Cytoskeleton of Mammalian Cells

*Klaus Weber and Mary Osborn*

## Introduction

Some progress has been made towards the understanding of the organisation and dynamics of the cytoplasm by concentrating on the three fibrous systems: microfilaments, microtubules and intermediate filaments. During the last ten years biochemical and structural studies have greatly expanded our knowledge of the function, composition and turnover of these structures. Two whole-mount techniques have made a major impact. The high voltage electron microscope has strongly emphasised the three-dimensionality of interconnecting fibrous organisations. The use of immunofluorescence microscopy using antibodies specific for the individual structural proteins has been a very rewarding way to do structural analysis on the light microscopical level.

The ability to retain a good deal of the structured cytoplasm in whole-mounts extracted with non-ionic detergents has led to preparations, often described as the *cytoskeleton*. As suitable as cytoskeletons are for structural, immunological and biochemical studies, they necessarily emphasise a rather static picture. The live cell, however, is characterised by dynamics and a high degree of ordered turnover and transition, which are not conveyed by the term *cytoskeleton*. Thus it is important to remember that the true cellular structure is poorly described by the word cytoskeleton. Here we concentrate on some novel aspects of microfilaments, microtubules and intermediate filaments as the major part of the cytoskeleton.

## Microfilaments

### Cells in Culture

Microfilaments were clearly identified by electron microscopical analysis as F-actin based structures, since they could be specifically labelled by heavy meromyosin in permeable cell models (Ishikawa *et.al.* 1969). Since then an ever increasing number of experiments showed a complex structure of F-actin filaments together with a variety of important associated proteins (see Table 1). Probably the major impact in the continuing attempt to unravel the 'proteinchemical anatomy' of the microfilament organisation has come from the introduction of immunofluorescence microscopy into cell biology (Lazarides and Weber 1974). This procedure provided the possibility of recognising the typical features of a cytoplasmic organisation in many cells simultaneously at the light microscopical level and was quickly exploited. Thus the often dominant microfilament bundles of various cultured cells ('stress fibres') were shown to contain myosin, the intracellular organisation of which had not been found in previous electron microscopical studies (Weber and Groeschel-Stewart 1974). In agreement with a possible function as 'cytomuscular structures' immunofluorescence microscopy revealed the presence of tropomyosin, $\alpha$-actinin, filamin, vinculin and fimbrin (Lazarides 1976; Lazarides and Burridge 1975; Wang et.al. 1975; Geiger 1979; Bretscher and Weber 1980a) as constituents of the stress fibres, which show ATP-dependent shortening in membrane-free cell models (Isenberg et.al. 1976).

Immunofluorescence microscopy, and later also biochemical studies, showed distinct differences for various microfilament organisations in the number and type of associated proteins present. Thus upon transition from the stress fibres to the highly motile ruffling edge one observes a wealth of filamin, $\alpha$-

**Table 1**

Proteinchemical anatomy of different microfilament types (March 1980)

| Protein | Tissue Culture Cells | | Intestinal Epithelium | | |
|---|---|---|---|---|---|
| | Stress fibres | Ruffles | Vaccinia-induced specialised 'macrovilli' | Terminal web | Microvilli |
| Filamin (250K) | + | + | + | + | — |
| Myosin (heavy chain 220K) | + | — | — | + | — |
| Vinculin (130K) | + | ? | ? | + | ? |
| Microvillus cross-bridge (110K) | ? | ? | ? | — | + |
| $\alpha$-actinin (100K) | + | + | + | + | — |
| Villin (95K)? | | | | | |
| Gelsolin? | —? | —? | — | + | + |
| Fimbrin (65K) | (+) | + | + | + | + |
| Actin (43K) | + | + | + | + | + |
| Tropomyosin (30K) | + | — | — | + | — |
| Calmodulin (16K) | +? | ? | ? | ? | + |

Gelsolin (95K)
Actinogelin (95K) } not determined
Profilin (16K)

actinin and fimbrin, and an at least relative loss of myosin and tropomyosin (Heggeness *et.al.* 1977; Lazarides 1976; Bretscher and Weber 1980a). This may reflect the importance of gel-sol transitions as the basis of mechanochemical events in addition to normal acto-myosin dependent undirectional shortening (for a review see Stossel 1978; Taylor and Condeelis 1979).

*Microvilli*
The intestinal epithelium is a particularly rewarding system for the study of microfilaments. The polarized cells carry on their apical side some thousand microvilli, each containing a highly oriented bundle of some 20 parallel F-actin filaments. The filaments extend from the tip of the microvillus (end-on attachment to the membrane) deep into the perpendicularly oriented terminal web microfilament system, which is associated with the *zonula adherens* junctions. The upper part of the cell (the 'brush border') is therefore dominated by two microfilament organisations: the terminal web system and the microvillus core organisation (for a review see Hull and Staehelin 1979).

The brush border can be isolated and membrane-enclosed microvilli can be derived from them. These microvilli still show lateral membrane association of the core filaments via slender sidearms or crossbridges (side-on attachment) as well as end-on association at the tip). Use of non-ionic detergents provides a clean preparation of ultrastructurally intact core filament bundles (Bretscher and Weber 1978). These contain F-actin and four major associated proteins (Matsudaira and Burgess 1979; Bretscher and Weber 1980a,b; Howe *et.al.* 1980). The actin is composed of the two cytoplasmic actin species $\beta$ and $\alpha$, typically found in all non-muscle cells. Thus both forms can participate in bundle formation. The 110K protein, although not yet purified, is assumed to be responsible for the 20-30nm crossbridges connecting the F-actin bundle with the inner side of the plasma membrane (Matsudaira and Burgess 1979). The 95K protein (villin) has been purified using its ability to bind in a $Ca^{++}$-dependent fashion to monoeric actin. It is a $Ca^{++}$-binding protein (dissociation constant $\mu M$) which, in the absence of $Ca^{++}$, bundles F-actin into structures reminiscent of the core filament bundle. Upon addition of $Ca^{++}$ villin shows a conformational transition and acts phenotypically as a F-actin 'severing' protein giving rise to short individual F-actin filaments (Bretscher and Weber 1980b; Glenney *et.al.* 1980). This $Ca^{++}$-dependent transition between 'severing' and 'bundling' will be discussed below. The third major associated protein of the core filament bundle is fimbrin with a molecular weight of 68,000. Although its functional role remains unknown, it is the first microfilament-associated protein found predominantly in motile cellular protrusions such as ruffles, microvilli and microspikes (Bretscher and Weber 1980a). The fourth associated protein has been identified as calmodulin (Howe *et.al.* 1980; Glenney *et.al.* 1980), the general eukaryotic $Ca^{++}$ regulatory protein of various key enzymatic processes including adenylate cyclase, cyclic AMP phosphodiesterase and various protein kinases among which is myosin light chain kinase (reviewed by Cheung 1980). Several ideas about the importance of calmodulin in core filament bundles are entertained. One approach (Howe *et al.* 1980) discusses the possibility that calmodulin may be translocated to the terminal web, where it activates myosin kinase. This enzyme could activate the F-actin dependent myosin ATPase activity, which should be intimately related with microfilament contractility (Yerna *et. al.* 1979). Alternatively calmodulin may display some of its usual enzyme-related functions and in addition, as a strong $Ca^{++}$-binding protein, may modulate the free cytosolic $Ca^{++}$ concentration around the core filament bundle. Such a function seems necessary, since otherwise $Ca^{++}$ influx into the cell could activate the severing function of villin thus leading to destruction of the highly $Ca^{++}$ sensitive structure of the core filament bundle (Glenney *et.al.* 1980). In addition, calmodulin seems to interact with the 110K crossbridge protein of the microvillus (Glenney and Weber 1980). The 110K protein could also have an ATPase activity, however, this possibility has so far not been explored (Matsudaira and Burgess 1979).

The small number of major structural proteins of the microvillus core makes this system especially attractive for reconstitution experiments and a study of microfilament-membrane anchorage. That the system reveals $Ca^{++}$ control and contains at least two $Ca^{++}$-binding proteins is a further advantage. The insertion of the microvillus cores into the terminal web microfilaments, which intermingle with intermediate filaments (cytokeratins; see below) inserting at desmosomal junctions, results in an impressive supramolecular structure. This organisation extends from the outside of the membrane with its numerous bound enzymes deep into the cellular cytoplasm. It should be a rewarding field for a molecular understanding of cytoskeleton-membrane interaction. In contrast to the microvilli the microfilament organisation of the terminal web contains the normal associated proteins also found in stress fibres (Bretscher and Weber 1978).

## *Ca++-Dependent Regulatory Factors*

Local changes in the free $Ca^{++}$ concentration are assumed to regulate the morphology and locomotion of non-muscle cells. Because these processes are intimately connected with the organisation and turnover of microfilaments, much interest has focussed on $Ca^{++}$ control. At least two $Ca^{++}$-dependent targets have been discussed (Table 2). The first is the action of the specific calmodulin-dependent myosin kinase, which phosphorylates a myosin light chain and thereby regulates the activity of the F-actin activated myosin ATPase considered to be the basis of microfilament contractility (see for instance Yerna *et al.* 1979). The second seems to be the organisation of the F-actin itself. $Ca^{++}$-dependent F-actin severing is a novel mechanism characterised so far by the properties of three proteins isolated from cell types as diverse as macrophages, intestinal epithelial cells and *Physarum poly-cephalum* (Yin and Stossel 1979; Yin *et al.* 1980; Bretscher and Weber 1980b; Hasegawa *et al.* 1980). All three proteins are $Ca^{++}$-binding proteins (dissociation constant $\mu M$). They restrict F-actin filaments at $\mu M$ free $Ca^{++}$ resulting, depending on their concentration, in short F-actin filaments or even stoichiometric complexes. They seem to promote $Ca^{++}$-dependent nucleation of actin assembly and may indeed 'sever' or 'break' preformed F-actin. The combined properties of these proteins (see Table 3) and the fact that they are major components in their respective cells opens several new avenues to certain puzzles of cellular architecture and locomotion. Local fluxes of free $Ca^{++}$ at $\mu M$ level could result in either a shortening or even dissolution of F-actin or alternatively in a new polymerization. In addition intracellular transport of actin does not necessarily have to rely on G-actin and its complexes with profilin-like molecules (Carlson *et.al.* 1976) but could be based on a $Ca^{++}$-dependent *F-actin shuttle* of shortened filaments. In addition at least villin changes its regulatory properties when depleted of $Ca^{++}$. It now

**Table 2**
$Ca^{++}$-Regulation of microfilaments

1 Myosin activation by calmodulin-dependent myosin kinase (specific light chain phosphorylation). Regulation of ATPase activity and contraction.

2a Transition of calcium-dependent actin binding proteins like villin from the gelation and bundling state ($Ca^{++} < 10^{-7}$ M) to the severing state ($Ca^{++} > 10^{-7}$ M) i.e. bundles, short filaments (F-actin shuttle) and complex with monomeric actin.

2b Ca-dependent severing but not bundling: gelsolin, fragmin.

**Table 3**
Proteins associated with microfilaments, and their functions

| | |
|---|---|
| 1 Ca-independent gelation | ABP, filamin (250K) |
| 2 Ca-dependent severing | villin, gelsolin, fragmin other 90-95 K |
| 3 Ca-inhibited bundling (gelation) | villin, actinogelin |
| 4 Ca-independent bundling | $\alpha$-actinin (?) |
| 5 Ca-independent depolymerisation | profilin (1:1), DNase 1, vit-D protein |
| 6 Ca-dependent depolymerisation | villin (1:2), fragmin (1:1) |
| 7 Contraction | myosin |
| 8 Others | vinculin (?), MV-110K, tropomyosin |
| 9 Indirectly bound proteins | calmodulin, fimbrin (?) and others (?) |

acts as a F-actin bundling factor giving rise to parallel-oriented F-actin bundles related to the core filament bundle of the microvillus (Bretscher and Weber 1980b). It remains to be seen if this property is also shared by other 'severing proteins'. If indeed F-actin severing and bundling are coupled in the same molecule one can expect a new outlook on F-actin transport and polarity.

*Membrane Anchorage and Other Structures*

This is not the place to discuss microfilament-membrane interaction in detail. However, it seems pertinent to mention one point briefly. It is often assumed that $\alpha$-actinin is the general membrane anchorage protein (Mooseker and Tilney 1975; Lazarides and Burridge 1975). Although there is no question that immunofluorescence pictures of cultured cells indicate a relative wealth of $\alpha$-actinin close to the plasma membrane, there are several difficulties to a unified concept. *First*, the few known biochemical properties of $\alpha$-actinin give no obvious clue why this should be the case. Indeed it seems more likely that $\alpha$-actinin may bundle F-actin filaments rather than insert them directly into the plasma membrane. *Second*, in the case of the microvillus core filament structure, $\alpha$-actinin is absent (Geiger *et.al.* 1979; Bretscher and Weber 1979; Craig and Lancashire 1980) and side-on membrane anchorage occurs via the 100K crossbridge protein (Matsudaira and Burgess 1979). End-on attachment at the tip has not yet been explained. *Third*, the possibility has been raised that other proteins, such as vinculin, are closer to the attachment points than $\alpha$-actinin (Geiger 1979).

Microfilamentous structures seem to interact with other cellular components. Examples include microtubules (Griffith and Pollard 1978), polyribosomes (Lenk *et.al.* 1977), at least certain membrane proteins (Ben-Ze'ev *et.al.* 1979), and possibly various glycolytic enzymes (Arnold and Pette 1968; Clarke and Morton 1976). Some of these results indicate not only an increasing complexity of microfilaments but also show the possibility that cytoplasmic dynamics may integrate different structures previously thought of as separate entities.

**Microtubules**

Although basically a light microscopic technique, immunofluorescence micro-scopy has greatly enhanced our knowledge of microtubular organisation in interphase cells (for a review see Weber and Osborn 1979; Brinkley *et.al.* 1980), and many of the features revealed are also apparent in whole amounts used by high voltage electron microscopy (Wolosewick and Porter, 1976 1979).

Microtubule visualisation by immunofluorescence has technically been improved since it was first achieved in 1975 (Weber *et.al.* 1975; Brinkley *et.al.* 1975a). These improvements involve the use of antigen affinity purified specific IgGs and better protocols in fixation involving both the use of the

$Ca^{++}$ chelator EGTA and glutaraldehyde (Fuller *et al.* 1975; Weber *et al.* 1976; Osborn and Weber 1977; Osborn *et.al.* 1978a; Small and Celis 1978; Weber *et al.* 1978). This allowed a direct comparison of the same cytoskeleton first in the fluorescence microscope and then after negative staining in the electron microscope. Such experiments proved that immunofluorescence microscopy can in principle record individual microtubules when well-spread cultured cellsa are used (Osborn *et.al.* 1978a). Direct visualisation at the three dimensional level has become possible by the use of stereo immunofluorescence microscopy (Osborn *et.al.* 1978b). In addition immunocytochemical studies have been extended to the level of the electron microscope using the peroxidase (DeMey *et.al.* 1976; De Brabander *et.al.* 1977; Henderson and Weber 1979) or the ferritin technique (Webster *et.al.* 1978).

*General Display of Cytoplasmic Microtubules*
The following features are generally recognised:

1) Microtubules traverse the cytoplasm as continuous structures for very long distances between the perinuclear space and the plasma membrane.
2) Microtubules are continuous fibers without breaks or branches and can in appropriate cells span distances as long as 50 $\mu$m.
3) Microtubules generally relate to cell morphology. Although they enter major cellular processes they seem to stop before the ruffling edges, which are characterised by a wealth of microfilaments (see above).
4) Microtubules often display gentle bends. In closer proximity with the cellular margin microtubules may stop abruptly sometimes nearly at right angles with the margin or they may bend and follow the margin in parallel alignment for longer distances.
5) Microtubules are present at all levels of the cell and not restricted to the adhesive side of the cell or to the flattened cytoplasmic areas. Stereo immunofluorescence microscopy reveals microtubules both above and below the nucleus. They appear to cascade at rather steep angles around the nucleus as they traverse from the perinuclear area through the endoplasm into the ectoplasm, where they are especially easy to record in the flattened parts of the cell.
6) Although the majority of microtubules seem to originate in the perinuclear area, direct visualisation of the unifocal origin at the centrosphere with its centrioles is not always possible because of the high number of microtubules involved and the blurring superposition of the structure.
7) The complex radial pattern of microtubules in interphase cells does not reveal directly the polarity present in these structures. Micro tubules reassemble from the cytocentre and not from the plasma membrane or randomly in the cytoplasm (Osborn and Weber 1976a,b; Brinkley *et.al.* 1975; Frankel 1976). Repolymerisation is a spatially ordered process with the

cytocentre acting as a microtubule organising centre (MTOC). This process can be seen in cells recovering from colcemid treatment or in cells respreading on a substratum. The preferred directionality of *in vivo* polymerisation is directly linked with the function of MTOCs. Regrowth indicates in general 1-2 major centres in the case of several cell types (references above) although the possibility of multiple sites for certain special cell types like neuroblastoma has been documented (Spiegelman *et al.* 1979a,b; Marchisio *et al.* 1979; Sharp *et al.* 1980a).

8) Probably the most striking rearrangement of microtubules is the dramatic loss of cytoplasmic microtubules with the onset of mitosis and the construction of the spindle microtubular apparatus (for reviews see McIntosh 1979; Weber and Osborn 1979).

Although there is general agreement on the display of microtubules in a predominantly radial complex, there has been some discussion on the organisation of microtubules in transformed cells, tumour cells (Brinkley *et.al.* 1976; Edelman and Yahara 1976; Miller *et.al.* 1977) or cells derived from animals suffering from either muscular dystrophy (Shay and Fuseler 1979) or the Chediak-Higashi-like syndrome (Oliver 1976). For these cases it was proposed that cells show major defects in their microtubular organisation. Total absence of microtubules, strikingly diminished profiles and broken microtubules have been described both by immunofluorescence microscopy and electron microscopy. In all these cases, however, later independent studies have been unable to substantiate the earlier reports (Osborn and Weber 1977; De May *et.al.* 1978; Tucker *et.al.* 1978; Watt *et.al.* 1978; Connolly *et.al.* 1979; Frankel *et.al.* 1978). Although it is difficult to assess the reasons for the original observations (for a discussion see Weber and Osborn 1979, and Brinkley *et.al.* 1980) it can be assumed that extensive cytoplasmic networks of microtubules are typical for all interphase cells attached to a substratum. Thus microtubles are a necessary part of the cytoskeleton.

*Associated Proteins and Interactions*

Microtubules purified from brain tissue contain not only tubulin but at least two classes of associated proteins which stimulate *in vitro* both the nucleation and the elongation of microtubule assembly (Murphy and Borisy 1975; Cleveland *et.al.* 1977; Herzog and Weber 1978). One protein, MAP$_2$, is a polypeptide of an exceedingly high molecular weight (approximately 300,-000) whereas the other (Tau protein), is composed of several polypeptides in the molecular weight region of 55-65,000. Immunofluorescence microscopy revealed both proteins as components of cytoplasmic and mitotic microtubules (Sherline and Schiavone 1977; Connolly *et.al.* 1977 1978). Since MAP$_2$ is responsible for the expression of wispy fibres protruding in a regular arrangement up to 30nm from the microtubular wall proper (Herzog and

Weber 1978; Kim *et.al.* 1979) the protein is an obvious candidate for a direct link between microtubules and other structures. Such structures may include intermediate filaments (Goldman and Knipe 1973), mitochondria (Heggeness *et.al.* 1977) or even individual F-actin fibres (Griffith and Pollard 1978).

**Intermediate Filaments**
The expression of intermediate filaments (diameter 7-11 nm) either as single fibres or laterally aggregated bundles in numerous vertebrate cells is now well established. Very little, however, is known about the true function of inter- mediate or 10 nm filaments (for reviews see Lazarides 1980; Weber and Osborn 1980). They seem to serve a cytoskeletal function and in fact may be the true cytoskeletons of numerous cell types, although they may be not present in certain embryonic cells (Paulin *et.al.* 1980). They could be involved in nuclear anchorage (Lehto *et.al.* 1977; Small and Celis 1978) and act in muscle cells as 'mechanical integrators of cellular space' (Lazarides 1980). In certain cell types, such as in intestinal epithelial cells, they may form an underlying cytoskeleton dominating the part of the cell below the brush border (see above) and may thus be responsible for the shape of the cell (Franke *et.al.* 1979d). In addition many intermediate filaments seem to be in a state of inter- dependence with microtubular expression. Depolymerisation of cytoplasmic microtubules as well as rearrangement of tubulin into spindle micro tubules is accompanied by dramatic bundling of certain but not all intermediate filament types (see for instance Goldman and Knipe 1973; Aubin *et.al.* 1980; Blose 1979). The molecular mechanism of this interdependence has remained unknown but seems in line with the rather similar radial organisation of the two filamentous systems (for references see above and Geiger and Singer 1980).
During the last two years an increasing body of evidence has documented the astonishing polymorphism of 10 nm filaments. Although rather similar in ultra- structure and morphology, differences in molecular weights and isoelectric points have been found. More importantly several laboratories have been able to elicit antibodies, which clearly distinguish several subclasses which are in general line with histologically distinct cell types according to known schemes of differentiation (Bennett *et.al.* 1978; Franke *et.al.* 1978a; Lazarides and Balzer 1978; Sun *et.al.* 1979).

*Subclasses of 10nm Filaments (see Table 4)*
1) *Cytokeratin filaments.* Antibodies to various epidermal keratin pre- parations used on frozen sections of adult mammalian tissues reveal cyto- keratins in a wide variety of well-known epithelia (Sun *et.al.* 1979; Franke *et al.* 1978a 1979e). These include all stratified squamous epithelia, lining epithelia, myoepithelial cells of various glands and the thymus reticular epithelium. Thus cytokeratins are clearly not restricted to keratinizing epithelia but appear to be a reliable marker of keratins characterised by true

desmosomes. In agreement, the earliest cell sheet of the mouse embryo, i.e. the trophoectoderm of the blastocyst, expresses cytokeratins (Paulin *et.al.* 1980) at a time when the proliferating cells of the inner cellular mass seem without any recognizable 10nm filaments. A wide variety of established cell lines reveal their original epithelial origin by cytokeratin expression. Examples include the human HeLa (Franke *et.al.* 1979a) and rat kangaroo PtK cell lines (Franke *et.al.* 1979a) and rat kangaroo PtK cell lines (Franke *et.al.* 1978b). 2) *Vimentin filaments.* Vimentin is the major intermediate filament protein found *in situ* in various mesenchymal cells. Examples include endothelial cells fibroblasts, lymphocytes, macrophages and chondrocytes (Franke *et. al.* 1978a). In addition some putative epithelia lacking both cytokeratins and desmosomes are rich in vimentin (Ramaekers *et.al.* 1980). Vimentin is expressed in many if not all cultured cells (Hynes and Destree 1978; Gordon *et.al.* 1978; Franke *et.al.* 1978a 1979c), which show permanent growth *in vitro*. These include not only mesenchymally derived cells but in addition cell lines derived from tissues known to have *in situ* a different 10nm filament system. Examples are epithelial cell lines (Franke *et al.* 1978a; Sun and Green 1978; Osborn *et.al.* 1980) and some glial cell lines (Paetau *et.al.* 1979). The reason for the expression of vimentin in the latter cells is unknown but may be related to permanent growth.
3) *Desmin filaments.* These are the dominant 10nm filament system of smooth muscle tissues such as stomach (Lazarides and Hubbard 1976; Small and Sobieszek 1977). Desmin is typical for Z-lines in sarcomeric muscles (Lazarides and Hubbard 1976). The reason for the occasional expression of desmin in certain cultured cell lines (Tuszynski *et.al.* 1979; Gard *et.al.* 1979) remains unknown.

**Table 4**
Sub-classes of intermediate filaments

| Protein | MW | Tissue/cell type | Remarks |
|---|---|---|---|
| 1 Keratins (Cytokeratins) | 40-60K | epithelial cells (keratinising or non-keratinising) | generally not lost upon growth; trophectoderm of blastocyst |
| 2 Desmin | 53K | muscle (Z line and IF) | lost upon growth? present in some but not all fibroblastic cells |
| 3 Neurofilaments | 50-220K | neuronal | lost upon growth? |
| 4 Glial filaments | 53K | glial and derived | lost upon growth |
| 5 Vimentin | 58K | 'mesenchymal cells' | acquired by permanent growth of epithelial, neuronal and glial cells |

4) *Neurofilaments*. Throughout the peripheral and central nervous system neurofilaments are found in axons and neurones (Bignami and Dahl 1977; Liem *et.al.* 1978). Neurofilament polypeptides are generally much higher in molecular weight than the other intermediate filament polypeptides (Schachner *et.al.* 1977; Schlaepfer 1977; Liem *et al*. 1978) potentially indicative of a possible functional difference.

5) *Glial filaments*. These are expressed as glial fibrillar acidic protein *in situ* only in astrocytes (Bignami and Dahl 1977) and not found in neurones.

Only sequence studies will reveal the degree of similarity of the different subclasses indicated by the similar ultrastructure of the filaments. The degree of difference implicated by the immunological data is impressive and may reflect a cytoskeletal difference in histologically distinct cell types. Attention should be drawn to the dramatic rearrangement of vimentin filaments with the onset of mitosis (Aubin *et.al.* 1980; Blose 1979) and the immunofluorescence studies showing distinct differences in the profiles of vimentin and cytokeratin in the same epithelial cells (Osborn *et.al.* 1980a).

## References

Arnold, H. and Pette, D. 1968. *Binding of glycolytic enzymes to structural proteins of the muscle.* Eur. J. Biochem. *6*, 163-171.

Aubin, J.E., Osborn, M., Franke, W.W. and Weber, K. 1980. *Intermediate filaments of the vimentin-type and the cytokeratin-type are distributed differently during mitosis.* Expl. Cell Res. *129*, 149-165.

Bennett, G.S., Fellini, S.A., Croop, J.M. *et al*. 1978. *Differences among 100 A filament subunits from different cell types.* Proc. natn. Acad. Sci. USA. 75, 4364-4368.

Ben-Ze'ev, A., Duerr, A., Solomon, F. and Penman, S. 1979. *The outer boundary of the cytoskeleton: a lamina derived from plasma membrane proteins.* Cell, *17*, 59- 865.

Bignami, A. and Dahl, D. 1977. *Specificity of glial fibrillary acidic protein for astrocytes.* J. Histochem. Cytochem. *25*, 466-469.

Blose, S.H. 1979. *Ten nanometer filaments and mitosis: maintenance of structural continuity in dividing endothelial cells.* Proc. natn. Acad. Sci. USA. *76*, 3372-3376.

Bretscher, A.P. and Weber, K. 1978a. *Localisation of actin and microfilament-associated proteins in the microvilli and terminal web of the intestinal brush border by immnofluorescence microscopy.* J. Cell Biol. *79*,839-845.

Bretscher, A.P. and Weber, K. 1978b. *Purification of microvilli and an analysis of the protein components of the microfilament core bundle.* Expl. Cell Res. *116*, 397-407.

Bretscher, A.P. and Weber, K. 1979. *Villin: the major microfilament-associated protein of the microvillus.* Proc. natn. Acad. Sci. USA. *75*, 2321- 2325.

Bretscher, A.P. and Weber, K. 1980a. *Fimbrin: a new microfilament-associated protein present in microvilli and other cell surface structures.* J. Cell Biol. *86*, 335-340.

Bretscher, A.P. and Weber, K. 1980b. *Villin is a major protein of the micro-villus cytoskeleton which binds both G- and F-actin in a calcium-dependent manner.* Cell, *20*, 839-847.

Brinkley, B.R., Fistel, S.H., Marcum, J.M. and Pardue, R.L. 1980. *Micro-tubules in cultured cells: indirect immunofluorescence microscopy with cultured cells.* Int. Rev. Cytol. *63*, 59-95.

Brinkley, B.R., Fuller, G.M. and Highfield, D.P. 1975. *Cytoplasmic micro-tubules in normal and transformed cells in culture. Analysis by tubulin antibody immunofluorescence.* Proc. natn. Acad. Sci. USA. *72*, 4981-4985.

Brinkley, B.R., Fuller, G.M. and Highfield, D.P. 1976. *Tubulin antibodies as probes for microtubules in dividing and non-dividing mammalian cells.* In *Cell Motility* (eds. R.D. Goldman, R. Pollard and J. Rosenbaum), Book A, pp. 435-456. New York: Cold Spring Harbor Laboratory.

Carlsson, L., Nystroem, L.E., Lindberg, U. *et.al.* 1976. *Crystallisation of a non-muscle actin.* J. molec. Biol. *105*, 353-366.

Cheung, W.Y. 1980. *Calmodulin plays a pivotal role in cellular regulation.* Science, *207*, 19-27.

Clarke, F.M. and Morton, D.J. 1976. *Aldolase binding to F-actin filaments.* Biochem. J. *159*, 797-798.

Cleveland, D.W., Hwo, S.-Y. and Kirschner, M.W. 1977. *Purification of tau, a microtubule-associated protein that induces assembly of microtubules from purified tubulin.* J. molec. Biol. *116*, 207-225.

Connolly, J.A., Kalnins, V.I., Cleveland, D.W. and Kirschner, M.W. 1977. *Immunofluorescent staining of cytoplasmic and spindle microtubules in mouse fibroblasts with antibody to tau protein.* Proc. natn. Acad. Sci. USA. *74*, 2437-2440.

Connolly, J.A., Kalnins, V.I., Cleveland, D.W. and Kirschner, M.W. 1978. *Intracellular localisation of the high molecular weight microtubule accessory protein by indirect immuno-fluorescence.* J. Cell Biol. *76*, 781-786.

Connolly, J.A., Kalnins, V.I. and Barber, B.H. 1979. *Microtubule organisation in fibroblasts from dystrophic chickens and persons with Duchenne muscular dystrophy.* Nature, *282*, 511-513.

Craig, S.W. and Lancashire, C.L. 1980 *Comparison of intestinal brush border 95K dalton polypeptide and alpha actinins.* J. Cell Biol. *84*, 755-667.

De Brabander, M., De Mey, J. Joniau, M. and Gueuens, G. 1977. *Immunocyto-chemical visualisation of microtubules and tubulin at the light and electron microscopic level.* J. Cell Sci. *28*, 283-301.

De Mey, J., Hoebeke, I., de Brabander, M. *et al.* 1976. *Immunoperoxidase visualisation of microtubules and microtubular proteins.* Nature, *264*, 273- 275.

De Mey, J., Joniau, M., de Brabander, M. *et al.* 1978. *Evidence for unaltered structure and in vivo assembly of microtubules in transformed cells.* Proc. natn. Acad. Sci. USA. *75*, 1339-1343.

Edelman, G.M. and Yahara, I. 1976. *Temperature sensitive changes in surface modulating assemblies of fibro blasts transformed by mutants of Rous sarcoma virus.* Proc. natn. Acad. Sci. USA. *73*, 2047-2051.

Franke, W.W., Appelhans, B., Schmid, E. *et al.* 1979a. *The organisation of cytokeratin filaments in the intestinal epithelium.* Eur. J. Cell Biol. *19*, 255-268.

Franke, W.W., Appelhans, B., Schmid, E. *et al.* 1979b. *Identification and characterisation of epithelial cells in mammalian tissues by immuno-fluorescence microscopy using antibodies to pre keratin.* Differentiation, *15*, 7-25.

Franke, W.W., Schmid, E., Breitkreutz, D. *et al.* 1979c. *Simultaneous expression of two different types of intermediate-sized filaments in mouse keratinocytes proliferation in vitro.* Differentiation, *14*, 35-50.

Franke, W.W., Schmid, E., Osborn, M. and Weber, K. 1978a. *Different intermediate-sized filaments distinguished by immunofluorescence microscopy.* Proc. natn. Acad. Sci. USA. *75*, 5034- 5038.

Franke, W.W., Schmid, E., Weber, K. and Osborn, M. 1979d. *HeLa cells contain intermediate-sized filaments of the prekeratin type.* Expl. Cell Res. *118*, 95-109.

Franke, W.W., Schmid, E., Winter, S. *et al.* 1979e. *Widespread occurrence of intermediate-sized filaments of the vimentin-type in cultured cells from diverse vertebrates.* Expl. Cell Res. *123*, 25-46.

Franke, W.W., Weber, K., Osborn, M. *et.al.* 1978b. *Antibody to prekeratin: decoration of tonofilament-like arrays is various cells of epithelial character.* Expl. Cell Res. *116*, 429-445.

Frankel, F.R. 1976. *Organisation and energy dependent growth of microtubules in cells.* Proc. natn. Acad. Sci. USA. *73*, 2798-2802.

Frankel, F.R., Tucker, R.W., Bruce, J. and Stenberg, R. 1978. *Fibroblasts and macrophages of mice with the Chediak-Higashi syndrome have microtubules and actin cables.* J. Cell Biol. *79*, 401-408.

Fuller, G.M., Brinkley, B.R. and Boughter, M.J. 1975. *Immunofluorescence of mitotic spindles using monospecific antibody against bovine brain tubulin.* Science, *187*, 948-950.

Gard, D.L., Bell, P.B. and Lazarides, E. 1979. *Coexistence of desmin and the fibroblastic intermediate filament subunit in muscle and non-muscle cells.* Proc. natn. Acad. Sci. USA. *76*, 3894-3898.

Geiger, B. 1979a. *A 130K protein from chicken gizzard: its localisation at the termini of microfilament bundles in cultured chicken cells.* Cell, *18*, 193-205.

Geiger, B. and Singer, S.J. 1980. *Association of microtubules and intermediate filament in chicken gizzard cells as detected by double immunofluorescence.* Proc. natn. Acad. Sci. USA. *77*, 4769-4773.

Geiger, B., Tokuyasu, K.T. and Singer, S.J. 1979b. *Immunocytochemical localisation of α-actinin in intestinal epithelial cells.* Proc. natn. Acad. Sci. USA. *76*, 2833-2837.

Glenney, J. Jr., Bretscher, A. and Weber, K. 1980. *Calcium regulation in the intestinal microvillus; implications for control of microfilament organisation.* Proc. natn. Acad. Sci. USA. *77*, In press.

Glenney, J. Jr. and Weber, K. 1980. *Calmodulin-binding proteins of the microfilaments present in brush borders and microvilli of intestinal epithelial cells.* J. Biol. Chem. *255*, 10551-10554.

Goldman, R.D. and Knipe, D.M. 1973. *Functions of cytoplasmic fibres in non-muscle cell motility.* Cold Spring Harbor Symp. Quant. Biol. *37*, 523-534.

Gordon III, W.E. Bushnell, A. and Burridge, K. 1978. *Characterisation of the intermediate (10nm) filaments of cultured cells using an autoimmune rabbit antiserum.* Cell, *13*, 249-261.

Griffith, L.M. and Pollard, T.D. 1978. *Evidence for actin filament-microtubule interaction mediated by microtubule associated proteins.* J. Cell Biol. *78*, 958-965.

Hasegawa, T., Tokahashi, S., Hayashi, H. and Hatano, S. 1980. *Framin: a calcium ion sensitive regulatory factor on the formation of actin filaments.* Biochemistry, *19*, 2677-2683.

Heggeness, M.H., Simon, M. and Singer, S.J. 1978. *Association of mitochondria with microtubules in cultured cells.* Proc. natn. Acad. Sci. USA. *75*, 3863-3866.

Heggeness, M.H., Wang, K. and Singer, S.J. 1977. *Intracellular distribution of mechanochemical proteins in cultured fibroblasts.* Proc. natn. Acad. Sci. USA. *74*, 3883-3887.

Henderson, D. and Weber, K. 1979. *Three-dimensional organisation of micro-filaments and microtubsles in the cytoskeleton.* Expl. Cell. Res. *124*, 301-316.

Herzog, W. and Weber, K. 1978. *Fractionation of brain microtubule-associated proteins. Isolation of two different proteins which stimulate tubulin polymerisation in vitro.* Eur. J. Biochem. *92*, 1-8.

Howe, C., Mooseker, M.S. and Graves, T.A. 1980. *Brush border calmodulin.* J. Cell Biol. *85*, 916-923.

Hull, B.E. and Staehelin, L.A. 1979. *The terminal web.* J. Cell Biol. *81*, 67-82.

Hynes, R.O. and Destree, A.I. 1978. *10nm filaments in normal and transformed cells.* Cell, *13*, 151-163.

Isenberg, G., Rathke, P.C., Hulsmann, N. *et al.* 1976. *Cytoplasmic acto myosin fibrils in tissue culture cells - direct proof of contractility by visualisation of ATP-induced contraction in fibrils isolated by laser microbeam dissection.* Cell Tiss. Res. *166*, 427-443.

Ishikawa, H., Bischoff, R. and Holtzer, H. 1969. *Formation of arrowhead complexes with heavy meromyosin in a variety of cell types.* J. Cell Biol. *43*, 312-328.

Kim, H., Binder, L.I. and Rosenbaum, J.L. 1979. *The periodic association of MAP2 with brain microtubules in vitro.* J. Cell Biol. *80*, 260-276.

Lazarides, E. 1976a. *Actin, α-actinin and tropomyosin interaction in the structural organisation of actin filaments in non-muscle cells.* J. Cell Biol. *68*, 202-219.

Lazarides, E. 1980. *Intermediate filaments as mechanical integrators of cellular space.* Nature, *283*, 249-256.

Lazarides, E. and Balzer, D.R. 1978, *Specificity of desmin to avian and mammalian muscle cells.* Cell, *14*, 429- 438.

Lazarides, E. and Burridge, K. 1975. *α-Actinin: immunofluorescent localisation of a muscle structural protein in nonmuscle cells.* Cell, *6*, 289-298.

Lazarides, E. and Hubbard, B.D. 1976b. *Immunological characterisation of the subunit of the 100 A filaments from muscle cells.* Proc. natn. Acad. Sci. USA. *73*, 4344-4348.

Lazarides, E. and Weber, K. 1974. *Actin antibody: the specific visualisation of actin filaments in non-muscle cells.* Proc. natn. Acad. Sci. USA. *71*, 2268-2272.

Lehto, V.P., Virtanen, I. and Kurki, P. 1978. *Intermediate filaments anchor the nuclei in nuclear monolayers of cultured human fibroblasts.* Nature, *272*, 175-177.

Lenk, R., Ramson, L., Kaufman, Y. and Penman, S. 1977. *A cytoskeletal structure with associated polyribosomes obtained from HeLa cells.* Cell, *10*, 67-78.

Liem, K.H., Yen, S.-H., Salomon, G.D. and Shelanski, M.L. 1978. *Intermediate filaments in nervous tissues.* J. Cell Biol. *79*, 637-645.

Marchisio, P.C., Weber, K. and Osborn, M. 1979. *Identification of multiple microtubule initiating sites in mouse neuroblastoma cells.* Eur. J. Cell Biol. *20*, 45-50.

Matsudaira, P.T. and Burgess, D.R. 1979. *Identification and organisation of the components in the isolated microvillus skeleton.* J. Cell Biol. *83*, 667-673.

McIntosh, J.R. 1979. *Cell Division. In Microtubules* (ed. K. Roberts and J.S. Hyams), pp 382-442. London, New York: Academic Press.

Miller, C.L., Fuseler, J.W. and Brinkley, B.R. 1977. *Cytoplasmic microtubules in transformed mouse and non-transformed human cell hybrids: correlation with in vitro growth.* Cell, *12*, 319-331.

Mooseker, M.S. and Tilney, L.G. 1975. *Organisation of an actin filament-membrane complex. Filament polarity and membrane attachment in the microvilli of intestinal epithelial cells.* J. Cell Biol. *67*, 725-743.

Murphy, D.B. and Borisy, G.G. 1975. *Association of high molecular weight protein with microtubules and their role in microtubular assembly in vitro.* Proc. natn. Acad. Sci. USA. *72*, 2696-2700.

Oliver, J.M. 1976. *Impaired microtubule function correctable by cyclic GMP and cholinergic agonists in the Chediak-Higashi syndrome.* Am. J. Path. *85*, 395-412.

Osborn, M., Born, T., Koitzsch, H.-J. and Weber, K. 1978a. *Stereo immunofluorescence microscopy. I: Three-dimensional arrangement of microfilaments, microtubules and tonofilaments.* Cell *14*, 477-488.

Osborn, M., Franke, W.W. and Weber, K. 1980. *Direct demonstration of the presence of two immunologically distinct intermediate-sized filament systems in the same cell by double immunofluorescence microscopy.* Expl. Cell Res. *125*, 37-46.

Osborn, M. and Weber, K. 1976a. *Cytoplasmic microtubules in tissue culture cells appear to grow from and organising structure towards the plasma membrane.* Proc. natn. Acad. Sci. USA. *73*, 867-871.

Osborn, M. and Weber, K. 1976b. *Tubulin specific antibody and the expression of microtubules in 3T3 cells after attachment to a substratum.* Expl. Cell Res. *103*, 331-340.

Osborn, M. and Weber, K. 1977. *The display of microtubules in transformed cells.* Cell, *12*, 561-571.

CYTOSKELETON

25

Osborn, M., Webster, R.E. and Weber, K. 1978b. *Individual microtubules viewed by immunofluorescence and electron microscopy in the same PtK2 cell.* J. Cell Biol. *77*, R27-R34.

Paetau, A., Virtanen, I., Stenman, S. *et al.* 1979. *Glial fibrillar acidic protein and intermediate filaments in human glioma cells.* Acta Neuropath. *47*, 71-74.

Paulin, D., Vabinet, C., Weber, K. and Osborn, M. 1980. *Antibodies as probes of cellular differentiation and cytoskeletal organisation in the mouse blastocyst.* Expl. Cell Res. In press.

Ramaekers, F.C.S., Osborn, M., Schmid, E. *et al.* 1980. *Identification of the cytoskeletal proteins in lens-forming cells, a special epitheloid cell type.* Expl. Cell Res. *127*, 309-327.

Schachner, M., Hedley-White, E.T., Hsu, D.W. *et al.* 1977. *Ultrastructural location of glial fibrillar acidic protein in mouse cerebellum by immunoperoxidase labeling.* J. Cell Biol. *75*, 67-73.

Schlaepfer, W.W. 1977. *Immunological and ultrastructural studies of neuro-filaments isolated from rat peripheral nerve.* J. Cell Biol. *74*, 226-240.

Sharp, G.A., Osborn, M. and Weber, K. 1980. *Ultrastructure of multiple microtubule initiating sites in mouse neuroblastoma cells.* J. Cell Sci. In press.

Shay, J.W. and Fuseler, J.W. 1979. *Diminished microtubules in fibroblast cells derived from inherited dystrophic muscle explants.* Nature *278*, 178-180.

Sherline, P. and Schiavone, K. 1977. *Immunofluorescence localisation of proteins of high molecular weight along intracellular microtubules.* Science *198*, 1038-1040.

Small, J.V. and Celis, J.E. 1978. *Direct visualisation of the 10-nm (100 A)-filament network in whole and enucleated cultured cells.* J. Cell Sci. *31*, 393-409.

Small, J.V. and Sobieszek, A. 2977. *Studies on the function and composition of the 10-nm (100 A)-filaments of vertebrate smooth muscle.* J. Cell Sci. *23*, 243-268.

Smith, D.S., Jarlfors, U. and Gayer, M.L. 1977. *Structural cross-bridges between microtubules and mitochondria in central axons of an insect Periplaneta americana.* J. Cell Sci. *27*, 255-272.

Spiegelman, B.M., Lopata, M.A. and Kirschner, M.W. 1979. *Aggregation of microtubule initiation sites preceeding neurite outgrowth in mouse neuroblastoma cells.* Cell, *16*, 253-263.

Stossel, T.P. 1978. *Contractile proteins in cell structure and function.* Ann. Rev. Medicine, *29*, 427-457.

Sun, T.T. and Green, H. 1978. *Immunofluorescence staining of keratin fibres in cultured cells.* Cell, *14*, 469-476.

Sun, T.T., Shih, C. and Green, H. 1979. *Keratin cytoskeletons in epithelial cells of internal organs.* Proc. natn. Acad. Sci. USA. *76*, 2813-2817.

Taylor, D.L. and Condeelis, J.S. 1979. *Cytoplasmic structure and contractility in amoeboid cells.* Int. Rev. Cytol. *56*, 57-144.

Tucker, R.W., Sanford, K.K. and Frankel, F.R. 1978. *Tubulin and actin in paired nonneoplastic and spontaneously transformed neoplastic cell lines in vitro: fluorescent antibody studies.* Cell, *13*, 629-642.

Tuszynski, G.P., Frank, E.D., Dansky, C.H. *et al.* 1979. *The detection of smooth muscle desmin-like protein in BHK₂ᵥ/C13 fibroblasts.* J. Biol. Chem. *254*, 6138-6143.

Wang, K., Ash, J.F. and Singer, S.J. 1975. *Filamin, a new high-molecular weight protein found in smooth muscle and non-muscle cells.* Proc. natn. Acad. Sci. USA. *72*, 4483-4486.

Watt, F.M., Harris, H., Weber, K. and Osborn, M. 1978. *The distribution of actin cables and microtubules in hybrids between malignant and non-malignant cells and in tumours derived from them.* J. Cell Sci. *32*, 419-432.

Weber, K. and Groeschel-Stewart, U. 1974. *Antibody to myosin: the specific visualisation of myosin-containing filaments in non-muscle cells.* Proc. natn. Acad. Sci. USA. *71*, 4561-4564.

Weber, K. and Osborn, M. 1979. *The intracellular display of microtubular structures revealed by indirect immunofluorescence microscopy. In, Microtubules* (ed. K. Roberts and J.S. Hyams), pp. 279-313.

Weber, K. and Osborn, M. 1980. *Microtubules and intermediate filament networks in cells viewed by immunofluorescence microscopy. In Cell surface reviews* (ed. G. Post and G.L. Nicolson). Amsterdam, New York: Biomedical Press. In press.

Weber, K. and Osborn, M. 1981. *The cytoskeleton. In Muscle and non-muscle motility* (ed. A. Stracher). New York: Academic Press. In press.

Weber, K., Pollack, R. and Bibring, T. 1975. *Antibody against tubulin: the specific visualisation of cytoplasmic microtubules in tissue culture cells.* Proc. natn. Acad. Sci. USA. *72*, 459-463.

Weber, K., Rathke, P.C. and Osborn, M. 1978. *Cytoplasmic microtubular images in glutaraldehyde-fixed tissue culture cells viewed by electron microscopy and by immunofluorescence microscopy.* Proc. natn. Acad. Sci. USA. *75*, 1820-1824.

Weber, K., Wehland, J. and Herzog, W. 1976. *Griseofulvin interacts with microtubules both in vivo and in vitro.* J. molec. Biol. *102*, 817-829.

Webster, R.E., Henderson, D., Osborn, M. and Weber, K. 1978. *Three-dimensional electron microscopical visualisation of the cytoskeleton of animal cells: immunoferritin identification of actin- and tubulin-containing structures.* Proc. natn. Acad. Sci. USA. *75*, 5511-5515.

Wolosewick, J.S. and Porter, K.R. 1976. *Stereo high voltage electron microscopy of whole cells of the human diploid line, WT-38.* Am. J. Anat. *147*, 303-324.

Wolosewick, J.S. and Porter, K.R. 1979. *Microtrabecular lattice of the cytoplasmic ground substance.* J. Cell Biol. *82*, 114-139.

Yerna, M.J., Dabrowska, R., Hartshorne, D.J. and Goldman, R.D. 1979. *Calcium-sensitive regulation of actin-myosin interactions in baby hamster kidney (BHK21) cells.* Proc. natn. Acad. Sci. USA. *76*, 184-188.

Yin, H.L. and Stossel, T.P. 1979. *Control of cytoplasmic actin gel-sol transformation by gelsolin a calcium-dependent regulatory protein.* Nature *281*, 583-586.

Yin, H.L., Zaner, K.S. and Stossel, T.P. 1980. *Ca++ control of actin gelation.* J. Biol. Chem. *255*, 9499-9500.

## Questions

*Rees*

Can I set the ball rolling by asking about your ideas on the control of actomyosin activity. The idea that calcium simultaneously disorganises the structure and activates the myosin is very attractive. Could you speculate beyond that as to how it might actually work in some cellular function like, for example, cell division or locomotion.

*Weber*

I do not understand locomotion. I do not understand mitosis. So, saying that very truthfully I can however say the following: there are lots of experiments in the literature, for instance, Brinkley and Means have shown that microtubules have a certain calcium sensitivity which is unfortunately not quite in the micromolar range and which seems to be mediated by calmodulin. One of the major protein kinases, which is calcium-dependent, is found to be associated with the microtubule-associated protein which is responsible for the slender side-arms coming off the microtubule and may be localised there by immunofluorescence microscopy. Now, in that case there you would expect that calcium would be involved probably in *de*-polymerisation so if you get a flow of calcium and the end of the microtubule were free, then you may envisage a process of shortening. Now, in the case of the microvillus one has to be careful. The intestinal epithelium and its microvillus may not be identical with microvilli on certain tissue culture cells. There you have a special situation because you have to avoid calcium destruction. But it is very clear that drugs which work on calmodulin, like the phenothiazines, immediately have an effect as seen on cells in tissue culture. In the scanning EM it is seen that these cells immediately lose their microvilli.

*Lodish*

Do you have any indication as to whether beta and gamma actin serve different

functions or are in different structures.

*Weber*

There is indeed no indication. If you take isolated core filaments of the microvillus, they contain the same amount the of the 2 species beta and gamma as the total intestinal cell and if you make sub-complexes derived from that it is still the same - they do not seem to separate in function. I sometimes wonder if this hasn't something to do with regulation of expression under certain conditions because Penman's paper of 2-3 years ago which showed quiescent cells being offered a new substratum and serum and (if I remember correctly) showed a specific stimulation of gamma synthesis and not beta synthesis (if I am not mistaken). So I think it must be something like that rather than function.

*Grand*

In the case of smooth muscle at least, I think there is still not complete agreement that phosphorylation by myosin light chain kinase is the only controlling mechanism in contraction. Certainly, there seem to be other proteins involved and this view seems to be out of favour with smooth muscle biochemists.

*Weber*

I would agree with you. The data are not so clear that you can say it is an absolute necessity. There may be other controlling features in smooth muscle, especially via calcium.

*Hunt*

Could you comment on the finding (or the reported finding) that ribosomes are associated with the cytoskeleton. What could that mean?

*Weber*

Well, you have two views. One is that they structure what is so nicely called the cell sap. Now, the cell sap is a biochemical artifact (but it is a good artifact). If you look at whole counts of Keith

Porter by high voltage electron microscopy, then the amount of space, or, the diameter of the channels of non-fibrous or filamentous material is maximally about 1000 angstroms. So you can still have things trying make their way through there but the idea which especially Penman advanced is that under conditions of protein biosynthesis, polysomes (but not monosomes) are bound to whatever that matrix is. I think that some people who have repeated these experiments have seen that too by other methods.

*Hunt*

But do you think that has any functional prospects?

*Weber*

Well, I would not go so far as he goes. He says that one advantage of such a mechanism would be that you insert the proteins directly into the structure. But I think that at least those polysomes resent in the cytoplasm which have previously been considered free are anchored.

# Pericellular Matrix Glycoproteins in Cell Differentiation and in Malignant Transformation

*Antti Vaheri and Kari Alitalo*

## Introduction

With few exceptions adherent cells *in vivo*, are intimately surrounded by extracellular matrix. In differentiated tissues the matrix is classified as interstitial connective tissue when occurring between similar cells or basement membranes when between dissimilar cells. The principal function of such a matrix is to give mechanical support and to anchor cells in tissue type-specific structures, but it may also have other duties, such as a selective filter function. The composition of the matrix surrounding cells, the pericellular matrix, is closely dependent on the cell type and the degree of its differentiation. The matrix phenotype is largely retained even in cell culture and this has greatly facilitated studies on the biosynthesis of matrix components and on their function at the pericellular level. It is becoming evident that the pericellular matrix is an integral part of the differentiated normal cellular phenotype and that alterations or defects in cell surface-matrix interaction may be salient features of the malignant phenotype. In the following, we first describe some of the properties of the major defined matrix components before considering their role for the cell phenotype.

## Matrix Glycoproteins

The extracellular matrix contains collagenous and noncollagenous glyco-proteins, elastin, sulphated proteoglycans and hyaluronic acid (Table 1). Collagen, fibronectin and laminin are the major matrix glycoproteins identi-fied so far and are found in association with a variety of different cellular phenotypes.

### Collagen

Collagen (for reviews see Prockop *et al* 1979, Bornstein and Sage 1980) is one of the most abundant proteins in the vertebrate body, constituting more than a third of the total protein in many adult organisms.

On the basis of protein chemical analysis at least five different collagen

**Table 1**

Major defined matrix components

| Type | Chain composition | Distribution | Distinctive features |
|---|---|---|---|
| Interstitial collagen types | | | |
| 1 | $(\alpha1(1))_2\alpha2$ $(\alpha1(1))_{32})$ | skin, bone, dentin, tendon, cornea 1 | presence of $\alpha2$ chain, less than 10 hydroxylysines/chain, 0.1% carbohydrate |
| 2 | $(\alpha1(2))_3$ | cartilage, vitreous body, notochord | 1% carbohydrate, greater than 10 hydroxylysines/chain |
| 3 | $(\alpha1(3))_3$ | as type 1, prominent in fetal skin[1], arteries, amniotic membrane, not in bone or tendon | presence of cysteine, high levels of hydroxyproline, glycine, histidine |
| Basement membrane collagens | | | |
| 4 | at least 2 chain sub-types $\alpha1(4)$ $\alpha2(4)$ $\alpha3(4)$ | basement membranes (*lamina densa*) | greater than 20 hydroxylysines/chain, high 3-hydroxyproline, low alanine and arginine |
| Other | | | |
| 5 | $\alpha1, \alpha2, \alpha3$ $\alpha1(5)_3$ $\alpha1(5)_2 \alpha2(5)$ $\alpha2(5)_3$? | associated with membraneous structures? (Roll *et al* 1980) | slightly larger than $\alpha1(1)$, 0.3% 3-hydroxyproline |
| Fibronectin | $2\times220,000$ | loose connective tissue matrix, basement membranes, body fluids | interactions, see Table 3 |
| Laminin | subunits 200,000-220,000 400,000-440,000 | basement membranes (*lamina rara*) | ordered polypeptide structures ($\alpha$-chain, $\alpha$-sheet), disulfide knot |
| Tropoelastin-Elastin | 72,000 | elastic fibres (Uitto 1979) | high content of alanine, valine, glycine contains hydroxyproline, cross-linking |
| Microfibrillin? | | | |
| Proteoglycans | | | matrix (and body fluids) |
| Glyco-saminoglycans sulfated proteo-glycans hyauronic acid | | | |

1) A higher content of type 1 trimer and type 3 collagens is found in embryonic and foetal tissues (Epstein 1974, Jimenex *et.al.*1977).

2) On the basis of amino acid sequence heterogeneity, nonallelic subtypes have been postulated to exist (Butler *et.al.*1977).

isotypes have been defined in man (Table 1). The isotypes differ in their primary structure and, therefore, are apparently products of different genes. While the interstitial collagen (types 1-3) fibres display a periodicity of 60-70 nm, basement membrane collagen (type 4) do not. As implicated by the nomenclature, the collagen isotypes differ in their distribution in tissues (see Gay and Miller 1978, Bornstein and Sage 1980). This is also reflected in the relatively specific expression by a given cellular phenotype *in vitro* (discussed below).

A soluble biosynthetic precursor, procollagen, is secreted by collagen-producing cells (Fessler and Fessler 1978). Coordinate action of at least eight enzymes is needed to complete the pathway to collagen fibril (Table 2). In the case of interstitial procollagens, the mostly nontriple-helical propeptides at both ends of the molecule are, after secretion, cleaved by specific enzymes: the procollagen aminoprotease and carboxyprotease (see Fessler and Fessler 1978, Prockop et. al. 1979). Conventional two-dimensional oligolayer cell culture conditions do not favour propeptide cleavages, and depending on the

**Table 2**
The biosynthesis of collagen

| Biosynthetic step | Collagen-specific enzymes involved |
|---|---|
| Transcription | |
| Processing to mRNA | |
| Translation | |
| Cleavage of pre-pieces | |
| Hydroxylation of prolyl and lysyl residues | prolyl 3-hydroxylase, 4-hydroxylase and lysyl hydroxylase* |
| Glycosylation of hydroxylysyl residues | hydroxylysyl glactosyltransferase, galactosyldroxylysyl glucosyltransferase (see Kivirikko and Myllyla 1980) |
| Chain association and disulfide bonding | |
| Regulated and controlled intracellular degradation? | |
| Triple helix formation | |
| Secretion of procollagen into the intracellular matrix | |
| Conversion of procollagen into collagen | aminoproteases, carboxyproteases (distinct procollagen types) |
| Aggregation of collagen molecules | |
| Cross-linking formation | lysyl oxidase, transglutaminase? |

*Enzymes are present also in collagen non-producing cells, such as lymphocytic cells (Chen-Kiang et.al 1978) and in macrophages (Myllyla and Seppa 1979) and the smaller enzymatically inactive subunit in great amounts in tissues (Chen-Kiang et.al. 1977, Kivirikko 1980).

source of cells (Taubman and Goldberg 1976), the pericellular *in vitro* matrix is therefore a mixture of collagenous molecules at different stages of propeptide cleavage. Further enzymatic processing of the maturing collagen fibrils involves covalent cross-linking of lysyl and hydroxylysyl residues by lysyl oxidase (Siegel 1979). Although inhibition of lysyl oxidase by lathyrogenic compounds, such as $\beta$-aminopropionitrile fumarate increases the extractable pool of collagen in cell culture (Layman *et al.* 1971), the extent of cross-linking in the pericellular *in vitro* matrix is poorly known (Bissell *et al* 1980). Cross-linking of collagen to fibronectin is catalysed by plasma transglutaminase (factor 13a ) *in vitro* (Mosher *et al* 1980).

*Fibronectin*

Fibronectins (Vaheri *et al.* 1980) are antigenically and biochemically partly defined glycoproteins, characteristically present both in interstitial and basement membrane matrices, in plasma and other body fluids. *In vivo* the soluble form of fibronectin has been found in all extracellular fluids studied and the relative protein concentrations suggest local synthesis by cells surrounding a particular anatomical compartment. In contrast to collagen, fibronectin possesses less higher order structure and no post-translational modifications or enzymes specific for fibronectin are known. Biosynthetic experiments have shown that both sulphate (Dunham and Hynes 1978) and phosphate (Teng and Rifkin 1979) are covalently incorporated into fibronectin. The fibronectin molecule is a dimer, apparently a heterodimer (Kurkinen *et al* 1980a), of 210,000-240,000 subunits linked near the carboxyl terminus by disulphide bonds. Ordinary asparagine-linked carbohydrate chains in fibronectin seem to protect it from proteolysis. Purified fibronectin is characterised by its multiple interactions (Table 3), tendency to polymerise (Vuento *et al* 1980) and sensitivity to proteolysis (Vartio *et al.* 1981). These properties and biological data suggest a more dynamic role for fibronectin than for collagen in connective tissues.

Soluble fibronectin can be purified by virtue of its specific affinity to denatured collagen (gelatin) (Engvall and Ruoslahti 1977) but it is not clear whether binding of fibronectin to collagen as observed *in vitro* actually occurs *in vivo*. However, fibronectin is able to promote the adhesion of many types of cells to various substrates, eg. gelatin (Pearlstein 1976) *in vitro* and so a role for it in adhesion of cells to collagen has been proposed to occur also *in vivo*. The adhesion of some cells to fibrin is mediated by fibronectin that may be covalently linked to the clot by plasma transglutaminase (Grinnell *et al.* 1980, Mosher 1980). Therefore, fibronectin may also function as a temporary organising matrix in wound healing before collagen is laid down. Mediation of cell-substrate interaction may be also involved in the stimulatory effects of fibronectin on cell migration (Ali and Hynes 1978) and on cell growth in defined media (Barnes and Sato 1980).

Whilst the principal binding sites have been identified of both parts of the fibronectin-collagen interaction, virtually nothing is known about the fibronectin receptors on the cell surface (see Vaheri *et.al.*1980) although sulphated proteoglycans and certain sialoglycolipids have been proposed as the putative receptors. Alternatively, the former molecules may regulate the deposition of matrix fibres since it has been shown that sulphated polysaccharides enhance the rate of binding of fibronectin to collagen (Johansson and Hook 1980), stabilize the fibronectin-collagen complex (Ruoslahti and Engvall 1980), induce the precipitation of fibronectin and subsequently collagen and promote the filamentous assembly of fibronectin (Jilek and Hormann 1979).

It should be noted though, that not all cells depend on fibronectin for their adhesion. For instance, adhesion of chondrocytes to type 2 collagen is stimulated by another protein present in serum called chondronectin (Hewitt *et al.*1980) and also epidermal cells attach to type 4 collagen in the absence of

**Table 3**
Interactions of fibronectin

| | |
|---|---|
| Binding of soluble fibronectin to: | |
| Fibronectin | Assembly into filamentous polymers (Vuento *et.al.*1980) |
| Collagen | Defined binding sites in collagen: strong binding to gelatin (Engvall and Ruoslahti 1977) |
| Clq component (Ruoslahti *et.al.* 1980) | Clq also found on fibroblast surface (Al-Adnani and McGree 1976) |
| Glycosaminoglycans | (Jilek and Hormann 1979, Ruoslahti and Engvall 1980, Yamada *et.al.* 1980) |
| Fibrin (in the cold) | Bound to fibrin clot (see Mosher 1980) |
| Cell surfaces | Not usually to suspended cells see (Pearlstein *et.al.* cell-cell adhesion, Speigel *et.al.* 1980) |
| Certain bacteria (Kuusela 1978) | Agglutinates *S.aureus* |
| Actin | Binds to actin-agarose (Keski-Oja *et.al.*) |
| DNA | Binds to DNA-agarose (Zardi *et.al.*1979) |
| Polyamines | Promote fibronectin assembly in a filamentous form (Vuento *et.al.* 1980), dissociation of fibronectin-gelatin complexes (Vuento and Vaheri 1979) |
| Susceptible to: | |
| Disuphide bonding | Soluble fibronectin is a dimer, in matrix more extensively disulphide-bonded (McConnell *et.al.*1978) |
| Proteinases | Sensitive cleavage sites (Vaheri *et.al.*1980) |
| Transglutaminase (factor 13a) | Both soluble and matrix forms get cross-linked Keski-Oja *et.al.* 1976, Mosher *et.al.* 1980, Mosher and Proctor 1980). |

serum factors or exogenous fibronectin (Murray et.al.1979) probably through laminin (Terranova et.al. 1980).

## Laminin

Laminin (Timpl 1981) is a 850,000 molecular weight glycoprotein originally isolated from mouse tumours producing great amounts of basement membrane matrix material (Chung et.al. 1979, Robey 1979, Timpl et.al. 1979). It has a four stranded elongated structure and is shown to be composed of at least two disuphide-bonded polypeptide chains ($M_r$=200,000-440,000).

Laminin contains about 12-15% carbohydrate (Chung et.al. 1979, Timpl et al. 1979) and is rich in sialic acid (4-6%). Laminin binds to heparin (Sakashita et.al. 1980) suggesting that it may interact with basement membrane heparan sulphate proteoglycan in vivo (Kanwar and Farquhar 1979, Hassell et.al 1980). In vivo, laminin antigen is found in all basement membranes studied (Rohde et.al. 1979, Timpl et.al. 1979), has been localised to the lamina rara of epidermal basement membranes (Foidart et. al. 1980) and is the most conspicuous component of Reichert's membrane of the mouse embryo (Hogan et.al. 1980, Leivo et.al. 1980).

In the early mouse embryo, laminin is the first matrix glycoprotein detected by immunofluorescence. It is found, for instance, in the compacted mouse embryo as early as the 16-cell preimplantation morula stage whereas fibronectin and type 4 collagen are first found after implantation in the inner cell mass of the blastocyst and interstitial (pro)collagen is only detected several days later during differentiation of the mesoderm, (Leivo et.al. 1980b). A striking induction of laminin synthesis is obtained upon differentiation of teratocarcinoma stem cells in vitro by retinoic acid and dibutyryl cyclic AMP (Strickland et.al. 1980).

### The Pericellular Matrix In vivo and In vitro

Most individual cells in vivo are in contact with extracellular matrix material; the exceptions including blood cells (which are mostly protected from connective tissue surrounding the vascular bed) and certain terminally-differentiated cells such as neurons and epidermal ketatinocytes. In culture conditions, adherent cells - perhaps all of them - synthesise matrix glyco-proteins and glycosaminoglycans. Even in adherent monocytes, the induction of fibronectin synthesis has been detected when they differentiate into macrophages (Alitalo et. al. 1980a). Furthermore, the matrix material pro-duced by a given cell, at least in primary culture, has a composition similar to that found in its tissue of origin, ie. it represents the differentiated phenotype of the cells as found in vivo.

The simple extraction of the cell layers with detergents, as introduced by Hedman et.al.(1979), leaves the integral matrix structure intact, attached to the substratum and amenable for analysis and has shown that both sulphated and nonsulphated glycosaminoglycans are constituents of the matrix (Hedman *et. al.* 1979, 1981a).

Most of the fibronectin synthesised by adherent cells is secreted into the culture medium. Only a small proportion is therefore deposited in a pericellular matrix (see Vaheri and Mosher 1978). Fibronectin must interact with a substratum in order to show the cell adhesion-promoting activity (Pearlstein 1978). Possibly a conformational change upon adsorption of fibronectin to the culture substratum exposes new sites for interaction. After secretion, matrix fibronectin is rapidly polymerised (McConnell *et. al.* 1978, Choi and Hynes 1979) and that its fibrillogenesis may be independent of collagenous matrix components is suggested by the spontaneous polymerisation of soluble fibronectin (Vuento *et al* 1980) as well as by the resistance of the pericellular fibronectin-containing structures to bacterial collagenase (Vaheri *et.al.*1978). In contrast, collagenase treatment releases some fibronectin from tissues (Bray 1978) from which it appears that in the matrix, fibronectin interacts with other components. For example in fibroblast matrix fibronectin, interstitial procollagens and sulphated glycosaminoglycans codistribute at the light microscopy level (Vaheri *et.al.*1978, Hedman *et.al.*1981a). Added cell surface fibronectin can also be chemically cross-linked to sulphated cell surface proteoglycans suggesting a close topographical neighbourhood (Perkins *et. al* 1979). In chondrocyte cultures, the distribution of fibronectin depends on the stage of chondrocyte differentiation; the protein is deposited in sizeable fibrils only in the periphery of type 1 procollagen-producing (de-differentiated) cells (Dessau *et. al.* 1978).

As for the degree of collagen processing in cell culture, it seems to be dependent on both species and cell type as well as on the procollagen type (Goldberg 1977a, Taubman and Goldberg 1976), and varies with other culture parameters. In human fibroblast cultures, mainly procollagen is deposited in the matrix before propeptide proteinases have cleaved it to collagen (Hedman *et. al.* 1979). The general assumption has been that the propeptides must be removed for fibrillogenesis to occur. Both pC and pN collagens (lacking the amino- and carboxyl propeptides, respectively) may be cross-linked by lysyl oxidase suggesting association with native-type fibrils (see Siegel 1979). *In vivo* procollagen type 3 antigenicity often codistributes with that of the respective collagen moiety, and partially-processed type 3 collagen can be extracted from skin tissue, suggesting that the fibril assembly may involve procollagen deposition *in vivo* (see Timpl *et.al.*1977, Bornstein and Traub 1980). In cultures of human amniotic epithelial cells, the partly processed $pN\alpha(3)$ molecules are deposited into periodic fibrils and subsequently cleaved to the collagen form (Hedman *et.al.*1981b).

## Pericellular Matrix Glycoproteins and Cell Differentiation

It has long been recognised in vertebrate development that the differentiation of epithelium and mesenchyme depends upon interactions between them and that the intercellular matrix probably plays an important part in this. Cell migration, cell proliferation and cell differentiation are all thought to be influenced by the type of matrix with which cells are in contact and *in vivo* studies are beginning to have an impact in this area.

In appropriate culture conditions, primary avian tendon cells synthesise extraordinarily large amounts of collagen (Schwarz and Bissell 1977; Schwarz *et. al.* 1978) and have been used as a source of procollagen in biosynthetic studies on type 1 collagen. But apart from this, they may be one of the best of the reported cells for studies on matrix glycoprotein metabolism in virus transformation since they are derived from a single organ containing mainly fibroblasts.

In general, cultured fibroblast cell strains show a relatively stable pattern of procollagen isotype production (Hance and Crystal 1977) but some fibroblastic cells such as chick embryo fibroblasts from tendon (Herrman *et. al* 1980) or cornea (Conrad *et.al.*1980) begin to synthesise procollagen type 3 only when released from their tissue matrices and passaged *in vitro*. Smooth muscle cells and chondrocytes (Mayne *et.al.*1976 1978, Burke *et.al.*1977) also show a phenotypic convergence towards fibroblast-like cells exhibiting common features of cell shape, pattern, and of fibronectin and procollagen production (see also Table 4). However, cell cloning experiments are needed to decide whether the fibroblastic phenotype is selected among the cells of the primary culture or whether a true derepression of synthetic programs occurs *in vitro*. This is highlighted by the common use of cultured rodent cells which undergo spontaneous 'transformation'. Their lower rate of collagen synthesis apparently reflects their degree of de-differentiation or transformation (see Green and Goldberg 1963 1965; Peterkofsky and Prather 1974) but this might also be explained by their genetically unstable behaviour upon prolonged cultivation *in vitro* (Ponten 1976). The labile nature of murine cells in culture is also reflected by specific changes which occur in collagen isotypes when 3T3 cells are transformed by sarcoma viruses or a chemical carcinogen (Hata and Peterkofsky 1977).

When chondrocytes are liberated from their *in vivo* matrix, synthesis of fibronectin ensues (Dessau *et.al.*1978). The freshly-plated cells do, however, still show a procollagen of type 2 and when grown in suspension culture, control of type 2 collagen production is maintained. But depending on culture conditions, some chondrocytes, when adherent, do acquire a fibroblastic morphology and begin to synthesise collagen types 1 and 3 (Cheung *et. al* 1976). Similarly, when exogenous fibronectin is added, the phenotype is switched towards fibroblastic morphology and collagen isotype production (West *et.al.*1979). The process is sensitive to a variety of factors, even to calcium or phosphate ion concentrations and calcitonin (Desmukh and Kline 1976, Desmukh et.al.1976 1977, Desmukh and Sawyer 1978), and the de-differentiation may be reversed in old cultures as seen by cartilage matrix production. This is probably in response to the influence of the deposited fibrillar fibronectin-type 1 procollagen matrix (Dessau et.al.1978).

Dibutyryl cAMP, together with retinoic acid, also causes changes in the matrix proteins secreted by chondrocytes (Desmukh and Sawyer 1977, Hassell et.al.1979), and teratocarcinoma cells (Strickland et.al.1980) and recent evidence indicates that intracellular cAMP levels also regulate the amounts of collagen degraded before secretion (Baum et.al.1980).

The cartilage phenotype is clearly labile in vitro and this has been used to explain degenerative articular diseases in man. Proliferating chondrocytes in osteoarthritis produce mainly type 1 collagen instead of cartilage-specific type 2 (Gay et.al.1976). It is of interest to note that a similar switch from type 2 to type 1 collagen occurs physiologically at the site of chondrocyte hypertrophy

Table 4
Pericellular matrix glcoproteins from cultures of human* and chick* cells

| Culture | Organ | Fibronectin | (Pro)collagen types |
|---|---|---|---|
| Human | | | |
| Fibroblasts | skin | + | 1, 3 |
| | lung | + | 1, 3, 4 |
| | gingiva | + | 1, 3 |
| Smooth muscle cells | human uterus | nd | 3, 1 |
| Endothelial cells | human umbilical vein | + | 4 |
| Epithelial cells | glomeruli | nd | 4 |
| | amniotic fluid | + | 1₃, 4 |
| | amnion | + | 3 (4, 5) |
| Chick | | | |
| Embryo fibroblasts | body wall | + | 1, 3 |
| | tendon | + | 1, 3, 5 |
| | cornea | + | 1, 3, 5 |
| Chondrocytes | sternal | + | 2 or 1 and 3 (labile) |
| Myoblasts | thigh muscle | | 1, 3, 5 |
| Organ cultures | corneal epithelium | nd | 1, 2 |
| | neural retina | - | 2, unknown (type 5?) |
| | cartilage | | 2 |
| | blood vessels | | 3 |
| | cranial bones | | 1 |

nd-not determined
*'stable' species in vitro (see Ponten 1976)
For references see text and Alitalo 1980b.

in the epiphyseal growth plate (Gay *et.al.*1976, Gay and Miller 1978) and during bone formation (Reddi *et. al.* 1977) and both are synthesised in fibrocartilage (Eyre and Muir 1977). In addition, repair processes, especially via granulation tissue in the body, are heralded by deposition of type 3 and type 1 collagens (Gay and Miller 1978).

Long before advanced culture techniques were available it was recognised by embryologists that the extracellular matrix was important for the acquisition and maintenance of the differentiated phenotype. These early studies (see Lash and Burger 1977) established that epithelial-mesenchymal interactions (in some cases, of the homologous tissues; Hata and Slavkin 1978) are needed for deposition of the basal lamina during embryogenesis. In muscle development, too, these early studies pointed to a role for collagen in myoblast fusion (Hauschka and Konigsberg 1966; see also de la Haba *et.al.*1975). It is now known that fibronectin is also involved (Furcht *et.al.*1978) and that cytoplasmic intermediate filaments play a role (Gard and Lazarides 1980). Postmitotic myoblasts and myotubes apparently do not synthesise fibronectin themselves (Ehrismann *et.al.*1980) but may need to attach to an extracellular matrix in order to respond to growth factors present in the culture medium (Gospodarowicz *et. al.* 1980). That the minimal requirement for an extracellular matrix is satisfied by fibronectin is exemplified by the growth of many cell lines and by the differentiation of the F9 teratocarcinoma cells in defined media supple mented with purified fibronectin (Rizzino and Crowley 1980).

A further example of cellular phenotype being modified in culture, has been described by Schwartz (1978) and others (Gospodarowicz *et.al.*1978; Mueller *et.al.*1980) in cultures of bovine aortic endothelial cells. In this process, called 'sprouting' some cells in the pavement-like strict endothelial cell monolayer acquire fibroblastic morphology and undermine the monolayer. There is some indication that instead of producing mainly type 3 procollagen (Sage *et. al* 1979), these cells start producing both types 1 and 3 (Cotta-Pereira *et. al* 1980). Bovine aortic endothelial cells plated between layers of collagen lose their characteristic configuration, separate from each other and assume a growth pattern similar to the sprouting pattern. The shape changes can also be induced by allowing collagen to gel over a confluent endothelium (Delvos *et.al* 1980). Clearly, the phenomenon of sprouting may be relevant to the pathogenesis of myointimal plaques.

**Production of Basement Membrane Matrix Proteins by Epithelial Cells in Culture**

The histogenesis and structure of basal laminal under most epithelia is poorly known. It is known, though, that collagen is produced in organ cultures of isolated epithelia (Dodson and Hay 1971; Hay and Dodson 1973, Cohen and Hay 1971) but only if opposed to a substratum of extracellular matrix. One of the major obstacles to further characterise these matrix proteins is that it has been difficult to maintain epithelial cell cultures from species that are genetically stable *in vitro*. It has been shown possible to identify the collagen isotypes synthesised in organ cultures of chick embryo corneal epithelium (types 1 and 2; Linsenmayer *et.al.*1977) and of visceral epithelial cells from human glomeruli (Killen *et.al.*1979) and our recent results on the biosynthesis and deposition of matrix glycoproteins in cultures of human epithelial cells are relevant here.

### Human Amniotic Epithelial Cells
Amniotic epithelium provides a unique source of large quantities of pure human epithelial cells and when supplied with epidermal growth factor these cells have been passaged serially for several generations. Prepared from the postpartal amniotic membranes (Valle and Penttinen 1962) the cultures exhibit typical characteristics of epithelial cells and grow initially as small islands of cells which stain positively for cytokeratin filaments.

Using a variety of biochemical techniques. (Alitalo *et.al.*1980a,b; Krieg *et.al* 1979; Hedman *et.al.* 1981b) fibronectin, type 3 procollagen, laminin and basement membrane collagen types 4 and 5 were all detected in the amniotic epithelial cell cultures and the same components were identified in the *in vivo* basement membranes by immunohistology. This indicates that aspects of the differentiated state *in vivo* are retained also in primary cultures of these cells, although some features, such as procollagen type 4 production may be under hormonal control as is the case in cells of the rat mammary gland (Salomon *et al.*1981). Even processing of type 3 collagen *in vivo* seems to be slow as seen by the retention of antigenic determinants of the propeptides in reticular structures of the compact layer. That the epithelial cells of the membrane survive in organ culture (unpublished) makes the model even more attractive in terms of basement membrane biosynthesis. But why only minute amounts of basement membrane collagen were produced is an enigma. Perhaps the postpartal amniotic epithelial cells may have already performed their function as part of a genetically regulated programme for effecting the easy rupture of membranes?

### Human Keratinocytes and Feeder Layer 3T3 Cells
The differentiation of epithelial cells *in vivo* is promoted by the basal lamina on which they rest (Grobstein 1967; Hay 1968; Kefalides *et.al.* 1979). Remodelling of tissue-type specific structures also requires an intact basement membrane (Vracko 1978) but although the formation of basal lamina structures by cultured epithelia requires contact with mesenchymal tissues, the biosynthetic origin of macromolecules specific to the basal lamina is known for only a few normal epithelia (Linsenmayer *et.al.*1977; Killen *et.al.*1979; Alitalo *et.al.*1980c; Quaroni and Trelstad 1980).

In view of this, it is interesting that culture conditions have recently been developed which promote the growth and differentiation of human epidermal keratinocytes (Rheinwald and Green 1977). The conditions developed by Green (1978) and his co-workers involve the use of 3T3 feeder cell layers as well as epidermal growth factor, hydrocortisone and cholera toxin as hormone supplements.

We grew human epidermal cells into colonies and eventually to stratified cell layers in co-culture with mouse 3T3 feeder cells and found them to synthesise and secrete fibronectin into their culture medium (Alitalo et. al. 1981). In contrast, little of laminin and only minor amounts of collagen types 4 and 5 were produced by the keratinocytes. The widely used Balb/3T3 feeder cells were found to produce basal lamina glycoproteins; type 4 procollagen and laminin in addition to the previously identified connective tissue matrix components of fibroblasts: interstitial procollagens and fibronectin.

It was of interest to find intracellular fibronectin staining largely confined to the outermost cells of the epidermal cell islands. A centripetal gradient of differentiation is known to form in the growing colonies with the least differentiated cells at the expanding periphery and terminally differentiating cells exfoliating on top of the colonies at their central parts (Sun and Green 1976). Thus, the synthesis of fibronectin may be lost early in keratinocyte differentiation. The mobile marginal cells in epithelial colonies are the most sensitive to the flattening and spreading effects of EGF (Keski-Oja et. al 1980a), whereas mitoses also occur in other parts of the keratinocyte islands. Furthermore, the production of fibronectin by the keratinocytes or by 3T3 cells was not found to be dependent on the presence of hormones reported to promote fibronectin deposition in cultures of epithelial (Marceau et al 1980) and of malignant cells (Furcht et.al.1977) and by the feeder layer 3T3 cells in serum-starved conditions (Chen et.al.1977).

The significance of the fibronectin production by the epidermal cells is unclear. It may just reflect the tendency of cells to dedifferentiate as part of a proliferative response. However, there is no apparent selection for fibronectin production in co-culture conditions, where both murine fibronectin from 3T3 cells from many other sources do produce fibronectin in culture (Quaroni et.al 1978, Smith et.al.1979).

The production of basal lamina proteins by the 3T3 feeder cells may facilitate adhesion and spreading of the keratinocytes since epithelial cells adhere preferentially to type 4 collagen (Murray et. al. 1979) probably through laminin. This cell-matrix interaction may also promote the effect of mitogens as has been reported in other cell cultures (Gospodarowicz et.al.1980), and thus explain the augmenting effect of medium conditioned by 3T3 cells on growth of the keratinocytes (Green 1978). Propagation for limited generations of human epidermal keratinocytes has been reported even in the absence of feeder layer or of medium supplements other than serum and hydrocortisone (Eisinger et.al.1978, Hawley-Nelson et.al.1980, Peehl and Ham 1980a,b). It may be that in these conditions of dense seeding the attachment of the keratinocytes to their growth substratum can occur through the matrix components they produce themselves. Interestingly, fibronectin coating of the growth substratum facilitates the growth of keratinocytes in culture (Gilchrest *et.al*.1980).

The old controversy about the phenotype of 3T3 cells (Porter *et.al*. 1973, Boone 1975) was thought to be clarified by the results of Goldberg (1977b) who showed that the cells produce collagen types 1 and 3 characteristic to fibroblasts. However, since then, it has been demonstrated that cells with a normal (human) fibroblast phenotype can produce simultaneously procollagens of both basement membrane and interstitial types (Alitalo 1980a). We have now noted procollagen type 4 and laminin in cultures of pure clonal fibroblastic A31 3T3 cells.

The results obtained with epidermal cells were recently extended to explant cultures of human ectocervical cells (Halila *et. al*. submitted) that are also derived from a stratified squamous epithelium (Vesterinen *et.al*.1980a). In comparison, endocervical cell cultures that are derived from a columnar epithelium and also grow unstratified *in vitro* (Vesterinen *et.al*.1980b), have a greater proportion of fibronectin synthesising cells (Halila *et.al*. submitted).

*Fibronectin-Collagen Matrix is Lost in Malignant Transformation*
Fibronectin is clearly an important constituent of the extracellular matrix and as such is involved in tissue organisation. The loss of fibronectin upon malignant transformation coincides with a disturbance of normal tissue structure and this is discussed here in as much as it reflects upon the role of fibronectin in determining the differentiated phenotype.

The great interest in fibronectin dates back to 1973 when it was first noted that a polypeptide was greatly reduced from the surface of virally transformed fibroblastic cells as compared to normal cells (see Vaheri and Mosher 1978). At about this time it was also convincingly shown that a reduction of collagen production occurred in virus-transformed fibroblasts (Levinson *et.al*. 1975). The role of the transforming viral genes in the loss of the pericellular matrix (Gahmberg *et.al*.1974, Vaheri and Ruoslahti 1974, Hynes and Wyke 1975, Adams *et.al*.1977, Arbogast *et.al*.1977, Vaheri *et.al*.1978) was established using virus mutants temperature sensitive for transformation.

The mechanism of the secondary loss of the pericellular matrix includes about five-fold reduction in the biosynthesis of both fibronectin and procollagen due to a corresponding reduction in the copy number of their messenger RNAs (Adams *et.al*.1977 1979, Howard *et.al*.1978, Rowe *et.al* 1978, Fagan *et.al*.1979, Sandmeyer and Bornstein 1979, Parker and Fitschen 1980, Sandmeyer *et.al*. 1981b). Indeed, this seems to be due to coordinate decrease in transcription of the procollagen genes (Sandmeyer *et.al*.1981a). In addition, in RSV-transformed chick embryo fibroblast cultures there is also an increased degradation of fibronectin (Olden and Yamada 1977), procollagen post-translational modifications are increased (Myllyla *et.al.*1981), and in transformed chick fibroblast cultures probably even less of the procollagen polypeptide cleavages are completed than in cultures of normal cells (Arbogast *et.al.*1977). It is also clear that malignantly transformed mesenchyme-derived cells have a reduced capacity to deposit the fibronectin they synthesise synthesise. The reduction in the amount of matrix fibronectin upon transformation has been measured by many methods in both viral, spontaneous and chemical transformation and there are few contrary reports (see Vaheri and Mosher 1978).

The proportions of different glycosaminoglycans are changed in transformed cells and the overall tendency is for a shift from complex sulphated glycosaminoglycans (eg. heparan sulfate) to hyaluronic acid production (see Roden 1980, Glimelius 1977). This could affect the distribution of fibronectin for as mentioned above, sulphated glycosaminoglycans interact with fibronectin and may be receptor molecules for fibronectin on the cell surface.

Altered patterns of glycosylation of cell surface proteins and of glycolipids in transformed cells have been also offered to explain the difference (see Atkinson and Hakimi 1980, Steiner and Steiner 1978, Tuszynski *et.al.*1978, Vaheri 1978). In addition, cytoskeletal structures are disturbed in transformed cells (Nicolson 1976ab). Experimental disruption of the microfilament bundles by cytochalasin B caused partial loss of the fibronectin matrix from the surface of normal cells (Kurkinen *et.al.*1978). On the other hand, addition of cell surface fibronectin restores a more normal morphology supported by pronounced microfilament bundles which implies some reciprocal interaction between the two systems. (Yamada *et.al.*1976a b, Ali *et.al.*1977, Willingham *et.al.*1977). Not only does such interaction between matrix and cytoskeleton suggest how cell morphology may be responsive to the nature of the substratum but offers a mechanism by which the anchorage requirement for the growth of normal cells in culture is fulfilled.

### Cell-Matrix Interaction and Anchorage-dependance of Normal Cells

A fundamental requirement for *in vitro* growth of normal non-hematopoietic cells is their anchorage to a substratum. Adherent cells in general produce components of the pericellular matrix that also are involved in their substrate-adhesion (Kurkinen *et. al.* 1980b, Penttinen *et. al.* 1980) and exogenous fibronectin present in culture media functions as an adhesive glycoprotein for a variety of cells (Vaheri *et.al.*1980). Recently, other molecules have been found that may be required to mediate the tissue type-specific adhesion of eg. epithelial cells to basement membranes (Terranova *et.al.*1980). In the case of human keratinocytes, one of the functions of the so-called feeder cells or of conditioned medium may be to supply these adhesion molecules for proper growth of the cells (Alitalo *et.al.*1981b).

The formation and ultrastructure of adhesive contacts *in vitro* have been studied in cultures of mesenchymal cells. A close association seems to exist between actin-containing microfilament bundles and extracellular fibronectin-containing fibers during cell spreading or at the termini of the microfilament bundles in adhesion plaques of the fully spread cells (Mautner and Hynes 1977, Hynes and Destree 1978).

Actin seems only to interact directly with fibronectin under experimental conditions (Keski-Oja *et.al.* 1980b) and an indirect, transmembrane linkage has been proposed to occur at local sites of cell-cell and cell-matrix interaction. Actin microfilaments are formed into bundles at these points of contact but the cytoplasmic components of these junctions are not yet fully resolved and the resolution of structural studies (Singer 1979) does not allow us to say where fibronectin is situated at the extracellular face of such trans-membrane complexes. Recent studies have begun to identify some of the components of the adhesion plaques such as $\alpha$)actinin and a 130,000 protein termed vinculin (Geiger 1979, Burridge and Feramisco 1980). Both are detected on the inner aspect of the plasma membrane at sites of contact of actin microfilaments with the membrane.

## The Transforming Kinases of Tumour Viruses and their Cellular Location

Recent studies show (see Hynes 1980; Langan 1980) that at lease some of the transforming kinases of tumour viruses are located at these adhesion plaques. Here, the kinases may catalyse phosphorylation of proteins which mediate microfilament bundle formation which further suggests that phosphorylation of plasma membrane-associated proteins could be a general mechanism for affecting cell-matrix interactions and be responsible for their changes brought about by malignant transformation.

The transforming proteins of several of both RNA and DNA tumour viruses are phosphoproteins and apparently most of them also behave as cyclic AMP-independent protein kinases (ATP:protein phosphotransferases). The pp60src protein kinase activity is temperature-sensitive when derived from viruses which have a ts mutation in the *src* gene (Erikson *et.al.* 1979), Maness *et.al* 1979). The specificity of phosphotransferase reaction is novel in having substrate tyrosine residues as acceptors (Hunter and Sefton 1980) and is possibly also inhibited by N-$\alpha$-tosyl-L-lysyl chloromethyl ketone (TLCK) (Richert *et. al.* 1979). While uninfected normal cells also contain a gene product homologous to that of pp60src (Collett *et.al.* 1978, Oppermann *et.al* 1979, Sefton *et.al.* 1980), transformation of ASV-infected cells may result from an enzyme-amplified increase in the reaction product.

Indirect immunofluorescence and immunoelectron microscopy using seemingly specific anti-pp60src antisera prepared from tumour-bearing animals has located this plasma membrane associated protein to areas of cell-cell

(Willingham *et.al*.1979) and cell-substratum contacts at the adhesion plaques (Rohrschneider 1979). Possibly in this latter location pp60src is associated with cytoskeletal structures as evidenced by resistance of the enzyme activity to solubilization by non-ionic detergens (Burr *et. al*. 1980, Shriver and Rohrschneider 1980). In this respect it is of interest to note that vinculin located in the detergent-exposed adhesion plaques of cultured cells is also phosphorylated at tyrosine residues in such structures and is a substrate for pp60src (Shriver and Rohrschneider 1980). There is evidence from sequence analysis of the *src* gene and from analysis of the transforming protein domain structure that the *src* protein has a hydrophobic N-terminus embedded within the plasma membrane, the carboxyl terminus being accessible (Czernil ofsky *et.al*. 1980, Levinson *et.al*. 1981) and phosphorylated at tyrosine residues (Purchio *et.al*.1980) on the cytoplasmic aspect of the plasma membrane. The catalytic activity of pp60src residues in the carboxyl terminus and may thus be directly exposed to the cytoplasm of the cell. It is of interest to recognise that the effects of the temperature-sensitive kinase on cell morphology, actin microfilament bundles and fibronectin are also observed in the absence of the nucleus (enucleated cells; Beug *et.al*.1978). The transforming protein pp60src thus exerts many if not all of its effects at the periphery of the cell and most if not all of the aberations in the neoplastic cell may eventually be traced to these effects at the cell periphery (Levinson *et.al*.1981). The transforming protein pp60src thus exerts many if not all of its effects at the periphery of the cell and most if not all of the aberrations in the neoplastic cell may eventually be traced to these effects at the periphery (Levinson *et.al*.1981).

**Cell-Substratum Interaction in Relation to Growth Factors**
There is evidence suggesting that cell-substratum contact is needed for maintenance of protein synthesis in anchorage-dependent cells (Ben-Ze'ev *et al*.1980) and that the degree of cell spreading is directly proportional to the synthesis of DNA (Folkman and Moscona 1978) which suggest that cell-substratum interactions affect growth control as well as cell morphology.

The effect of certain growth factors may be enhanced by supplying cultures with substrate-adhesion proteins or by growing cells on prepared extracellular matrices or feeder layers instead of plastic (Gospodarowicz *et. al*.1980). Tyrosine phosphorylation of membrane proteins by an EGF-enhanced (receptor- associated) membrane protein kinase has been recently reported (Ushiro and Cohen 1980). A number of human and animal carcinoma and sarcoma cells secrete 'growth factor' activity (Todaro *et. al*, 1980, and phospho-proteins; Senger *et.al*.1980) that acts via the EGF receptors in an analogous manner. Sarcoma growth factor strongly stimulates anchorage-independent growth of cells that will not multiply or form clones in soft agar in its absence (DeLarco and Todaro 1978). Thus the intriguing possibility exists that the requirement of a pericellular matrix for growth of normal cells is based on regulatory signals mediated through phosphorylation reactions at the cell surface membrane, while the autonomous growth of tumour cells is uncoupled from this requirement by autocrine secretion mechanisms or by transforming kinase-catalysed reactions also occurring at the plasma membrane.

## Acknowledgements

Original contributions from this laboratory were supported by grants from the National Institutes of Health, NCI, grant no. CA 24605, The Academy of Finland, and the Finnish Cancer Foundation.

## References

Adams, S.L., Sobel, M.E., Howard, B.H., Olden, K., Yamada, K.M., de Crommbrugghe, B. and Pastan, I. 1977. *Levels of translatable mRNAs for cell surface protein precursors and two membrane proteins are altered in Rous sarcoma virus-transformed chick embryo fibroblasts.* Proc. Natl. Acad. Sci. USA *74*, 3399-3403.

Adams, S.L., Alwine, J.C., de Crombrugghe, B. and Pastan, I. 1979. *Use of recombinant plasmids to characterise collagen RNAs in normal and transformed chick embryo fibroblasts.* J. Biol. Chem. *254*, 4945-4938.

Al-Adnani, M.S. and McGee, J.O'D. 1976. *C1q production and secretion by fibroblasts.* Nature, *263*, 145-146.

Ali, I.U. and Hynes, R.O. 1978. *Effects of LETS glycoprotein on cell motility.* Cell, *14*, 439-446.

Ali, I.E., Mautner, V. and Lanza, R. *et al.* 1977. *Restoration of normal morphology, adhesion and cytoskeleton in transformed cells by addition of a transformation-sensitive surface protein.* Cell, *11*, 847-857.

Alitalo, K. 1980a. *Production of both interstitial and basement membrane procollagens by fibroblastic WI-38 cells from human embryonic lung.* Biochem. Biophys. Res. Commun. *93*, 873-880.

Alitalo, K. 1980b. *Connective tissue glycoproteins of normal differentiated and of malignant human cells.* Thesis. Helsinki.

Alitalo, K., Hovi, T. and Vaheri, A. 1980a. *Fibronectin is produced by human macrophages.* J. Exp. Med. *151*, 602-613.

Alitalo, K., Kurkinen, M., Vaheri, A., Krieg, T. and Timpl,R. 1980b. *Basement membrane components synthesised by human amniotic epithelial cells in culture.* Cell, *19*, 1053-1062.

Alitalo, K., Kuismanen, E., Myllyla, R., Kiistala, U., Asko-Seljavaara, S. and Vaheri, A. 1981a. *Human epidermal keratinocytes synthesise and deposit collagen 1(5) chains and secrete together with feeder 3T3 cells fibronectin, type 4 collagen and laminin.* Submitted for publication.

arbogast, B.W., Yoshimura, M., Kefalides, N.A., Holtzer, H. and Kaji, A. 1977. *Failure of cultured chick embryo fibroblasts to incorporate collagen into their extracellular matrix when formed by Rous sarcoma virus.* J. Biol. Chem. *252*, 8863-8868.

Atkinson, P.H. and Hakimi, J. 1980. *Alterations in glycoproteins of the cell surface. In: The Biochemistry of Glycoproteins and Proteoglycans* (ed. W.J. Lennartz) Plenum Press, New York, pp. 191-240.

Barnes, D. and Sato, G. 1980. *Serum-free cell culture: a unifying approach.* Cell, *22*, 649-655.

Baum, B.J., Moss, J., Breul, S.D., Berg, E.A. and Crystal, R.G. 1980. *Effect of cyclic AMP on the intracellular degradation of newly synthesised collagen.* J. Biol. Chem. *255*, 2843-2847.

Ben-Ze'ev, A., Farmer, S.R. and Penman, S. 1980. *Protein synthesis requires cell-surface contact while nuclear events respond to cell shape in anchorage-dependent fibroblasts.* Cell, *21*, 365-372.

# 46 CELLULAR CONTROLS IN DIFFERENTIATION

Beug, H., Claviez, M., Jockusch, B.M. and Graf, T. 1978. *Differential expression of Rous sarcoma virus-specific transformation parameters in enucleated cells.* Cell, *14*, 843-856.

Bissell, M.J., Orne, A. and Schwarz, R. 1980. *Analysis of collagen containing extracellular matrix from primary avian tendon cells (PAT) in culture.* J. Cell Biol. *87*, 125a.

Boone, C.W. 1975. *Malignant haemagioendotheliomas produced by subcutaneous inoculation of Balb/3T3 cells attached to glass beads.* Science, *188*, 68-70.

Bornstein, P. and Sage, H. 1980. *Structurally distinct collagen types.* Ann. Rev. Biochem. *49*, 957-1003.

Bornstein, P. and Traub, W. 1980. *The Chemistry and Biology of Collagen. In: The Proteins,* vol. *4* (ed. H. Neutath and R.L. Hill) Academic Press, New York, pp. 411-462.

Bray, B.A. 1978. *Cold-insoluble globulin (fibronectin) in connective tissues of adult human lung and in trophoblast basement membrane.* J. Clin. Invest. *62*, 745-752.

Burke, J.M.,Balian, G., Ross, R. and Bornstein, P. 1977. *Synthesis of types I and III procollagen and collagen by monkey aortic smooth muscle cells in vitro.* Biochemistry, *16*, 3243-3249.

Burr, J.G., Dreyfuss, G., Penman, S.H. and Buchanan, J.M. 1980. *Association of the src gene product of Rous sarcoma virus with cytoskeletal structures of chicken embryo fibroblasts.* Proc. Natl. Acad. Sci. USA. *77*, 3483-3488.

Burridge, K. and Feramisco, J.R. 1980. *Microinjection and localisation of a 130K protein in living fibroblasts: a relationship to actin and fibronectin.* Cell, *19*, 587-595.

Butler, W.T., Finch, J.E. Jr. and Miller, E.J. 1977. *The covalent structure of cartilage collagen.* J. Biol. Chem. *252*, 639-643.

Chen, L.B., Gudor, R.C., Sun, T.-T., Chen, A.B. and Mosesson, M.W. 1977. *Control of a cell surface major glycoprotein by epidermal growth factor.* Science, *19*, 776-778.

Chen-Kiang, S., Cardinale, G.J. and Undenfriend, S. 1977. *Homology between a prolyl hydroxylase subunit and a tissue protein that cross-reacts immunologically with the enzyme.* Proc. Natl. Acad. Sci. USA. *74*, 4420-4424.

Chen-Kiang, S., Cardinale, G.J. and Udenfriend, S. 1978. *Expression of collagen biosynthetic activities in lymphocytic cells.* Proc. Natl. Acad. Sci. USA. *75*, 1379-1383.

Cheung, H.S., Harvey, W., Benya, P.D. and Nimni, M.E. 1976. *New collagen markers of derepression synthesised by rabbit articular chondrocytes in culture.* Biochem. Biophys. Res. Commun. *68*, 1371-1378.

Choi, M.G. and Hynes, R.O. 1979. *Biosynthesis and processing of fibronectin in NIL 8 hamster cells.* J. Biol. Chem. *254*, 12050-12055.

Chung, A.E., Jaffe, R., Freeman, J.L., Vernes, J.P., Graginski, J.E. and Carlin, B. 1979. *Properties of a basemewnt membrane-related glycoprotein synthesised in culture by mouse embryonal carcinoma-derived cell line.* Cell, *16*, 277-287.

Cohen, A.M. and Hay, E.D. 1971. *Secretion of collagen by embryonic neuro-epithelium at the time of spinal cord-somite interaction.* Devel. Biol. *26*, 578-605.

Collett, M.S., Brugge, J.S. and Erikson, R.L. 1978. *Characterisation of a normal avian cell protein related to the avian sarcoma virus transforming gene product.* Cell, *15*, 1363-1369.

Conrad, G.W., Dessau, W. and von der Mark, K. 1980. *Synthesis of type III collagen by fibroblasts from the embryonic chick cornea.* J. Cell. Biol. *84*, 501-512.

Cotta-Pereira, F., Sage, H., Bornstein, P., Ross, R. and Schwartz, S. 1980. *Studies of morphologically atypical ('sprouting') cultures of bovine aortic endothelial cells. Growth characteristics and connective tissue protein synthesis.* J. Cell. Physiol. *102*, 183-191.

Czernilofsky, A.P., Levinson, A.D., Varmus, H.E., Bishop, J.M., Tischer, E. and Goodman, H.M. 1980. *Nucleotide sequence of an avian sarcoma virus oncogene (src) and proposed amino acid sequence for gene product.* Nature, *287*, 198-203.

de la Haba, G., Kamall, H.M. and Tiede, D.M. 1975. *Myogenesis of avian striated muscle in vitro: Role in collagen myofiber formation.* Proc. Natl. Acad. Sci. USA. *72*, 2729-2732.

De Larco, J.E. and Todaro, G.J. 1978. *Growth factors from murine sarcoma virus-transformed cells.* Proc. Natl. Acad. Sci. USA. *75*, 4001-4005.

Delvos, U., Gajdusek, C., Harker, L.A. and Schwartz, S.M. 1980. *Growth of vascular wall cells in and on collagen.* Fed. Proc. *39*, 770.

Desmukh, K. and Sawyer, B.D. 1977. *Synthesis of collagen by chondrocytes in suspension culture: Modulation by calcium, 3':5'-cyclic AMP, and prosta-glandins.* Proc. Natl. Acad, Sci. USA. *74*, 3864-3868.

Desmukh, K. and Kline, W.G. 1976. *Characterisation of collagen and its precursors synthesised by rabbit articulage cartilage cells in various culture systems.* Eur. J. Biochem. *69*, 117-123.

Desmukh, K., Kline, W.F. and Sawyer, B.D. 1976. *Role of calcium in the phenotypic expression of rabbit articular chondrocytes in culture.* FEBS Letters, *67*, 58-51.

Desmukh, K., Kline, W.G. and Sawyer, B.D. 1977. *Effects of calcitonin and parathyroid hormone on metabolism of chondrocytes in culture.* Biochim. Biophys. Acta. *499*, 28-35.

Desmukh, K. and Sawyer, B.D. 1978. *Influence of extracellular pyrophosphate on the synthesis of collagen by chondrocytes.* FEBS Letters, *89*, 230-232.

Dessau, W., Sasse, J., Timple, R., Jilek, F. and von der Mark, K. 1978. *Synthesis and extracellular deposition of fibronectin in chondrocyte cultures.* J. Cell Biol. *79*, 342-355.

Dodson, J.W. and Hay, E.D. 1971. *Secretion of collagenous stroma by isolated epithelium grown in vitro.* Exp. Cell Res. *65*, 215-220.

Dunham, J.S. and Hynes, R.O. 1978. *Differences in the sulphated macromolecules synthesised by normal and transformed hamster fibroblasts.* Biochim. Biophys. Acta. *506*, 242-255.

Ehrismann, R., Chiquet, M. and Turner, D.C. 1980. *Fibronectin: Mode of action and possible role in muscle morhpogenesis.* Proc. IX Meeting of the British Society of Cell Biology.

Eisinger, M., Lee, S.J., Hefton, J.M., Darzynkiewica, Z., Chiao, J.W. and de Harven, E. 1978. *Human epidermal cell cultures: Growth and differentiation in the absence of dermal components or medium supplements.* Proc. Natl. Acad. Sci. USA. *76*, 5340-5344.

Engvall, E. and Ruoslahti, E. 1977. *Binding of soluble form of fibroblast surface protein, fibronectin to collagen.* Int. J. Cancer. *20*, 1-5.

Epstein, E.H. Jr. 1974. *1(III)3 human skin collagen.* J. Biol. Chem. *249*, 3225-3231.

Erikson, R.L., Collett, M.S., Erikson, E. and Purchio, A.F. 1979. *Evidence that the avian sarcoma virus transforming gene product is a cyclic AMP-independent protein kinase.* Proc. Natl. Acad. Sci. USA. *76*, 6260-6264.

Eyre, D.R., and Muir, H. 1977. *Quantitative-analysis of type-1 collagen and type-2 collagen in human intervertebral discs at various ages.* Biochim. Biophys. Acta. *494*, 29-42.

Fagan, J.B., Yamada, K.M., de Crombrugge, B. and Pastan, I. 1979. *Partial purification and characterisation of the messenger-RNA for cell fibronectin.* Nucl. Acids Res. *6*, 3471-3480.

Fessler, J.H. and Fessler, L.I. 1978. *Biosynthesis of procollagen.* Ann. Rev. Biochem. *47*, 129-162.

Foidart, J.M., Bere, E.W., Yaar, M., Rennard, S.I., Cullino, M., Martin, G.R. and Katz, S.I. 1980. *Distribution and immunoelectron microscopic localisation of laminin, a noncollagenous basement membrane glycoprotein.* Lab. Invest. *42*, 336-342.

Folkman, J. and Moscona, A. 1978. *Role of cell shape in growth control.* Nature *273*, 345-349.

Furcht, L.T., Mosher, D.F., and Wendelschafer-Crabb, G. 1978. *Immunocytochemical localisation of fibronectin (LETS protein) on the surface of L6 myoblasts: Light and electron microscopic studies.* Cell, *13*, 263-271.

Furcht, L.T., Mosher, D.F., Wendelschafer-Crabb, G., Woodbridge, P.A. and Foidart, J.M. 1977. *Dexamethasone-induced accumulation of a fibronectin and collagen extracellular matrix in transformed human cells.* Nature, *271*, 393-395.

Gahmberg, C.G., Kiehn, D. and Hakomori, S.-I. 1974. *Changes in a surface-labelled galactoprotein and in glycolipid concentrations in cells transformed by a temperature-sensitive polyoma virus mutant.* Nature, *248*, 413-415.

Gard, D.L. and Lazarides, E. 1980. *The synthesis and distribution of desmin and vimentin during myogenesis in vitro.* Cell, *19*, 263-275.

Gay, S. and Miller, E.J. 1978. Collagen in the Physioogy and Pathology of Connective Tissue (ed.) Gustav Fischer Verlag, Stuttgart, New York.

Gay, S., Martin, G.R., Muller, P.K., Timpl, R. and Kuhn, K. 1976. Simultaneous synthesis of types I and III collagen by fibroblasts in culture. Proc. Natl. Acad. Sci. USA. 73, 4037-4040.

Geiger, B. 1979. A 130K protein from chicken gizzard; Its localisation at the termini of microfilament bundles in cultured chicken cells. Cell, 18, 193-205.

Gilchrest, B.A., Nemore, R.E. and Maciag, T. 1980. Growth of human keratinocytes on fibronectin-coated plates. Cell Biol. Int. Reports. 4, 1009-1016.

Glimelius, B. 1977. Thesis. Almquist and Wiksell, Stockholm.

Goldberg, B. 1977a. Kinetics of processing of types I and type III procollagens in fibroblast cultures. Proc. Natl. Acad. Sci. USA. 74, 3311-3325.

Goldberg, B. 1977b. Collagen synthesis as a marker for cell type in mouse 3T3 lines. Cell, 11, 169-172.

Gospodarowicz, D. and Tauber, J.P. 1980. Growth factors and the extracellular matrix. Endocrine Rev. 1, 201-227.

Gospodarowicz, D., Mescher, A.L. and Birdwell, C.R. 1978. Control of cellular proliferation by the fibroblast and epidermal growth factors. Natl. Cancer Inst. Monogr. 48, 109-130.

Gospodarowicz, D., Delgado, D. and Vlodavsky, I. 1980. Permissive effect of the extracellular matrix on cell proliferation in vitro. Proc. Natl. Acad. Sci. USA. 77, 4094-4098.

Green, H. 1978. Cyclic AMP in relation to proliferation of the epidermal cells: a new view. Cell, 15, 801-811.

Green, H. and Goldberg, B. 1963. Kinetics of collagen synthesis by established mammalian cell lines. Nature, 4911, 1097-1098.

Green, H. and Goldberg, B. 1965. Synthesis of collagen by mammalian cell lines of fibroblastic and nonfibroblastic origin. Proc. Natl. Acad. Sci. USA. 53, 1360-1365.

Grinnell, F., Feld, M. and Minter, D. 1980. Fibroblast adhesion to fibrinogen and fibrin substrate: Requirement for cold-insoluble globulin (plasma fibronectin). Cell, 19, 517-525.

Grobstein, C. 1967. Mechanisms of organogenetic tissue interaction. Natl. Cancer Inst. Monogr. 26, 279-299.

Halila, H., Vesterinen, E., Vaheri, A., and Alitalo, K. 1981. Fibronectin production and keratinisation distinguish endo- and ectocervical human uterine epithelial cells in culture. (Submitted for publication).

Hance, A.J. and Crystal, G.R. 1977. Rigid control of synthesis of collagen types I and III by cells in culture. Nature, 268, 151-154.

Hassell, J.R., Pennypacker, J.P., Kleinman, H.K., Pratt, R.M. and Yamada, K.M. 1979. Enhanced cellular fibronectin accumulation in chondrocytes treated with vitamin A. Cell, 17, 821-826.

Hassell, J.R., Robey, P.G., Barrach, H.J., Wilczek, J., Rennard, S.J. and Martin, G.R. 1980. Isolation of heparin sulphate containing proteoglycan from basement membrane. Proc. Natl. Acad. Sci. USA. 77, 4494-4498.

Hata, R.I. and Peterkofsky, B. 1977. Specific changes in the collagen phenotype of BALB 3T3 cells as a result of transformation by sacroma viruses or a chemical carcinogen. Proc. Natl. Acad. Sci. USA. 74, 2933-2937.

Hata, R.I. and Slavkin, H. 1978. De novo induction of a gene product during heterologous epithelial-mesenchymal interactions in vitro. Proc. Natl. Acad. Sci. USA. 75, 2790-2794.

Hauschka, S.D. and Konigsberg, I.R. 1966. The influence of collagen of the development of muscle clones. Proc. Natl. Acad. Sci. USA. 55, 119-126.

Hawley-Nelson, P., Sullivan, J.E., Kung, M., Hennings, H. and Yuspa, S.H. 1980. Optimised conditions for the growth of human epidermal cells in culture, J. Invest. Dermatol. 75, 176-182.

Hay, E.D. 1978. *Role of basement membranes in development and differentiation. In: Biology and Chemistry of Basement Membranes* (ed. N.A. kefalides) Academic Press, New York, pp. 119-136.

Hay, E.D. and Dodson, J.W. 1973. *Secretion of collagen by corneal epithelium. I. Morphology of the collagenous products produced by isolated epithelia grown on frozen-killed lens.* J. Cell Biol. *57*, 190-213.

Hedman, K., Kurkinen, M., Alitalo, K., Vaheri, A., Johansson, S., and Hook, M. 1979. *Isolation of the pericellular matrix of human fibroblast cultures.* J. Cell Biol. *81*, 83-91.

Hedman, K., Johansson, S., Vartio, T., Kjellen, L., Vaheri, A. and Hook, M. 1981 a. *Structures of the pericellular matrix in human fibroblast cultures: Association of sulphated glycosaminoglycans with the fibronectin-procollagen fibres.* Submitted for publication.

Hedman, K., Alitalo, K., Lehtinen, S., Timpl, R. and Vaheri, A. 1981b. *Deposition of procollagen type III PN° molecules into periodic fibrils in the matrix of amniotic epithelial cells.* Submitted for publication.

Herrmann, H., Dessau, W., Fessler, L.I. and von der Mark, K. 1980. *Synthesis of types I, III and AB₂ collagen by chick tendon fibroblasts in vitro.* Eur. J. Biochem. *105*, 63-74.

Hewitt, A.T., Kleinman, H.K., Pennypacker, J.P. and Martin, G.R. 1980. *Identification of an adhesion factor for chondrocytes.* Proc. Natl. Acad. Sci. USA. *77*, 385-388.

Hogan, B.L.M. Ashley, A.R. and Kurkinen, M. 1980. *Incorporation into Reichert's membrane of laminin-like extracellular proteins synthesised by parietal endoderm cells of the mouse embryo.* Devel. Biol. (in press).

Howard, B.H., Adams, S.L., Sobel, M.E., Pastan, I. and de Crombrugghe, B. 1978. *Decreased levels of collagen mRNA in Rous sarcoma virus-transformed chick embryo fibroblasts.* J. Biol. Chem. *253*, 5869-5874.

Hunter, T. and Sefton, B.M. 1980. *Transforming gene product of Rous Sarcoma virus phosphorylates tyrosine.* Proc. Natl. Acad. Sci. USA. *77*, 1311-1315.

Hynes, R.O. 1980. *Cellular location of viral transforming proteins.* Cell, 601-602.

Hynes, R.O. and Destree, A.T. 1978. *Relationship between fibronectin and actin.* Cell, *15*, 875-886.

Hynes, R.O. and Wyke, J.A. 1975. *Alterations in surface proteins in chicken cells transformed by temperature-sensitive mutants of Rous sarcoma virus.* Virology, *64*, 492-504.

Jilek, F. and Hormann, H. 1979. *Fibronectin (cold-insoluble globulin): Influence of heparin and hyealuronic acid on the binding of native collagen.* Hoppe Seyler's Z. Physiol. Chem. *360*, 597-603.

Jimenez, S.A., Bashey, R.J., Benditt, M. and Yankowsky, R. 1972. *Identification of collagen 1 (I) trimer in embryonic chick tendons and calvaria.* Biochem. Biophys. Res. Commun. *78*, 1354-1361.

Johansson, S. and Hook, M. 1980. *Heparin enhances the rate of binding of fibronectin to collagen.* Biochem. J. *187*, 521-524.

Kanwar, Y.S. and Farquhar, M.G. 1979. *Isolation of glycosaminoglycans (heparan sulphate) from glomerular basement membranes.* Proc. Natl. Acad. Sci. USA. *76*, 4493-4497.

Kefalides, N.A., Alper, R. and Clark, C.C. 1979. *Biochemistry and metabolism of basement membranes.* In: Int. Rev. Cytol. vol. *61* (ed. G.H. Bourne, F. Danielli, and K.W. Jeon) Academic Press, New York, pp. 167-228.

Keski-Oja, J., Mosher, D.F. and Vaheri, A. 1976. *Cross-linking of a major fibroblast surface-associated glycoprotein (fibronectin catalysed by blood coagulation factor XIII.* Cell, *9*, 29-35.

Keski-Oja, J., Heine, U.I., Rapp, U.R. and Wetzel, B. 1980a. *Epidermal growth factor-induced alterations in proliferating mouse epithelial cells.* Exp. Cell Res. *128*, 279-290.

Keski-Oja, J., Sen, A. and Todaro, G.J. 1980b. *Direct association of fibronectin and actin molecules in vitro.* J. Cell Biol. *83*, 527-533.

Killen, P.D., Striker, G.E. and Byer, P.H. 1979. *Human glomerular visceral epithelial cells synthesise a basal lamina collagen in vitro.* Proc. Natl. Acad. Sci. USA. *76*, 3518-3522.

Kivirikko, K.I. 1980. *Post-translational modifications of collagen. In: Gene Families of Collagen and Other Proteins* (ed. Prockop, D.J. and Champe, P.C.) Elsevier North Holland, New York, pp. 107-119.

Kivirikko, K.I. and Myllyla, R. 1980. *Collagen glycosyltransferases.* Int. Rev. Conn. Tissue Res. *8*, 23-72.

Krieg, T., Timpl, R., Alitalo, K., Kurkinen, M. and Vaheri, A. 1979. *Type III procollagen is the major collagenous component produced by a continuous rhabdomyosarcoma cell line.* FEBS Letters, *104*, 405-409.

Kurkinen, M., Wartiovaara, J. and Vaheri, A. 1978. *Cytochalasin B releases a major surface-associated glycoprotein, fibronectin, from cultured fibroblasts.* Exp. Cell Res. *111*, 127-137.

Kurkinen, M., Vartio, T. and Vaheri, A. 1980a. *Polypeptides of human plasma fibronectin are similar but not identical.* Biochim. Biophys. Acta. *624*, 490-498.

Kurkinen, M., Alitalo, K., Hedman, K. and Vaheri, A. 1980b. *Fibronectin, procollagen and the pericellular matrix in normal and transformed fibroblast cultures. In: Biology of Collagen* (ed. Viidik, A. and Vuust, J.) Academic Press, London, pp. 223-235.

Kuusela, P. 1978. *Fibronectin binds to Staphylococcus aureus.* Nature, *273*, 718-720.

Langan, T. 1980. *Malignant transformation and protein phosphorylation.* Nature, *286*, 329-330.

Lash, J.W. and Burger, M.M. 1977 (eds.) *Cell and Tissue Interactions.* Raven Press, New York.

Layman, D.I., McGoodwin, E.B. and Martin, G.R. 1971. *The nature of the collagen synthesised by cultured human fibroblasts.* Proc. Natl. Acad. Sci. USA. *68*, 454-456.

Leivo, I., Vaheri, A., Timpl, R. and Wartiovaara, J. 1980. *Appearance and distribution of collagens and laminin in the early mouse embryo.* Devel. Biol. *76*, 100-114.

Levinson, W., Bhatnagar, R.S. and Liu, T.Z. 1975. *Loss of ability to synthesise collagen in fibroblasts transformed by Rous sarcoma virus.* J. Natl. Cancer Inst. *55*, 807-810.

Levinson, A.D., Courtneidge, S.A. and Bishop, J.M. 1981. *Structural and functional domains of the Rous sarcoma virus transforming protein (pp60 src ).* Proc. Natl. Acad. Sci. USA.

Linsenmayer, T.F., Smith, G.N. and Hay, E.D. 1977. *Synthesis of two collagen types of embryonic chick corneal epithelium in vitro.* Proc. Natl. Acad. Sci. USA. *74*, 39-43.

Maness, P.F., Engeser, H., Greenberg, M.E., O'Farrel, M., Gall, W.E. and Edelman, G.M. 1979. *Characterisation of the protein kinase activity of avian sarcoma virus src gene product.* Proc. Natl. Acad. Sci. USA. *76*, 5028-5032.

Marceau, N., Goyette, R., Valet, J.P. and Deschenes, J. 1980. *The effect of dexamethasone on formation of a fibronectin extracellular matrix by rat hepatocytes in vitro.* Exp. Cell Res. *125*, 497-502.

Mautner, V. and Hynes, R.O. 1977. *Surface distribution of LETS protein in relation to the cytoskeleton of normal and transformed cells.* J. Cell Biol. *75*, 743-768.

Mayne, R., Vail, M.S., Mayne, P.M. and Miller, E.J. 1976. *Changes in type of collagen synthesised as clones of chick chondrocytes grow and eventually lose division capacity.* Proc. Natl. Acad. Sci. USA. *73*, 1674-1678.

Mayne, R., Vail, M.S. and Miller, E.J. 1978. *Characterisation of the collagen chains synthesised by cultured smooth muscle cells derived from rhesus monkey thoracic aorta.* Biochemistry, *17*, 446-452.

McConnell, M.R., Blumberg, P.M. and Rossow, P.W. 1978. *Dimeric and high molecular weight forms of the large external transformation sensitive protein on the surface of chick embryo fibroblasts.* J. Biol. Chem. *253*, 7522-7530.

Mosher, D.F. 1980. *Fibronectin.* Progr. Hemost. Thromb. 5, 111-151.

Mosher, D.F. and Proctor, R.A. 1980. *Binding of factor XIII a mediated cross linking of a 27 kilodalton fragment of fibronectin to Staphylococcus aureus.* Science. *209*, 927-929.

Mosher, D.F., Schad, P.E. and Vann, J.M. 1980. *Cross linking of collagen and fibronectin by factor XIIIa. Localisation of participating glutaminyl residues to a tryptic fragment of fibronectin.* J. Biol. Chem. *155*, 1181-1188.

Mueller, S.N., Rosen, E.M. and Levine, E.M. 1980. *Cellular senescence in a cloned strain of bovine fetal aortic endothelial cells.* Science. *207*, 889-890.

Murray, J.C., Stingl, G., Kleinman, H.K., Martin, G.R. and Katz, S.I. 1979. *Epidermal cells adhere preferentially to type IV basement membrane collagen.* J. Cell. Biol. *80*, 197-202.

Myllyla, R. and Seppa, H. 1979. *Studies in enzymes of collagen biosynthesis and the synthesis of hyroxyproline in macrophages and mast cells.* Biochem. J. *182*, 311-316.

Myllyla, R., Alitalo, K., Vaheri, A. and Kivirikko, K.I. 1981. *Regulation of collagen quality in transformed human and chick embryo cells.* Biochem. J. (in press).

Nicolson, G.L. 1976a. *Surface changes associated with transformation and malignancy.* Biochem. Biophys. Acta. *458*, 1-72.

Nicolson, G.L. 1976b. *Transmembrane control of receptors on normal and tumour cells. Cytoplasmic influence over cell surface components.* Biochim. Biophys. Acta. *457*, 57-108.

Olden, K. and Yamada, K. 1977. *Mechanism of the decrease in the major cell surface protein of chick embryo fibroblasts after transformation.* Cell, *11*, 957-969.

Oppermann, H., Levinson, A.D., Varmus, H.E., Levintow, L. and Bishop, J.M. 1979. *Uninfected vertebrate cells contain a protein that is closely related to the product of the avian sarcoma virus transforming genes (src).* Proc. Natl. Acad. Sci. USA. *76*, 1804-1808.

Parker, I. and Fitschen, W. 1980. *Procollagen mRNA metabolism during the fibroblast cell cycle and its synthesis in transformed cells.* Nucleic Acids Res. *8*, 2823-2833.

Pearlstein, E. 1976. *Plasma membrane glycoprotein which mediates adhesion of fibroblasts to collagen.* Nature, *262*, 497-500.

Pearlstein, E. 1978. *Substrate activation of cell adhesion factor as a prerequisite for cell attachment.* Int. J. Cancer, *22*, 32-35.

Pearlstein, E., Gold, L.I. and Garcia-Pardo, A. 1980. *Fibronectin: a review of its structure and biological activity.* Mol. Cell. Biochem. *29*, 103-128.

Peehl, D.M. and Ham, R.G. 1980a. *Growth and differentiation of human keratinocytes without feeder layer or conditioned medium.* In vitro. *16*, 516-525.

Peehl, D.M. and Ham, R.G. 1980b. *Clonal growth of human keratinocytes with small amounts of dialyzed serum.* In vitro. *16*, 526-538.

Penttinen, R., Frey, H., Aalto, M., Vuorio, E. and Marttala, T. 1980. *Collagen synthesis in cultured cells. In: Biology of collagen* (eds. Viidik, A. and Vuurst, J.) Academic Press, New York, pp. 87-103.

Perkins, M.E., Ji, T.H. and Hynes, R.O. 1979. *cross-linking of fibronectin to sulphated proteoglycans at the cell surface.* Cell, *16*, 941-952.

Peterkofsky, B. and Prather, W.B. 1974. *Increased collagen synthesis in Kirsten sarcoma virus-transformed BALB 3T3 cells grown in the presence of dibutyryl cyclic AMP.* Cell, *3*, 291-299.

Ponten, J. 1976. *the relationship between in vitro transformation and tumour formation in vivo.* Biochim. Biophys. Acta. *458*, 397-422.

Porter, K.R., Todaro, G.J. and Fonte, V. 1973. *A scanning electron microscope study of surface features of viral and spontaneous transformants of mouse BALB/3T3 cells.* J. Cell Biol. *59*, 633-642.

Prockop, D.J., Kivirikko, K.I., Tuderman, L. and Guzman, N.A. 1979. *The biosynthesis of collagen and its disorders.* New Engl. J. Med. *301*, 13-23, 77-85.

Purchio, A.F., Erikson, E., Collett, M.S. and Erikson, R.L. 1980. *Properties of the src protein kinase from ASV transformed and normal cells. Abstracts of the meeting on Protein Phosphorylation.* Cold Spring Harbor, p. 82.

Quaroni, A., Isselbacher, K.J. and Ruoslahti, E. 1978. *Fibronectin synthesis by epithelial crypt cells of rat small intestine.* Proc. Natl. Acad. Sci. USA. *75*, 5548-5552.

Quaroni, A. and Trelstad, R.L. 1980. *Biochemical characterisation of collagen synthesised by intestinal epithelial cell cultures.* J. Biol. Chem. 255, 8351-8361.

Reddi, A.H., Gay, R., Gay, S. and Miller, E.J. 1977. *Transitions in collagen types during matrix induced cartilage, bone, and bone marrow formation.* Proc. Natl. Acad. Sci. USA. 74, 5589-5592.

Rheinwald, J.G. and Green, H. 1977. *Epidermal growth factor and the multiplication of human epidermal keratinocytes.* Nature, 265, 421-424.

Richert, N., Davies, P.J.A., Jay, G. and Pastan, I. 1979. *Inhibition of the transformation specific kinase of ASV transformed cells by N-tosyl L-lysyl chloromethyl ketone.* Cell, 18, 369-374.

Rizzino, A. and Crowley, C. 1980. *Growth and differentiation of embryonal carcinoma cell line F₉ in defined media.* Proc. Natl. Acad. Sci. USA. 77, 457-461.

Robey, P.G. 1979. Thesis. Washington, D.C.

Roden, L. 1980. *Structure and metabolism of connective tissue proteoglycans. In: The Biochemistry of Glycoproteins and Proteoglycans* (ed. Lennarz, W.J.) Plenum Press, New York and London, pp. 267-371.

Rohde, H., Wick, G. and Timpl, R. 1979. *Immunochemical characteristion of the basement membrane glycoprotein laminin.* Eur. J. Biochem. 102, 195-201.

Rohrschneider, L.R. 1979. *Immunofluorescence on avian sarcoma virus transformed cells: Localisation of the src gene product.* Cell 16, 11-24.

Roll, F.J., Madri, J.A., Albert, J. and Furthmayer, H. 1980. *Codistribution of collagen types IV and AB₂ in basement membranes and mesangium of the kidney.* J. Cell Biol. 85, 597-616.

Rowe, D.W., Moen, R.C., Davidson, J.M., Byers, P.H., Bornstein, P. and Palmiter, R.D. 1978. *Correlation of procollagen mRNA levels in normal and transformed chick embryo fibroblasts with different rates of procollagen synthesis.* Biochemistry, 17, 1581-1590.

Ruoslahti, E. and Engvall, E. 1980. *Effect of glycosaminoglycans on complexing of fibronectin and collagen.* Biochim. Biophys. Acta. 631, 350-358.

Ruoslahti, E., Hayman, E.G. and Engvall, E. 1980. *Fibronectin. In: Cancer Markers: Developmental and Diagnostic Significance* (ed. S. Sell) Humana Press, San Francisco. pp. 485-505.

Sage, H., Crouch, E. and Bornstein, P. 1979. *Collagen synthesis by bovine aortic endothelial cells in culture.* Biochemistry, 18, 5433-5441.

Sakashita, S., Engvall, E. and Ruoslahti, E. 1980. *Basement membrane glycoprotein laminin binds to heparin.* FEBS Letters, 116, 243-246.

Salomon, D.S., Liotta, L.A. and Kidwell, W.R. 1981. *Differential response to growth factor by rat mammary epithelium plated on different collagen substrata in serum free medium.* Proc. Natl. Acad. Sci. USA. 78, 382-386.

Sandmeyer, S. and Bornstein, P. 1979. *Declining procollagen mRNA sequences in chick embryo fibroblasts infected with Rous sarcoma virus.* J. Biol. Chem. 254, 4950-4953.

Sandmeyer, S., Gallis, B. and Bornstein, P. 1981a. *Coordinate transcriptional regulateon of type I procollagen genes by Rous sarcoma virus.* J. Biol. Chem. (in press).

Sandmeyer, S., Smith, R., Kiehn, D. and Bornstein, O. 1981b. *Correlation of collagen synthesis and procollagen messenger RNA levels with transformation in rat embryo fibroblasts.* Cancer Res. (in press).

Schwartz, S.M. 1978. *Selection and characterisation of bovine aortic endothelial cells, In vitro.* 14, 966-980.

Schwarz, R.I. and Bissell, M.J. 1977. *Dependence of the differentiated state on the cellular environment: Modulation of collagen synthesis in tendon cells.* Proc. Natl. Acad. Sci. USA. 74, 4453-4457.

Schwarz, R.I., Farson, D.A., Soo, W. J. and Bissell, M.J. 1978. *Primary avian tendon cells in culture.* J. Cell Biol. 79, 672-679.

Sefton, B.M., Hunter, T. and Beemon, K. 1980. *Relationship of polypeptide products of the transforming gene of Rous sarcoma virus and the homologous gene of vertebrates.* Proc. Natl. Acad. Sci. USA. *77,* 2059-2063.

Senger, D.R., Wirth, D.F., Bryant, C. and Hynes, R.O. 1980. *Transformation specific secreted proteins.* Cold Spring Harbor Symp. Quant. Biol. XLIV, pp. 651-658.

Shriver, K. and Rohrschneider, L.R. 1980. *Spatial and enzymatic interactions of the Rous sarcoma virus transforming protein with components of the cellular cytoskeleton. Abstracts of the meeting on Protein Phosphorylation.* Cold Spring Harbor, p. 85.

Siegel, R.C. 1979, *Lysyl oxidase.* Int. Rev. Conn. Tissue Res. *8,* 73-118.

Singer, I.I. 1979. *The fibronexus: a transmembrane association of fibronectin containing fibres and bundles of 5nm microfilaments in hamster and human fibro blasts.* Cell *16,* 675-685.

Smith, H.S., Hackett, A., Riggs, J.L., Mosesson, M.W., Walton, J.R. and Stampfer, M.R. 1979. *Properties of epithelial cells cultured from human carcinomas and nonmalignant tissues.* J. Supramolec. Struct. *11,* 147-166.

Spiegel, E., Burger, M. and Spiegel, M. 1980. *Fibronectin in the developing sea urchin embryo.* J. Cell Biol. *87,* 309-313.

Steiner, S. and Steiner, M.R. 1978. *Glycolipids in virus-transformed cells. In: Virus transformed Cell Membranes* (ed. Nicolau, C.) Academic Press, pp. 91-110.

Strickland, S., Smith, K. and Marotti, K. 1980. *Hormonal induction of differentiation in teratocarcinoma stem cells: generation of parietal endoderm by retinoic acid and dibutyryl cAMP.* Cell, *21,* 347-355.

Sun, T. T. and Green, H. 1976. *Differentiation of the epidermal keratinocyte in cell culture: formation of the cornified envelope.* Cell, *9,* 511-521.

Taubman, M.B. and Goldberg, B. 1976. *The processing of procollagen in cultures of human and mouse fibroblasts.* Arch. Biochem. Biophys. *174,* 490-494.

Teng, M. H. and Rifkin, D.B. 1979. *Fibronectin from chicken embryo fibroblasts contains covalently bound phosphate.* J. Cell Biol. *80,* 784-791.

Terranova, V.P., Rohrbach, D.H., Maurray, J.C., Martin, G.R. and Yuspa, S.H. 1980. *The role of laminin in epidermal cell attachment to basement membrane collagen.* Cold Spring Harbor Conf. on the Biology of the Vascular cell, p. 37.

Timpl, R. 1981. *Laminin.* Methods Enzymol. (in press).

Timpl, R., Rohde, H., Robey, P.G., Rennard, S.I., Foidart, J.M. and Martin, G.R. 1979. *Laminin - a glycoprotein from basement membranes.* J. Biol. Chem. *254,* 9933-9937.

Timpl, R., Wick, G. and Gay, S. 1977. *Antibodies to distinct types of collagens and procollagens and their application in immunohistology.* J. Immunol. Methods. *18,* 165-182.

Todaro, G.J., Fryling, C. and De Larco, J.E. 1980. *Transforming growth factors produced by certain human tumour cells: Polypeptides that interact with epidermal growth factor receptors.* Proc. natl. Acad. Sci. USA. *77,* 5258-5262.

Tuszynski, G.P., Baker, S.R., Fuhrer, J.P., Buck, C.A. and Warren, L. 1978. *Glycopeptides derived from individual membrane glycoproteins from control and Rous sarcoma virus-transformed hamster fibroblasts.* J. Biol. Chem. *253,* 6092-6099.

Uitto, J. 1979. *Biochemistry of elastic fibres in normal connective tissues and its alterations in diseases.* J. Invest. Dermatol. *72,* 1-10.

Ushiro, H. and Cohen, S. 1980. *Identification of phosphotyrosine as a product of epidermal growth factor-activated protein kinase in A-431 cell membranes.* J. Biol. Chem. *255,* 8363-8365.

Vaheri, A. 1978. *Surface proteins of virus-transformed cells. In: Virus- transformed Cell Membranes* (ed. C. Nicolau), Academic Press, London, pp. 1-90.

Vaheri, A. and Mosher, D.F. 1978. *High molecular weight, cell surface-associated glycoprotein (fibronectin) lost in malignant transformation.* Biochim. Biophys. Acta. *516,* 1-25.

Vaheri, A. and Ruoslahti, E. 1974. *Disappearance of a major cell-type specific surface antigen (SF) after transformation of fibroblasts by Rous sarcoma virus.* Int. J. Cancer. *13,* 579-586.

Vaheri, A., Keski-Oja, J., Vartio, T., Alitalo, K., Hedman, K. and Kurkinen, M. 1980. *Structure and functions of fibronectin. In: Gene Families of Collagen and Other Proteins* (ed. Prockop. D.J. and Champe, P.C.). Elsevier North Holland, New York, pp. 161-178.

Vaheri, A., Kurkinen, M., V.-P., Linder, E. and Timpl, R. 1978. *Codistribution of pericellular matrix proteins in cultured fibroblasts and loss in transformation: Fibronectin and procollagen.* Proc. Natl. Acad. Sci. USA. *75*, 4944-4948.

Valle, M. and Penttinen, K. 1962. *Routine culture of human amnion cells.* Ann. Med. Exper. Fenn. *40*, 342-351.

Vartio, T., Seppa, H. and Vaheri, A. 1981. *Susceptibility of soluble and matrix fibronectins to degradation by tissue proteinases, mast cell chymase and cathepsin G.J.* Biol. Chem. *256*, 471-477.

Vesterinen, E.H., Carson, J., Walton, L.A., Collier, A.M., Keski-Oja, J., Nedrud, J.G. and Pagano, J.S. 1980b. *Human ectocervical and endocervical epithelial cells in culture: A comparative ultrastructural study.* Am. J. Obstet. Gynelcol. *137*, 681-686.

Vesterinen, E.H., Nedrud, J.G., Collier, A.M., Walton, L.A., and Pagano, J.A. 1980a. *Explanation and subculture of epithelial cells from human uterine ectovervix.* Cancer Res. *40*, 512-518.

Vracko, R. 1978. *Anatomy of basal lamina scaffold and its role in maintenance of tissue structure. In: Biology and Chemistry if Basement Membranes* (ed. Sefalides, N.A.), Academic Press, New York, pp. 165-176.

Vuento, M. and Vaheri, A. 1979. *Purification of fibronectin from human plasma by affinity chromatography under nondenaturing conditions.* Biochem. J. *183*, 331-O337.

Vuento, M., Vartio, T., Saraste, J., von Bonsdorff, C.-H. and Vaheri, A. 1980. *Spontaneous and polyamine-induced formation of filamentous polymers from soluble fibronectin.* Eur. J. Biochem. *105*, 33-42.

Willingham, M., Yamada, K.M., Yamada, S.S., Pouyssegur, J. and Pastan, I. 1977. *Microfilament bundles and cell shape are related to adhesiveness and are dissociable from growth control in cultured fibroblasts.* Cell, *10*, 375-380.

Willingham, M.C., Jay, G. and Pastan, I. 1979. *Localisation of the ASV src gene product to the plasma membrane of transformed cells by electron microscopic immunocytochemistry.* Cell, *18*, 125-134.

Yamada, K.M., Kennedy, D.W., Kimata, K. and Pratt, R.M. 1980. *Characterisation of fibronectin interactions with glycosaminoglycans and identification of active proteolytic fragments.* J. Biol. Chem. *255*, 6055-6063.

Yamada, K.M., Ohanian, S.H. and Pastan, I. 1976a. *Cell surface protein decreases microvilli and ruffles on transformed mouse and chick cells.* Cell, *9* 241-245.

Yamada, K.M., Yamada, S.S. and Pastan, I. 1976b. *Cell surface protein partially restores morphology, adhesiveness, and contact inhibition of movement to transformed fibroblasts.* Proc. Natl. Acad. Sci. USA. *73*, 1217-1221.

Zardi, L., Siri, A., Carnemolla, B., Santi, L., Gardner, W.D. and Hoch, S.O. 1979. *Fibronectin: a chromatin-associated protein.* Cell, *18*, 649-657.

## Questions

*Sager*

I would just like to ask about this malignant phenotype. What cells were used in those experiments and was this transformation-promoting activity reversible and do you know whether those cells that were transformed in fact become tumour forming cells.

*Vaheri*

That was not really the purpose of the experiment. These were chick embryo fibroblasts and this is strictly an experimental system which had been injected with a Rous sarcoma virus mutant temperature-sensitive for transformation. You can detect a similar transformation-enhancing activity also using other models.

*Sager*

If you had used non-transformed cells to start with then.

*Vaheri*

That type of study is going on at the moment. So, what happens to normal cells, are these tumour promoters? These may be questions we have to face ultimately.

*Crumpton*

If you take the antibody against collagen and you get fibronectin, is that also active in enhancing transformation?

*Vaheri*

Well the answer is, no. We recently obtained monoclonal antibodies to these fragments and they can inhibit the activity of those fragments but that is no big news, and gelatin will certainly inhibit the activity of that gelatin- binding fragment. But the antibodies as such are not, as far as I know, doing anything.

*Crumpton*

So you do not look upon your fragments as being inhibitors of interaction between.

*Vaheri*

Well clearly that is the most plausible explanation that in the intact molecule you have multiple binding sites and then when you have a fragment it may interfere with one of those binding sites and thereby interfere with the assembly of the matrix. Please note that we are dealing here with a very small concentration - we are in the nanomolar range so we have to consider alternative possibilities such as enzymatic or hormonal action. But the mechanism is clearly open.

*Wolpert*

I want to ask a general question. You have mainly spoken about the extracellular matrix as an expression of the phenotype. What about the extracellular matrix changing?

*Vaheri*

Well, as I mentioned, there is no clear evidence that the matrix is acting like a signal for differentiation. There are experiments mainly using chondrocytes, but the chondrocyte system is a very flexible one, you give them almost anything and they do whatever you want and then you can publish that data but in the proper embryonic system of which you are very well aware, I do not find any informative properties for the matrix so far.

*Questioner*

When you mentioned that the macrophage also secretes fibronectin, I wonder if this activates or arrests the developmental phase.

*Vaheri*

These were human peripheral blood monocytes that have the capacity to differentiate into macrophages simply by adjusting the culture conditions. They are not activated, they are differentiated macrophages. You can further stimulate their activities, for instance, by using interferon.

*RM Brown Jr*
What is the secretory pathway of the...


*Vaheri*
Well that is a good question. You have these two sub-units initially. Kurkinen did some experiments suggesting that the two sub-units might be translated separately but then, the next step, you find it if you do intracellular immuno-EM (as Klaus Hedman did) you find the protein in the rough ER. It is notably absent from the flat stacked parts of the Golgi but so is pro-collagen, so what is the uniqueness here? In the next step, you find it in the vesicles on the way, probably, to the membrane and this is what is known about the protein. There is no evidence for assembly inside the cell. This has not been studied well so far.


*Bernfield*
In view of the binding of fibronectin to collagen as being of potential biological significance, could you comment on the much greater affinity of fibronectin for denatured collagen than native collagen?

*Vaheri*
Yes, this is indeed true. The affinity to gelatin makes it possible to purify fibronectin almost by a single step from human plasma and then one may ask whether there is any real binding at all to native collagen; you may criticise those who have made such claims that they are unable to purify collagen in native form. But I think a plausible explanation is that the mechanism would be used in the opsonic activity of fibronectin. Whenever you have denatured collagen in your circulation (which you certainly do, at least in experimental conditions) fibronectin interacts strongly and this complex is then able to interact with the cells of the reticuloendothelial system and this is a mechanism for clearance of fragments containing denatured collagen from the circulation. I do not think there is good evidence that the interaction of fibronectin with native collagen would be needed for the assembly of the collagen matrix. I think we are more inclined to think of the sulphated proteoglycans and other glycosamino glycans, hyaluronic acid, will be involved in such processes.

# 3
# Internalisation of
# Extracellular Factors

As social entities, tissue cells are responsive to signals which help co-ordinate their behaviour.

In the previous section, it was seen that the control is exerted by large assemblies such as matrices or other cells but cells are also sensitive to smaller signals such as growth substances and hormones which originate, not from neighbouring cells, but from more distant sites in the organism.

In this chapter, Drs Willingham & Pastan describe their studies on the mechanism by which certain biologically active molecules are internalised and processed by cells in culture.

# The Morphologic Pathway of Receptor-Mediated Endocytosis in Cultured Fibroblasts

*Mark C Willingham and Ira H Pastan*

## Introduction

*Non-Concentrative Endocytosis*

Endocytosis of many materials from the environment of animal cells occurs through non-specific surface invaginations and ruffles which deliver these non-receptor-bound substances into the lysosomal system within the cell. This process, originally termed pinocytosis (Lewis 1931) and more recently divided into macropinocytosis and micropinocytosis depending on the morphologic structure involved (Silverstein *et.al.* 1977) results in rapid degradation of the endocytosed material by lysosomal hydrolases. In cultured mammalian cells this degradation begins within seconds or only a few minutes after entry into the cell. Ligands which bind to the cell surface, but otherwise are not segregated into unique areas of the cell surface, are internalised by this pathway (reviewed in Pastan and Willingham 1981). The characteristics of this non-specific pathway are:

1) The morphologic structures involved include caveolae (small invaginations of the plasma membrane) which form micropinosomes., and surface ruffles which fold back fusing with an adjacent area of membrane, forming macropinosomes;

2) The internalised materials are rapidly delivered to mature lysosomes through fusion with the incoming micro- or macropinosomes (Willingham and Yamada 1978; Willingham *et.al.* 1979). Since the areas of the plasma membrane which participate in this process are relatively unspecialised, the entire plasma membrane will, with time, participate in this degradative pathway. The time course of these overall cell surface events are rather slow, however, requiring an hour or two to internalise all of the membrane in this fashion.

*Concentrative Receptor-Mediated Endocytosis*

A second pathway exists in animal cells which results in rapid endocytosis of

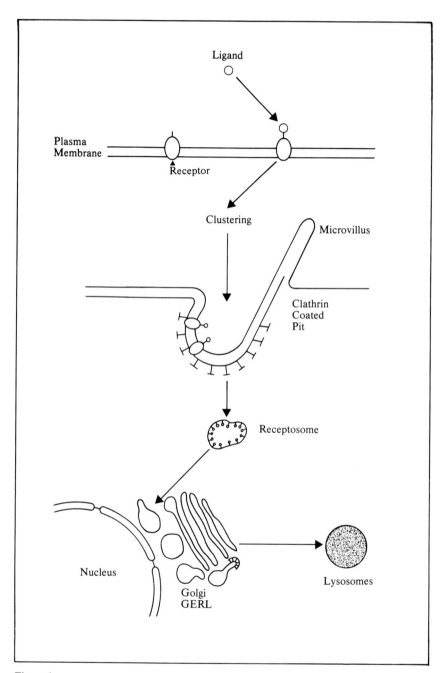

**Figure 1**
A diagrammatic summary of receptor-mediated endocytosis in cultered cells.

extracellular materials with a very different time course and fate for the internalised substances. (Summarised in Figures 1 and 2). Many physiological substances have specific receptors on the surface of cells, which bind these ligands tightly. For those which bind but have no other specialisation, such as artificial ligands or some plant lectins (reviewed in Pastan and Willingham 1981), the internalisation pathway will be only through the non-specific mechanisms described earlier. However, a large number of physiological ligands have receptors which are specialised to concentrate through lateral diffusion in the membrane at specific sites on the plasma membrane in response to binding of ligand. This initial concentrative step is the primary event to entry into the specialised pathway of endocytosis.

## Coated Pits on the Plasma Membrane
The plasma membrane mediates a number of physiological mechanisms such as nutrient transport and ionic equilibria. The majority of the membrane is uniformly smooth on its cytoplasmic face with a closely associated mat of actin-containing microfilaments. In less than 2% of this membrane, there are unique spots with a lattice coating on the cytoplasmic face, along with a discontinuity in the microfilament meshwork (Willingham *et.al.*1981c). This lattice coating was first described by Roth and Porter (1964) as a 'bristle coat'. These sites have the appearance of pits of varying degrees of invagination. They were originally identified on the basis of their morphology and their role in specific endocytosis of yolk protein in mosquito oocytes (Roth and Porter 1964). In 1974, Pearse identified the coat material as being predominantly composed of a single protein called 'clathrin'. The protein had the unique property of being able to form these lattice structures *in vitro*. Anderson *et.al* (1976) showed that these coated regions on the plasma membrane served as clustering sites for low density lipoprotein. Subsequently, many ligands have been found to cluster in these pits, including alpha$_2$-macroglobulin ($\alpha_2$M) and epidermal growth factor (Willingham *et.al.*1979; Willingham *et.al.*1981a). In all of these studies, the clustering of ligand-receptor complexes in coated regions has been seen to accompany and precede the specific endocytosis of the ligand.

## The Clustering of Ligands in Coated Pits
For some ligands, such as $\alpha_2$M, the process of receptor-ligand complex clustering in coated pits has been shown to occur at low temperature (4°C), whereas endocytosis itself following this clustering requires higher temperature (37°C). This property has allowed controlled experiments in which binding and clustering of ligands can be performed followed by short-term synchronous endocytosis by simply raising the temperature.

Other experiments can be performed, however, in which ligands are simply added at 37°C, and the cumulative endocytosis process including binding,

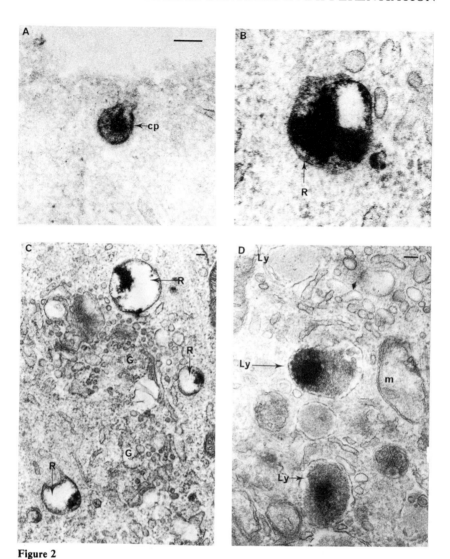

**Figure 2**

The morphologic features of receptor-mediated endocytosis in cultured fibroblasts. Swiss 3T3 cells were incubated at 4°C with $\alpha_2$-macroglobulin ($\alpha_2$M) and subsequently labelled with antibody coupled to horseradish peroxidase. Cells were either fixed in glutaraldehyde at 4°C (A) or warmed to 37°C for 5 minutes (B), 30 minutes (C), or 60 minutes (D). $\alpha_2$M clustered in coated pits (cp) at 40°C (A) appears in receptosomes (R) after the cells have been warmed to 37°C for 5 minutes (B). At later times (30 minutes) (C) after warming to 37°C, internalised $\alpha_2$M can be found in receptosomes in the Golgi region (G) in receptosomes (R). One hour after initial warming (D), the ligand appears in small homogeneous lysosomes (Ly-arrow) first evident in the Golgi region. Many other adjacent lysosomes can be seen (D) which do not contain the label (Ly) (mitochondrion). (Mags: A,B=X108,000; C=X36,000; D=X54,000; all bars-0.1$\mu$; lead citrate counterstain).

clustering, and endocytosis can be observed. Using fluorescent ligands, these experiments could be performed with light microscopy and the fluorescence of ligands in intracellular vesicles could be used to detect specific endocytosis (Willingham and Pastan 1978). In this manner, a number of chemical compounds were tested to determine their effects on specific endocytosis. Following the observations of the effects of ammonia on the specific uptake of lysosomal enzymes (reviewed in Pastan and Willingham 1981), primary amines were found to inhibit the endocytosis of many ligands. These compounds, along with other specific inhibitors, shared the property of being inhibitors of a family of enzymes called 'transglutaminases' (Davies et. al. 1980; Levitzki et. al. 1980). While some ligands, such as epidermal growth factor, are less affected in their endocytosis by these transglutaminase inhibitors (Haigler et. al. 1980), the pharma-cological similarity of the inhibition of endocytosis of other ligands and inhibition of transglutaminase was striking. In addition, electron microscopic experiments have shown that these compounds inhibit the clustering into coated pits as a primary effect (Maxfield et.al. 1979), thus, preventing the original entry of ligands such as $\alpha_2$M into the coated pit endocytic pathway.

Recently, Dickson et. al.( 1981) have found that these transglutaminase inhibitors have specific effects on the apparent affinity of the binding of $\alpha_2$M. Using $^{125}$I-$\alpha_2$M, the binding to cells at 4°C, or in isolated plasma membranes at 37°C, has been found to have two components with different affinities. The higher affinity component with a small number of sites is selectively inhibited by inhibitors of transglutaminase and endocytosis, while the lower affinity, majority of the sites is unaffected. This has led to the hypothesis that ligands clustered in coated pits acquire an apparent higher affinity, perhaps through a lower rate of dissociation. Preventing the clustering of these ligand-receptor complexes in pits by inhibitors of trans-glutaminase, thus, prevents the appearance of this higher affinity class. The existence of these properties in isolated membranes also points to the effects of these inhibitors on endocytosis being primarily on this process, and not through other factors that could occur in intact cells, such as receptor recycling. Further, this quantitative data has presented the surprising result that the amount of $\alpha_2$M internalised at 37°C is quite large, and that to account for the number of molecules taken in constantly at 37°C considering the known number of ligand molecules in coated pits at any one time, the coated pit must deliver its contents through endocytosis every 20-30 seconds. This points out the extremely rapid process this specialised pathway mediates. Another result discovered during experiments with fluorescent ligands was that during the time that primarily fluorescently-labelled ligands reside in coated pits, their fluorescence is decreased (Willingham et. al. 1981a). This was seen quantitatively by measuring the fluorescence output from cells incubated and fixed at 4°C with a labelled ligand such as rhodamine-$\alpha_2$M, and then measuring the fluorescent signal after endocytosis of the ligand, induced by warming to $37°C$, had occurred. From electron microscopic and $^{125}$I-labelled experiments, it was known that the same number of ligand molecules clustered in pits at $4°C$ were initially internalised into intracellular vesicles at $37°C$. This result could also be shown by labeling clustered ligands such as $α_2M$ or LDL using antibodies with the fluorochrome attached to the antibody molecule. In this case, the fluorochrome spaced away from the membrane showed normal fluorescence, whereas fluorochrome directly attached to the ligand did not (Anderson et.al. 1980; Willingham et. al. 1981a). The precise reason for the decrease in fluorescence of primarily labelled ligand is not known, but one possibility would be the insertion of the fluorochrome into a lipid environment when attached close to the membrane. The significance of this result is only that ligands directly labelled with fluorochrome may not be as suitable for observing their clustering in coated pits as they are for observing their endocytosis in intracellular vesicles.

### The Endocytic Process from Coated Pits:
### Do Coated Vesicles Exist?

The original observations of coated pits often seen in tangential section by electron microscopy, and the isolation of single coated vesicles on homogenisation of tissues, led to the logical conclusion that coated pits pinched off from the membrane to form isolated coated vesicles. However, the derivative vesicles in the cytoplasm from the coated pits, the receptosomes, do not have a clathrin coat (Willingham and Pastan 1980). This has required a re-evaluation of the endocytic process itself. Ultrastructural immunocytochemical studies (Willingham et.al. 1981b) have shown that the cytosol contains very little, if any, soluble clathrin. This makes the uncoating of endocytosed coated vesicles less likely. The observations from quantitative internalisation experiments that the coated pit must recycle in only a few seconds makes the pinching off of coated pits and re-coating of adjacent plasma membrane a more difficult hypothesis. Thus, the concept of a stable coated pit which cycles through a transient budding or extrusion of uncoated membrane to form an intra-cellular receptosome has become a more attractive possibility. Recent studies (Wehland et.al. 1981) have shown that microinjection of antibody to clathrin in the living cell decorates existing coated structures, but has no effect on the process of endocytosis over a period of hours. This again suggests that the coat is a stable structure which neither disassembles rapidly nor forms isolated coated vesicles. Other experiments have shown that under appropriate conditions all of the plasma membrane coated pits can be shown to be in continuity with the outside of the cell (Willingham and Pastan manuscript in preparation). Thus, the exact nature of the transition of coated pit containing ligand to receptosome containing ligand will have to await further study.

## The Receptosome:
## Morphologic Characteristics

The receptosome could be defined as the intracellular isolated vesicle which contains clustered ligand derived from the coated pits on the plasma membrane. Their original characterisation was through the use of fluorescently labelled ligands such as $\alpha_2M$ which were internalised through the coated pit pathway. The receptosomes could be visualised within minutes after formation, and their movements were followed using video intensification microscopy (Willingham and Pastan 1978). Similar experiments have been performed using fluorescent derivatives of insulin (Schlessinger et.al. 1978), epidermal growth factor (Maxfield et.al. 1978), and triiodothyronine (Cheng et.al. 1980). The pattern of motion of these vesicles is of a discontinuous jumping character, typical of many intracellular organelles including lysosomes and mitochonria. This motion, referred to as 'saltatory motion' (Rebhun 1972), is only found in intracellular organelles separated from other structures, demonstrating that the receptosomes were, indeed, separate vesicles in living cells.

The electron microscopic appearance of these vesicles was determined through cytochemical experiments, using electron dense markers coupled to specific ligands (Willingham and Pastan 1980). Once the morphologic appearance of these structures was determined, it was evident that they could in many cases, be detected on the basis of morphologic criteria alone, without cytochemical labels. In the past, these vesicles had been referred to as multivesicular bodies or lysosomal elements (reviewed in Pastan and Willingham 1981), but through the use of cytochemical labels they are clearly a separate organelle. Acid phosphatase and aryl sulfatase cytochemistry have shown that the newly formed receptosome lacks these lysosomal markers (MC Willingham unpublished data). While they are frequently seen without cytochemical labels, their life span is relatively short, usually less than 30 minutes. The pathway receptosomes take is through saltatory motion back to the Golgi-GERL region of the cell with delivery of the ligand into the Golgi system. Therefore, the number of receptosomes seen in cells at any one moment is restricted by their short life span.

Figure 3 demonstrates the morphologic features of receptosomes using a variety of ligand labels. The initial features of newly formed receptosomes are their early proximity to coated pits at the cell surface, their relatively empty internal appearance, and the frequent observation of a single small vesicular element in their lumen. Thus, these early receptosomes could be called 'monovesicular' bodies as a descriptive term. From ligand labeling experiments using quantifiable labels such as ferritin, the number of ligand molecules contained within these early receptosomes is identical with the number seen clustered in a single coated pit. This had led to the idea that each coated pit forms a single initial receptosome.

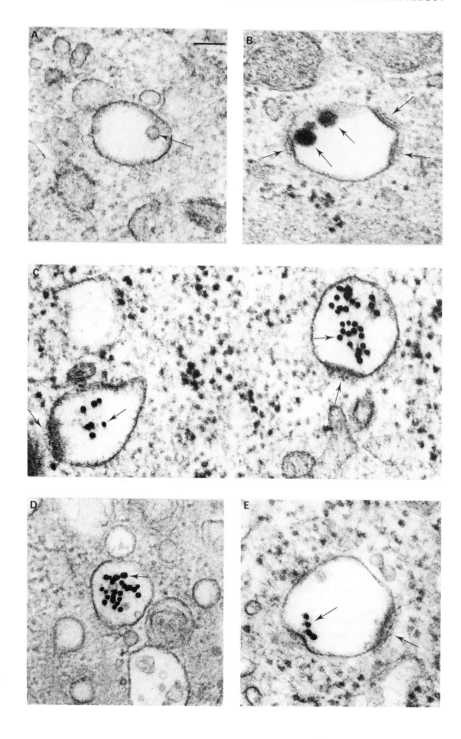

One of the characteristic features of these vesicles, seen by both light and electron microscopic methods, is their failure to fuse with mature lysosomes, in spite of their proximity to these organelles. This is quite different from the immediate fusion of micro- and macropinosomes with mature lysosomes (Willingham and Yamada 1978; Willingham et.al. 1979), and suggests that the receptosome must have special characteristics that make it unable to fuse with lysosomes. By immunocytochemistry, macropinosomes have been found often to be surrounded by bits of the microfilament mat after endocytosis (Willingham et.al. 1981c), but receptosomes characteristically have no actin or clathrin around them (Willingham and Pastan 1980). Thus, materials brought in through the coated pit pathway will not be exposed to lysosomal enzymes immediately, as they would through non-concentrative pinocytosis.

There is evidence which suggests, however, that receptosomes may fuse with each other. With time, the ligand-containing receptosomes appear to become larger in size and the amount of ligand they contain appears to increase. Usually, a ligand label will appear as a cluster at one edge of the receptosomal lumen, a cluster of the same size as when observed in the coated pit. Often, receptosomes that have been in the cytoplasm for 10-15 minutes will have two or three areas of membrane with clustered label at different spots in the lumen. Further, multiple monovesicular structures contained in the early receptosomes appear in older receptosomes, making them fit the descriptive term of 'multivesicular body'. The important point here is that while this morhologic descriptive term is appropriate, these later receptosomes do not fuse with mature lysosomes, a feature different from the reported fate for multivesicular bodies in other systems (reviewed in Pastan and Willingham 1981).

Another bit of evidence suggesting receptosomal fusion is that one would expect perhaps 1000 early receptosomes from each coated pit on the surface of a single cell, but after a few minutes at 37°C, the number of labelled

◄

**Figure 3**

Morphologic characteristics of receptosomes. In Swiss 3T3 cells, receptosomes can be identified by many unique morphologic features. In (A), the characteristic single small intraluminal vesicular element (arrow) can be seen in an unlabelled early receptosome. In (B), adenovirus particles (arrowheads) are seen in the lumen of a later receptosome, with three distinct lamellar structures on different parts of the cytosol face of the receptosomal membrane (arrows). In (C), two receptosomes containing $\alpha_2$M-colloidal gold (arrowheads) are seen which have the usual single dense lamellar peri-receptosomal structure (arrows). In (D), a receptosome labelled with $\alpha_2$M-colloidal gold is shown demonstrating the large number of concentrated ligand markers (arrowhead) that can be found in these structures. In (E), the characteristic features of the early receptosome are shown, with a membrane-associated cluster of ligand at one edge (arrowhead) and the lamellar peri-receptosomal structure on another part of the receptosome membrane (arrow). The small single intraluminal vesicular structure lies just beyond the plane of section, but can be barely seen in the upper left corner of this receptosome. (Mags: X108.000; bar=0.1$\mu$; A,D=lead citrate; B,C,E=uranyl acetate-lead citrate counterstained).

receptosomes seen by light microscopy are usually closer to 100 per cell. Even assumming that every coated pit might not be heavily labelled at any one time a finding supported by electron microscopy, one would still expect around 500 early receptosomes forming at any one time per cell. Thus, it is likely that multiple small early receptosomes may fuse to form a smaller number of larger sized receptosomes.

One of the striking features of receptosomes is a structure at their edge. The edge of receptosomes often show a straightened segment with dense material on the cytoplasmic face. At times this density appears laminated with fibrillar extensions into the adjacent cytoplasm (see Figure 3). While it is tempting to suggest that this area mediates either some specific fusion event or mediates saltatory motion, there is no direct evidence as to its function. This structure is another bit of evidence in favour of receptosome-receptosome fusion, however, since older receptosomes often have multiple dense edges. This dense material does not label with antibodies to clathrin, actin, myosin, filamin, or tubulin, so its exact nature is still unknown.

### Delivery of Ligand to the Golgi system

After 15-30 minutes, receptosomes formed all over the periphery of the cell accumulate near the nucleus in the Golgi region. Electron microscopy shows these vesicles in close approximation to elements of the GERL or acid-phosphatase positive region of the Golgi. This point is the last time at which receptosomes maintain their morphologic character. Soon after this time, the ligand can be found in small homogenous primary lysosomal elements in the GERL or in larger secondary lysosomes in an eccentric location (see Figure 4). At these times, biochemical experiments show that ligand degradation is well advanced. Whether some degradation can occur in the receptosomal system prior to delivery to lysosomes is not clear. The segregation of ligand into the lysosomes appears to be a specific process. Others have shown that other bound ligands can enter the coated pit pathway when present in large concentration and be delivered to the Golgi system, but that in the Golgi they may be delivered into the secretory, rather than the lysosomal, pathway (reviewed in Pastan and Willingham 1981; Herzog and Farquhar 1977; Ottosen *et.al.* 1980). The concept that segregation of ligands in the Golgi into secretory or lysosomal pathways is a receptor-dependent process has been proposed (Sly and Stahl 1978) (see below).

### The Physiologic Role of the Coated Pit Pathway

Since almost all cell types in mammals have been found to contain clathrin or to have bristle-coated pits, the process of receptor-mediated endocytosis through this pathway is likely to be ubiquitous throughout the body. One might assume that this implies that it serves some essential function in cell physiology. So far, this endocytic pathway has been shown to be involved in

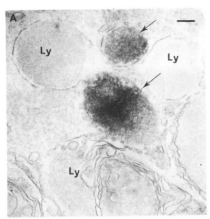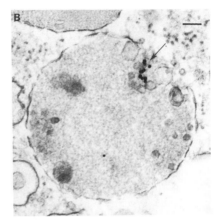

**Figure 4**

Lysosomal incorporation of labelled ligands. Cells incubated with either $\alpha_2$M-peroxidase (A) or $\alpha_2$M-colloidal gold (B) were incubated for one hour at 37°C following initial binding at 4°C. Label appears either homogeneously distributed in small primary lysosomes (arrows) as in (A), or eccentrically (arrow) in large, secondary lysosomes (B). Many other adjacent lysosomes (Ly) are unlabelled. (Mags: A=X60,000; B=X72,000; bars=0.1$\mu$; A=lead citrate; B=uranylacetate-lead citrate counterstained).

the processing of hormones (such as insulin, epidermal growth factor, and triiodothyronine) and molecules of probable metabolic function (such as LDL, asialoglycoproteins, lysosomal enzymes and, perhaps, $\alpha_2$-macroglobulin) (reviewed in Pastan and Willingham 1981; Wall *et al.* 1980). Since receptors for these ligands are likely to be endocytosed with the ligand through this process, the recycling or regulation of receptors may be a major function of this pathway.

Recently, it has also become clear that pathologic processes may utilize this pathway for their own purposes. A number of bacterial toxins (reviewed in Pastan and Willingham 1981) have been implicated in this process in one way or another. Pseudomonas toxin, for example, has been directly observed entering the cell through coated pits, and inhibition of this internalisation through the use of transglutaminase inhibitors has protected cells from its toxic effects (Fitzgerald *et. al.* 1980). Thus, for those toxins which utilize this pathway to exert their effects, the knowledge of the mechanisms of this process can be of therapeutic value.

In addition, a number of viruses have been shown to utilise the coated pit pathway to gain entrance into the cell, a process essential for their infectivity. The significant work of Dales in showing the selective presence of many different viruses in coated pits (reviewed in Dales 1973), recently extended by Helenius *et. al.* using Semliki forest virus (Helenius *et. al.* 1980), shows the remarkable morphologic segregation of many different viruses into this single common pathway. Recently, Schlegel *et. al.* (1981) have shown that treatment of cells with transglutaminase inhibitors, including some previously classified as antiviral drugs, has dramatic effects on the infectivity of vesicular stomatitis virus. This mechanistic approach provides significant new possibilities for the treatment of viral disease. The further delineation of the biochemical processes involved in this pathway will presumably give more insights into potentially valuable therapeutic agents.

### The Golgi-GERL System:
### A Mirror Image of the Plasma Membrane?

One cannot deal with the coated pits on the plasma membrane and their morphologic clathrin coat without realising that a second cell subcompartment contains clathrin-coated pits as well. The Golgi-GERL system in virtually all animal cells contain 'budding' clathrin-coated pits about half the diameter of those at the plasma membrane. Considering the evidence suggesting that coated pits on the plasma membrane may never pinch off to form coated vesicles, then the same possibility, though less well supported with data, may exist for the Golgi-GERL structures. If one assumes that these pits in the Golgi are, themselves, stable pits, then why would we not also assume that they can serve the same role as the plasma membrane pits; that is, could it not be possible that these regions serve as clustering sites for receptor-ligand complexes in the GERL system? Carrying the analogy further, where would the clustered ligands be delivered to?

The two major fates of materials from the Golgi-GERL system are likely to be either secretion out to the plasma membrane, or internal secretion into the lysosomal compartment. A number of experiments suggest that the Golgi-GERL system may be continuous, at least functionally. Ligands which enter the cell are often selectively concentrated into primary and secondary lysosomes after interactions with the Golgi-GERL region of the cell (Willingham and Pastan 1980). Some endocytosed materials which bind on the basis of charge, such as cationised ferritin (Farquhar 1978) enter the cell to some extent in the coated pit pathway and are delivered to the Golgi system. But once in the Golgi, the charge-mediated binding apparently can be transferred to secretory products. These experiments are the most direct evidence for the mixing of endocytic and secretory pathways in the Golgi. But we already know that ligands bound to specific receptors entering through this endocytic pathway can be selectively shuttled to lysosomes from the Golgi. Other intriguing evidence comes from studies on lysosomal enzymes. In I-cell disease, in which the lysosomal enzymes synthesised by the cell in the endoplasmic reticulum apparently lack their receptor recognition marker (mannoside-$PO_4$) the enzymes are secreted out of the cell, rather than being selectively segregated into the lysosomal system. The interesting thing about these cells, however, is that one can add lysosomal enzymes from normal cells that have the recognition marker, and they are endocytosed into the I cell in an apparently normal fashion. Eventually, the lysosomes in these mutant cells can regain a more normal enzyme content in their lysosomes through this manner. Thus, the segregation mechanism, which we would presume exists in the Golgi-GERL system, may still function in these cells. The determining factor for the delivery of these lysosomal enzymes to their proper compartment would then be specific receptor binding, presumably in the Golgi-GERL system (Sly and Stahl 1978). Another bit of evidence relating to the mixing of secretory and lysosomal pathways in the Golgi, is the finding that $\alpha_2$M-gold taken into the cell hours before, which had been segregated completely into the lysosomal compartment, can reappear in the Golgi in the small vesicular elements seen in other systems to mediate extracellular secretion (Dickson *et al.* 1981a). This agrees with previous biochemical evidence showing that cells (cultured in the absence of $\alpha_2$M) can secrete $\alpha_2$M from their lysosomes that had been taken up from their medium many hours earlier (Pastan *et.al.* 1977). In fact, $\alpha_2$M may be a uniquely useful marker for this purpose since its degradation in the lysosomal system is quite slow (Maxfield *et.al.* 1981), possibly because of its antiprotease properties.

**Hypothesis**
The hypothesis that emerges from these results might be summarised as follows:

1) The Golgi-GERL system mirrors the processing at the plasma membrane in that ligands in its lumen are segregated into coated pits through a receptor-dependent process;
2) The materials clustered in these coated regions are selectively delivered to the lysosomal system;
3) Materials not bound to receptors, or bound to receptors that do not cluster in coated regions, are secreted to the cell exterior;
4) The receptosomal endocytic system delivers internalised ligand directly into the Golgi system, where it is segregated into the lysosomal pathway if still bound to a clustering receptor, or to the secretory pathway if not.

While the specifics of this hypothesis must await further experiments, one group of results is compatible with it. Vesicular stomatitis virus produces a single major glycoprotein in the endoplasmic reticulum membrane (G protein), which concentrates in the Golgi region of the cell and is secreted to the plasma membrane as an integral membrane glycoprotein. Electron microscopic localisation of G-protein during this transition has shown that G-protein concentrates in the Golgi in uncoated small vesicles, and later appears on the plasma membrane. The coated pit regions in the Golgi-GERL system appear devoid of G-protein and no localisation has ever been seen in lysosomes (Willingham and Pastan Manuscript in preparation). This protein would then be an example of a strictly secretory protein. Similar results have been observed with the secretion of fibronectin, a luminal secretory protein in these fibroblastic cells (Yamada *et.al.*1980). More direct experiments testing the hypothesis of mixing in the Golgi of the secretory and lysosomal pathways using specific ligand-receptor markers, and of the participation and content of the coated pits in the Golgi system, will help elucidate the elements of this process.

## Conclusions

Receptor-mediated internalisation occurs by specific mechanisms in animal cells involving unique morphologic structures. The clathrin-coated pit at the plasma membrane, the receptosome, the Golgi-GERL system, and the lysosome all appear to play a part in this process. The ubiquity of these structural elements in multiple cells types and the conservation of the structure of clathrin throughout evolution, suggests that this pathway is of major importance in the functioning of the cell. The potential involvement of this pathway in pathological processes, such as viral infection, make the understanding of these events of long term significance and of potential therapeutic value.

## References

Anderson, R.G.W., Goldstein, J.L. and Brown, M.S. *Localisation of low-density lipoprotein receptors on plasma membrane of normal human fibroblasts and their absence in cells from a familid hyperchodesterolemia homozygote.* Proc. Natl. Acad. Sci. USA. *73* : 2434-2438, 1976.

Anderson, R.G.W., Goldstein, J.L. and Brown, M.S. *Fluorescence Visualisation of receptor-bound low density lipoprotein in human fibroblasts.* J. Receptor Res. *1* : 17-39, 1980.

Cheng, S., Maxfield, F.R., Robbins, J., Willingham, M.C. and Pastan, I.H. *Receptor-mediated uptake of 3,3', 5-Triiodo-L-Thyonine by cultured fibroblasts.* Proc. Natl. Acad. Sci. USA. *77*, 3425-3429, 1980.

Dales, S. *Early events in cell-animal virus interactions.* Bacteriol. Rev. *37*, 103-135, 1973.

Davies, P.J.A., Davies, D.R., Levitzki, A., Maxfield, F.R., Milhaud, P., Willingham, M.C. and Pastan, I.H. *Evidence that transglutaminase plays an essential role in the receptor mediated endocytosis of $\alpha_2$-macroglobulin and polypeptide hormones.* Nature, *283*, 162-167, 1980.

Dickson, R.B., Willingham, M.C. and Pastan, I. *$\alpha_2$-macroglobulin adsorbed to colloidal gold: a new probe in the study of receptor-mediated endocytosis.* J. Cell Biol. (in press), 1981a.

Dickson, R.B., Willingham, M.C. and Pastan, I. *Binding and internalisation of 125 I-$\alpha_2$ macroglobulin by cultured fibroblasts.* J. Biol. Chem. (in press), 1981b.

Farquhar, M.G. *Traffic of products and membranes through the Golgi complex In Transport of Macromolecules n Cellular Systems.* (S.C. Silverstein, ed.) Dahlem Konferenzen, Berlin, p. 341, 1978.

Fitzgerald, D., Morris, R.E., and Saelinger, C.B. *Receptor-mediated internalisation of Pseudomonas toxin by mouse fibroblasts.* Cell, *21*, 867-873, 1980.

Haigler, H.T., Willingham, M.C. and Pastan, I. *Inhibitors of 125 I- epidermal growth factor internalisation.* Biochem. Biophys. Res. Comm. *94*, 630-637, 1980.

Helenius, A., Kartenbeck, J., Simons, K. and Fries, E. *On the entry of Semliki forest virus into BHK-21 cells.* J. Cell Biol. *84*, 404-420, 1980.

Herzog, V. and Farquhar, M.G. *Luminal membrane retrieved after exo cytosis reaches most Golgi cisternae in secretory cells.* Proc. Natl. Acad. Sci. USA. *74*, 5073-5078, 1077.

Levitzki, A., Willingham, M.C. and Pastan, I. *Evidence for the participation of transglutaminase in receptor mediated endocytosis.* Proc. Natl. Acad. Sci. USA. *77*, 2706-2710, 1980.

Lewis, W.H. *Pinocytosis.* Bull. Johns Hopkins Hosp. *49*, 17-36, 1931.

Maxfield, F.R., Schlessinger, J., Shechter, Y., Pastan, I. and Willingham, M.C. *Insulin, epidermal growth factor, and $\alpha_2$-macroglobulin rapidly collect in the same patches on the surface of cultured fibroblasts and are internalised together.* Cell, *14*, 805-810, 1978.

Maxfield, F.R., Schlessinger, J., Shechter, Y., Pastan, I. and Willingham M.C. *Insulin, epdiermal growth factor, and $\alpha_2$-macroglobulin rapidly collect in the same patches on the surface of cultured fibroblasts and are internalised together.* Cell, *14*, 805-810, 1978.

Maxfield, F.R., Willingham, M.C., Davies, P.J.A. and Pastan, I. *Amines inhibit the clustering of $\alpha_2$-macroglobulin and EGF on the fibroblast cell surface.* Nature, *277*, 661-663, 1979.

Maxfield, F.R., Willingham, M.C., Haigler, H.T., Dragsten, P. and Pastan, I. *Binding, surface mobility, internalisation and degradation of rhodamine labeled $\alpha_2$-macroglobulin.* (submitted), 1981.

Novikoff, A.B. and Novikoff, P.M. *Cytochemical contributions to differentiating GERL from the Golgi apparatus.* Histochem. J. *9*, 525-551, 1977.

Ottosen, P.D., Courtoy, P.J. and Farquhar, M.G. *Pathways followed by membrane recovered from the surface of plasma cells and myeloma cells.* J. Exp. Med. *152*, 1-19, 1980.

Pastan, I.H. and Willingham, M.C. *Receptor-mediated endocytosis of hormones in cultured cells.* Ann. Rev. Physiol. *43*, 239-250, 1981.

Pastan, I., Willingham, M., Anderson, W. and Gallo, M. *Localisation of serum derived $\alpha_2$-Macroglobulin in cultured cells and decrease after Moloney Sarcoma virus transformation.* Cell, *12*, 609-617, 1977.

Rebhun, G.I. *Polarised intracellular particle transport: saltatory movements and cytoplasmic streaming.* Int. Rev. Cytol. *32*, 93-137, 1972.

Roth, T.F. and Porter, K.R. *Yolk protein uptake in the oocyte of the mosquito Aedes aegypti L.* J. Cell Biol. *20*, 330-332, 1964.

Schlegel, R., Dickson, R.B., Willingham, M.C. and Pastan, I.H. *Antiviral activities of amantadine and dansylcadaverine may be associated with the inhibition of receptor-mediated endocytosis.* (submitted), 1981.

Schlessinger, J., Shechter, Y., Willingham, M.C. and Pastan, I. *Direct visualisation of the binding, aggregation and internalisation of insulin and epidermal growth factor on fibroblastic cells.* Proc. Natl. Acad. Sci. *75*, 2659-2663, 1978.

Silverstein, S.C., Steinman, R.M. and Cohn, Z.A. *Endocytosis.* Ann. Rev. Biochem. *46*, 669-722, 1977.

Sly, W.S. and Stahl, P. *Receptor-mediated uptake of lysosomal enzymes. In Transport of Macromolecules in Cellular Systems,* S.C. Silverstein, ed. Berlin: Dahlem Konferenzen, pp. 229-244, 1978.

Wall, D.A., Wilson, G. and Hubbard, A.L. *The galactose-specific recognition system of mammalian liver: the route of ligand internalisation in rat hepatocytes.* Cell, *21*, 79-93, 1980.

Wehland, J., Willingham, M.C. and Pastan, I. *Microinjection of antibodies to clathrin does not interfere with receptor-mediated endocytosis.* (submitted), 1981.

Willingham, M.C., Haigler, H.T., Dickson, R.B. and Pastan, I. *Receptor-mediated endocytosis in cultured cells: coated pits, receptosomes, and lysosomes.* In International Cell Biology 1980-81. pp. 613-621, 1981a.

Willingham, M.C., Keen, J.H. and Pastan, I. *Ultrastructural immunocytochemical localisation of clathrin in cultured fibroblasts.* Exp. Cell Res. (in press), 1981b.

Willingham, M.C., Maxfield, F.R. and Pastan, I.H. *α₂-Macroglobulin binding to the plasma membrane of cultured fibroblasts: diffuse binding followed by clutering in coated region.* J. Cell Biol. *82*, 614-625, 1979.

Willingham, M.C. and Pastan, I. *The visualisation of fluorescent proteins in living cells by video intensification microscopy (VIM).* Cell, *13*, 501-507, 1978.

Willingham, M.C. and Yamada, S.S. *A mechanism for the destruction of pinosomes in cultured fibroblasts: Piranhalysis.* J. Cell Biol. *78*, 480-487, 1978.

Willingham, M.C. and Pastan, I. *The Receptosome: An intermediate organelle of receptor-mediated endocytosis in cultured fibroblasts.* Cell, *21*, 67-77, 1980.

Willingham, M.C., Yamada, S.S., Davies, P.J.A., Rutherford, A.V., Gallo, M.G. and Pastan, I. *The intracellular localisation of actin in cultured fibroblasts by electron microscopic immunocytochemistry.* J. Histochem. Cytochem. *29*, 17-27, 1981c.

Yamada, S.S., Yamada, K.M. and Willingham, M.C. *Intracellular localisation of fibronectin by immuno-electron microscopy.* J. Histochem. Cytochem. *28*, 953-960, 1980.

## Questions

*Crumpton*

Do you have any knowledge of the receptor for $\alpha_2M$ and in particular one might speculate that the apparent molecular size of that receptor might vary according to the amount of $\alpha_2M$ that you use as a ligand. In other words, if you use $\alpha_2M$ at very low concentration so that you are restricting it to bind in clusters and if transglutaminase is then putting in a cross link so that receptor it might have a larger apparent molecular weight than binding to the receptor in a non-catalytic way.

*Willingham*

We are in the process of isolating the receptor for $\alpha_2M$. It is not an easy job. Also, the apparent pharmacologic identity of this enzymatic activity as being transglutaminase is just that - it is pharmacologic. The enzyme has not been isolated from cells, it has not been ratified as being a transglutaminase, nor do we know that there is covalent bond formation going on. But pharmacologically it acts identically in its inhibitability to a trans glutaminase-like molecule. But really, the isolation of the receptor is going to help in this regard a lot.

*Crumpton*

But you do not need to isolate - you could use biosynthetically- labelled cells and with antibody.

*Willingham*

Yes, we have tried to make antibodies to a receptor-type material at the surface of cells; so far, unsuccessfully.

*Thorogood*

You talked about the internalisation of molecules destined for an intracellular fate. I wonder about systems in which molecules are transported across epithelia. For instance, colostral immunoglobulins bound by Fc receptors in the apical cell membrane are transported across the cell and released intact on the basal side of the cell and of course the integrity of the molecule is important for transferring immunity into the young animal. I wonder if the coated pit/receptosome system is relevant there.

*Willingham*

Some work has been done on that by Rodewald and his colleagues, and by others as well. It is not clear to me exactly what morphologic entities are involved. It is possible there may be a selective, special differentiated pathway that those molecules follow. It is clear there is some clustering in coated pits on the lumenal surface and there is material which appears to be clustered and there are coated things on the other surface of the cell and it is very complicated in between and I am not exactly sure what is going on.

*Lodish*

Some groups of investigators, particularly Anderson, Goldstein and Brown have described the involvement of coated vesicles in receptor-mediated endocytosis - which is to say vesicles that contain the ligand-receptor and are coated with clathrin - as an intermediate. I also believe there are several publications describing the isolation of coated vesicles with various receptor- ligands inside them. Yet, these are conspicuously absent from your model. Would you like to talk about it?

*Willingham*

I was afraid you were going to ask that question, but since you did. We have no evidence now which suggests there are no coated vesicles in these cells at all. The evidence goes something like this - we were initially shocked to find the receptosome had no clathrin associated with it so we tried to see when things were communicating with the outside of the cell. This is dealing now only with coated pits on the cell surface and not necessarily with the ones in the Golgi system. One thing we discovered is that if you cool cells to $4°C$, every coated structure near the plasma membrane is communicating with the outside of the cell, in which case you can label it with things like conA-peroxidase, ruthenium red - a variety of extracellular macromolecular labels. If you warm the cells to 37°C, about half of them were images of coated pits which had a narrowed neck which would not allow the label to get through but the neck was not in fact fused. So then we took those cells which we had cooled at 4°C and warmed them to 37°C and immediately cooled them back down to 4°C. One would expect that if you formed a coated vesicle by pinching off a coated pit from the plasma membrane, then the coated vesicle would be trapped in the cytoplasm and would not be able to refuse with the plasma membrane and so we went back, after that initial loss of communication with the outside, cooled down rapidly to 4°C and again, every coated structure (1,000 out of 1,000) was communicating with the outside of the cell. Now, some more recent data (and we have done this simultaneously with ligands which we can then follow into the receptosomes) show a lot of images which look like receptosome formation from the adjacent edge of what looks like a narrowed-neck coated pit. In collaboration with Jurgen Wehland, we have microinjected anti-clathrin antibodies into the cell. One would expect that if there was free clathrin, empty baskets, isolated coated vesicles, that you would see with time, with an excess of antibody, aggregation of these materials somewhere in the cell. Absolutely no aggregation is seen for hours on end with excess anti-clathrin. By EM, the antibody is coating the inside surface - the cytoplasmic face - of the coated pits on the cell surface and the coated regions in the Golgi. When we tried to use an extracellular ligand (like $\alpha_2$M) and see if it is internalised, it is internalised perfectly normally and the cells are running along just fine. In the image we then see (I will draw it) this kind of image where the neck is removed, and in which the ligand-receptor complexes in some images are here, in other images are over here. It seems to be that these things must close and internalise every 20 seconds and then there is an uncoated pit somewhere which is available for the clustering of another 10-50 molecules on the surface. If you count the number of molecules getting internalised you find it is happening with such rapidity. If these became coated vesicles, they would have to be going back up to the cell surface every 20 seconds and shuttling back and forth. Since when we cool these back down to 4°C and every thing is communicating with the outside (all the coated structures we see and we do not think they ever contract.

*Lodish*
If I can just follow that up. Four degrees is clearly an artificial circumstance. Are you also implying that under physiological conditions at 37°C, in cells which have never been cooled, that the coated vesicles are artifacts in this process?

*Willingham*
Artifacts in the sense that when you homogenise the cell you take coated pits, break them off from their membrane attachments and they close just like ER closes to form microsomes. Yes, I would say that is in fact what is going on. They never become isolated vesicles.

*Obrink*
I have a question that relates to Dr Lodish's and that concerns the uptake of LDL. It has been suggested for a long time that it is the binding to the receptor which triggers the clustering and the clustering triggers the uptake. But Anderson, Goldstein and Brown postulated that the receptors already are in the coated pits and the coated pits are an artifact caused by the LDL which happens to bind to the cell.

*Willingham*
Right, you have to go and look at the experimental data which support that

idea. One is that they made the assumption that at 4°C the LDL receptor was totally immobilised and that is not necessarily a safe assumption at all. In most of the experiments they did 4°C binding of LDL for 2 hours. We in fact see clustering of $\alpha_2M$ in 2 minutes at 4°C. The only way to deal with that issue is whether or not (in a pre-fixation experiment) the initial distribution of receptors is diffuse or clustered. It is possible that some of them could be pre-clustered. It is clear that for LDL bound to a cell surface, that many of those receptors are mobile - you can measure it with fluorescence photobleaching - they move around on the surface. Certainly, not all of them at any one time could be clustered anyway. No, the thing we found was that it seems that at 4°C much less of the LDL is clustered than when you warm it up to 37°C where you get a more rapid clustering. The same is true for EGF; when you initially label at 4°C there is much less clustering in the pits than when you warm it up then you get a progressive clustering right before the endocytic event. So, I think you have to look back at the data to figure that out. Really, the only way to know the native distribution of the receptor is if we had antibodies to the receptor so that we could directly label after fixing with glutaraldehyde.

*RM Brown Jr*
Are you saying that you have no evidence in your system for exocytosis. Is that right?

*Willingham*
There is an exocytotic process. We have in fact been studying it using VSPG protein as the model. We see an exclusion of G protein from all the coated structures in the Golgi system. It seems to be the only part of the Golgi where we cannot find G protein by immunocytochemistry and the concentrative vesicles which we see going to the outside of the cell are in fact not coated. Now, you have to remember of course that once it gets to the

plasma membrane, and if it is making virus, it can turn around and bind to its receptor and cluster in the coated pits selectively. So it is a complicated thing to measure biochemically but at least morphologically we can see no coating associated with the exocytosis of G protein.

*Hopkins*
McKanna's description of the fate of ferritin-EGF goes through (and this is in the A431 cell) the coated vesicle to a monovesicular body stage. Would you equate that with your receptosome?

*Willingham*
OK. Receptosomes have been seen for years and they have been called a variety of things. One of the things they have been called is multivesicular bodies although that is not exactly a very descriptive term. Most of our receptosomes are *mono* vesicular bodies and have a lumenal tiny vesicle on one edge. The A431 cells are very unusual - they have 3 million EGF receptors per cell; have a biological response to the addition of EGF so it ruffles like crazy when you add EGF for the first minute or so - almost all the plasma membrane goes in by macropinocytosis. So the majority of the internal isation of EGF you see is in the macropinocytotic pathway which then fuses with lysomes very quickly so the degradation is very fast. Then in a cell like a Swiss 3T3 which has perhaps 20,000 EGF receptors per cell, then almost all of it goes through the coated pit pathway and degradation begins much later. Twenty minutes is the first point we see any.

*Hopkins*
But the point was in that experiment that the ferritin-EGF was on the vesicles inside the multivesicular body. Now your label is also in the lumen of the body and it was possible to equate his pictures with the idea that the ferritin was actually showing where the receptor was and the receptor therefore has left the membrane which was immediately adjacent to the

cytoplasm. Now, in your receptosome, if you had to say where the receptor was where would you think it to be?

*Willingham*
Well, one has to be very careful about distribution of a ligand in an empty vesicle because if you fix with glutaraldehyde you would expect that a protein in the middle of the lumen might get dragged to the membrane and get cross-linked to another protein. What we see, prominently, is the ferritin-EGF lying at the membrane of the receptosome and later on in internalisation we will occasionally see it out in the lumen. The idea being that may be it is dissociated from its receptor. But those are very difficult interpretations to make from that kind of image.`

*Bernfield*
Do you see down-regulation of EGF receptors in your cells?

*Willingham*
Yes, EGF receptors down-regulate.

*Bernfield*
Could you suggest a way in which with co-internalisation of $\alpha_2$M you do not see down-regulation and with internalisation of EGF you do?

*Willingham*
It is the way we do the experiment, we put the cells at 4°C and we label them with both $\alpha_2$M and EGF at 4°C then warm them up. So you would not see any down-regulation because its the first chance they have to go in. You start off with a cell having all its EGF receptors sitting on the outside. If, for instance, we pre-treated them with EGF and then tried to do the double-label experiment we probably would not see any EGF binding because they would have all gone in. These are cells which aren't treated with EGF for hours and hours before the experiment.

# 4
# Internal Responses

The foregoing papers reflect the growing awareness of how extracellular information is presented to the cell and in the following section we can expect to see how this is translated into effects upon the biosynthetic machinery of the cell, for contained in 'Internal Responses' are two papers which address themselves to how the cytoplasm responds to signalling in a co-ordinate manner.

In his paper, Dr Coffino outlines the way in which genetic analysis of cyclic AMP mutants may be used to dissect out the response of cells to this regulatory molecule. That calcium and cyclic AMP are the second messengers in this line of communication across the cell has been known for some time but great advances are now being made towards seeing how these two systems dove-tail and this is the subject of Dr Cohen's contribution.

One connection to be made between this and the first two papers is that we are quickly moving to a position from which we can see how virus-encoded perturbations of phosphorylation can initiate those varied symptoms of the transformed state: from modified utilisation of glucose to derangements of cell contact properties.

# The Role of Protein Phosphorylation in the Neural and Hormonal Control of Intermediary Metabolism

*Philip Cohen*

## Introduction

Although it has been known for almost 100 years that proteins contain covalently bound phosphorus, it is only since the discovery of enzyme regulation by reversible phosphorylation that interest in protein phosphorylation has gathered momentum (figure 1). In 1956, Krebs and Fischer discovered that glycogen phosphorylase, the rate limiting enzyme in glycogenolysis, could be converted from a dephosphorylated '*b*' form which was only active in the presence of the allosteric effector 5' AMP to a phosphorylated '*a*' form which was almost fully active in the absence of 5'AMP. In 1959, Krebs *et al*, demonstrated that phosphorylase kinase, the enzyme which converted phosphorylase b to a, was itself an 'interconvertible' enzyme which could exist as a less active dephosphorylated state or a more active phosphorylated state. The third enzyme shown to be regulated by this mechanism was also in the field of glycogen metabolism. In 1963, Friedman and Larner showed that glycogen synthase, the rate limiting enzyme in glycogen synthesis, could be converted from a dephosphorylated form of high activity to a phosphorylated form which required the allosteric effector glucose-6P for activity.

The idea that this mechanism of regulation might exist in other systems was slow to take root. It was only following the discovery of cyclic AMP-dependent protein kinase (Walsh *et.al.*1968) (also during studies of the control of glycogen metabolism), and the realization that many hormones increased the intracellular concentration of cyclic AMP (5), that the field started to progress rapidly. There are now (Robison *et.al.*1971) some 25 enzymes (figure 1) and countless other proteins which have been reported to be regulated by phosphorylation-dephosphorylation, and protein phosphorylation can now be said to be the major general mechanism by which intracellular activities are controlled by external physiological stimuli. This area has now reached an exciting stage where unifying concepts are linking areas of research which were previously thought of as being quite separate (Cohen 1980a). This article

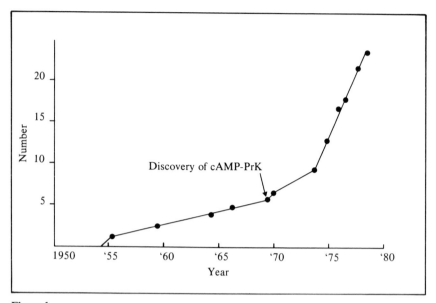

**Figure 1**
Enzymes reported as undergoing regulation by phosphorylation-dephosphorylation (reproduced by permission of Edwin G Krebs). cAMP-PrK-cyclic AMP-dependent protein kinase.

will summarise recent advances which are pointing to the existence of a relatively simple network of phosphorylation-dephosphorylation reactions which allow diverse metabolic pathways to be controlled in a synchronous manner by neural and hormonal stimuli.

## The Neural and Hormonal Control of Glycogen Metabolism in Mammalian Skeletal Muscle

The first three enzymes shown to be regulated by phosphorylation-dephosphorylation were those concerned with the regulation of glycogen metabolism in mammalian skeletal muscle (figure 1) and this system continues to act as the model to which all others are compared. It is therefore important to summarise briefly our current understanding of this system and its implications for other processes which respond to neural and hormonal stimuli.

Glycogen metabolism in skeletal muscle is regulated by the hormones adrenaline and insulin as well as by the contractile state of the tissue. These stimuli act by changing the activities of glycogen phosphorylase and glycogen synthase (the rate limiting reactions in glycogenolysis and glycogen synthesis respectively).

## Adrenergic Control of Glycogen Metabolism

The interaction of adrenaline with its $\beta$-receptors on the outer surface of the

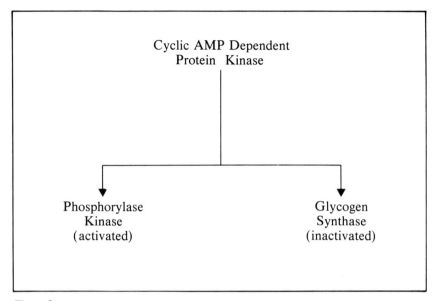

**Figure 2**
Co-ordinated control of glycogenolysis and glycogen synthesis by cyclic AMP-dependent protein kinase in response to adrenaline.

plasma membrane leads to an activation of adenylate cyclase located on the inner surface of the membrane. This elevates the intracellular level of cyclic AMP thereby activating cyclic AMP-dependent protein kinase. This enzyme possesses the subunit structure $R_2 C_2$ where R, the regulatory subunit, binds cyclic AMP and C is the catalytic subunit. The binding of cyclic AMP to the inactive $R_2 C_2$ complex causes it to dissociate to the active catalytic subunit.

$R_2 C_2 + 4$ cAMP → $R_2(cAMP)_4 + 2C$
(inactive)                    (active)
(Corbin *et.al.* 1978; Ogreid & Dosekeland 1980)

The catalytic subunit controls glycogen metabolism through the phosphorylation of three proteins, namely phosphorylase kinase, glycogen synthase and inhibitor-1 (reviewed in Cohen 1978). The phosphorylation of phosphorylase kinase and glycogen synthase increases and decreases the activity of these two enzymes respectively (figure 2). Thus the two opposing pathways of glycogenolysis and glycogen synthesis can be regulated in a synchronous manner in response to adrenaline.

These effects are amplified by inhibitor-1. This protein is phosphorylated on a single threonine residue by cyclic AMP-dependent protein kinase (Table 1), and in its phosphorylated state is a very powerful inhibitor of protein

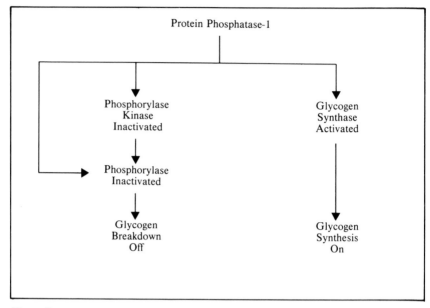

**Figure 3**
Role of protein phosphatase-1 in the control of glycogen metabolism.

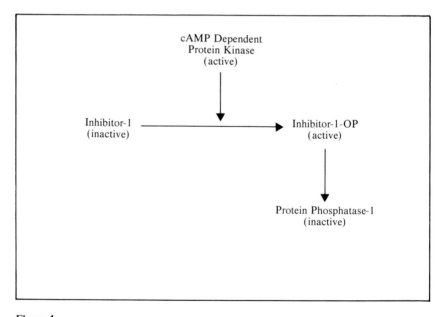

**Figure 4**
Cyclic AMP-dependent protein kinase inactives protein phosphatase-1 through the phosphorylation of inhibitor-1.

phosphatase-1, the major protein phosphatase involved in the regulation of glycogen metabolism (figures 3,4) (Cohen 1978; Foulkes and Cohen 1979). This provides a mechanism for amplifying the effect of cyclic AMP and for exerting a tight control over several protein kinase/protein phosphatase cycles.

Interestingly, inhibitor-1 does not inhibit its own dephosphorylation by protein phosphatase-1, even at concentrations 1,000 fold higher than those which inhibit the dephosphorylation of other substrates. Consequently there is no need to invoke the existence of a separate enzyme for the dephosphorylation of inhibitor-1 other than protein phosphatase-1 itself (Nimmo and Cohen 1978).

## Neural Control of Glycogen Metabolism

When muscle is stimulated electrically, calcium ions are released from the sarcoplasmic reticulum into the cytoplasm. The calcium ions not only activate actomyosin ATPase activity and initiate muscle contraction, but also activate phosphorylase kinase which is dependent on this divalent cation for activity (Brostrom et.al.1971). The activation of phosphorylase kinase promotes the conversion of phosphorylase $b$ to $a$, stimulating glycogenolysis and thereby

**Table 1**
Amino acid sequences at the phosphorylation sites of the enzymes of glycogen metabolism*

a) Sites phosphorylated by cyclic AMP-dependent protein kinase
(The roles of the basic amino acids just N-terminal to the phosphorylated residues in determining the specificity of this enzyme are discussed in Section 6a)

| Protein | Sequence |
|---|---|
| Phosphorylase kinase (α-subunit) | ala-arg-thr-lys-arg-ser-gly-ser(P)-val-tyr-glu-pro-leu-lys- |
| Glycogen synthase (site-1b) | gly-gly-ser-lys-arg-ser-asn-ser(P)-val-ser-ser-leu-ser-pro- |
| Phosphorylase kinase ( -subunit) | phe-arg-arg-leu-ser(P)-ile-thr-glu-ser-gln-pro |
| Glycogen synthase (site-1a) | pro-gln-trp-pro-arg-arg-ala-ser(P)-cys-thr-ser-ser-ser-gly |

b) Sites phosphorylated by phosphorylase kinase
(The numbers indicate distances from the N-terminus of each enzyme. Residues in identical positions are marked by a full line and in conservative differences by a broken line)

|  | 10    14        20 |
|---|---|
| Glycogen phosphorylase | glu-lys-arg-lys-gln-ile-ser(P)-val-arg-gly-leu-ala-gly-val-glu |
|  | 5   7    10      15 |
| Glycogen synthase (site-2) | pro-leu-ser-arg-thr-leu-ser(P)-val-ser-ser-leu-pro-gly-leu-glu |

c) Sites phosphorylated by glycogen synthase kinase-3

|  | 3a      3b      3c |
|---|---|
| Glycogen synthase (sites-3a, 3b, 3c) | arg-tyr-pro-arg-pro-ala-ser(P)-val-pro-pro-ser(P)-pro-ser-leu-ser(P)-arg |

*Cohen 1978; Yeaman et.al.1977; Parker et.al.1981; Cohen et.al.1977; Embi et.al.1979; Rylatt et.al.1980.

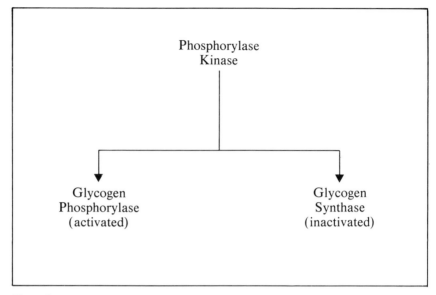

**Figure 5**
Co-ordinated control of glycogenolysis and glycogen synthesis by phosphorylase kinase during muscle contraction.

providing the ATP necessary to sustain muscle contraction. Recently, phosphorylase kinase has been shown to phosphorylate glycogen synthase and to decrease its activity (Embi *et.al.*1979; Roach *et.al.*1978; DePaoli-Roach *et al.*1979; Soderling *et.al.*1979; Walsh *et.al.*1979). Thus, the two opposing pathways of glycogenolysis and glycogen synthesis may be regulated in a synchronous manner during muscle contraction (figure 5). Glycogen phosphorylase is phosphorylated on a single serine residue 14 amino acids from the N-terminus of the protein which comprises 841 residues (Table 1), and glycogen synthase is phosphorylated by phosphorylase kinase on a serine residue (termed site-2) only seven amino acids from the N-terminus of this protein which comprises about 770 residues (Table 1). The sequences surrounding these two phosphoserine residues show considerable similarity (Table 1).

Phosphorylase kinase is composed of four different subunits and has the structure $(\alpha\beta\gamma\delta)_4$, where the molecular weights of the $\alpha$, $\beta$, $\gamma$ and $\delta$units are 145,000, 130,000, 45,000 and 17,000 respectively (Cohen *et. al.*1978; Shenoliker *et.al.*1979). The $\alpha$-and $\beta$-subunits are the components phosphorylated by cyclic AMP-dependent protein kinase (Table 1), the $\gamma$-subunit appears to be the catalytic subunit (Skuster *et.al.*1980) and the $\delta$-subunit is the calcium binding subunit (Cohen *et.al.*1978; Shenolikar *et al* 1979).

The $\delta$-subunit of phosphorylase kinase is identical to the calcium binding protein termed calmodulin (Cohen *et.al.*1978; Shenolikar *et.al.*1979; Grand *et* *al.* 1980). This protein, which was originally discovered as an activator of a quite different enzyme, is now implicated as the regulator of a number of calcium dependent enzymes (see section 6B). Calmodulin is 50% identical in amino acid sequence to troponin-C, the protein which confers calcium sensitivity to actomyosin ATPase in the muscle contractile apparatus, and like troponin-C can bind four molecules of $Ca^{2+}$ per mole with affinities in the range 1-20 $\mu$M (Watterson *et. al.* 1980; Klee *et. al.* 1980). The first and second molecules of $Ca^{2+}$ are bound to calmodulin at *ca* 10-fold lower concentrations of $Ca^2$ than are the third and fourth molecules.

It has recently been discovered that phosphorylase kinase can interact with a second molecule of calmodulin termed the $\delta'$-subunit, which activates the dephosphorylated form of the enzyme 5-fold at saturating $Ca^{2+}$. Troponin-C, the troponin complex, and even artificial thin filaments of muscle (made by mixing actin, tropomyosin and the troponin complex in physiological pro portions) can substitute for the $\delta'$-subunit in the activation of phosphorylase kinase (Shenolikar *et. al.* 1979; Cohen 1980b), and a number of lines of evidence suggest that troponin-C rather than the $\delta'$-subunit is really the physiological activator of phosphorylase kinase (Cohen 1980b). Since activation by the troponin complex occurs at lower concentrations of $Ca^{2+}$ than does activation by the $\delta'$-subunit, the dephosphorylated form of phosphorylase kinase is almost completely dependent on the troponin complex for activity at concentrations of $Ca^{2+}$ in the micromolar range.

Phosphorylation of phosphorylase kinase with cyclic AMP-dependent protein kinase increases the activity 15-fold at saturating $Ca^{2+}$ and also decreases the concentration of $Ca^{2+}$ required for half-maximal activation (from *ca* 20 $\mu$M to *ca* 1.5 $\mu$M). It therefore appears that phosphorylation of the $\alpha$ and $\beta$-subunits not only increases the catalytic activity of the $\gamma$-subunit, but allows it to be activated when only two molecules of $Ca^{2+}$ are bound to each $\delta$-subunit, whereas the binding of three or four molecules of $Ca^{2+}$ are required to activate the dephosphorylated enzyme. The phosphorylated enzyme can only be stimulated very slightly by either the $\delta'$-subunit or the troponin complex (Cohen 1980b).

Although it has been believed for some years that $Ca^{2+}$ is the link between glycogenolysis and muscle contraction it is only very recently that this concept has started to be placed on a firm molecular basis. The current ideas are summarised in figure 6. It appears that the regulation of phosphorylase kinase by $Ca^{2+}$ is determined by the two calcium binding proteins calmodulin and troponin-C and that their relative importance depends on the state of phosphorylation of the enzyme. An increase in the concentration of $Ca^2$ from $\leq 0.1$ $\mu$M (resting muscle) into the micromolar range (contracting muscle) would activate the dephosphorylated enzyme only 4-8 fold through the binding of $Ca^{2+}$ to calmodulin (the $\delta$-subunit) but a further 20-30 fold through the binding of $Ca^{2+}$ to troponin-C. Troponin-C rather than the $\delta$-subunit is

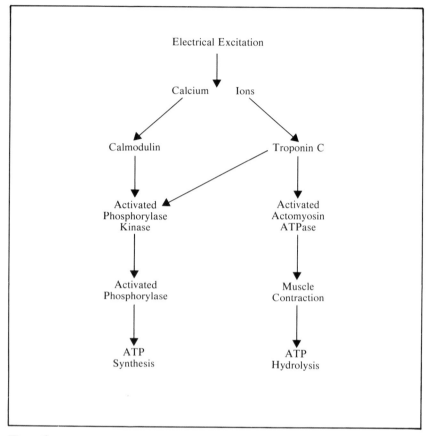

**Figure 6**
Calcium control of phosphorylase kinase through the combined action of calmodulin (the $\delta$-subunit) and troponin-C.

therefore the dominant calcium dependent regulator of the dephosphorylated form of the enzyme. This provides an attractive mechanism for coupling glycogenolysis and muscle contraction since both processes are activated by the same calcium binding protein. On the other hand the phosphorylated enzyme cannot be activated to a significant extent by troponin-C, although this form of the enzyme still has an absolute requirement for $Ca_{2+}$. Calmodulin (the $\delta$-subunit) rather than troponin-C is therefore the dominant calcium dependent regulator of phosphorylase kinase in its hormonally activated state (Cohen 1980b).

The $\delta$-subunit is complexed with the $\gamma$-subunit of phosphorylase kinase, whereas the $\delta'$-subunit (and therefore presumably troponin-c) interacts with both the $\alpha$ and $\beta$-subunits (Picton *et. al.* 1980).

## Multisite Phosphorylation of Phosphorylase
## Kinase and Glycogen Synthase

Phosphorylase kinase is phosphorylated *in vitro* on two serine residues, one on the $\alpha$ and one on the $\beta$-subunit (Table 1). The initial rate of phosphorylation of the $\beta$-subunit is 5-10 fold faster than the $\alpha$-subunit, and the activity of the enzyme correlates with the state of phosphorylation of the $\beta$-subunit (Cohen 1973; 1980c). The phosphorylation of the $\alpha$-subunit does not affect the activity directly (Cohen 1980c) and its function is unknown (Stewart *et.al* 1981), although the $\alpha$ as well as the $\beta$-subunit is phosphorylated *in vivo* in response to the adrenaline (Yeaman and Cohen 1975). Protein phosphatase-1 dephosphorylates the $\beta$-subunit specifically, and a separate enzyme (termed protein phosphatase-2) is required for the dephosphorylation of the $\alpha$-subunit (Cohen 1978; Antoniw and Cohen 1976).

Glycogen synthase is phosphorylated by cyclic AMP-dependent protein kinase on three serine residues *in vitro* termed site-1a, site-1b and site-2 (Table 1). The initial rate of phosphorylation of site-la is 7-10 fold faster than site-2 and 15-20 fold faster than site-1b. The activity of glycogen synthase is determined by the state of phosphorylation of site-2 and site-1a, but not site-1b (Embi *et.al*.1980a).

Cyclic AMP-dependent protein kinase and phosphorylase kinase are not the only glycogen synthase kinases in skeletal muscle. At least one further enzyme exists which has been termed glycogen synthase kinase-3 (Embi *et.al*.1980b). This enzyme, whose activity is unaffected by cyclic AMP, cyclic GMP, $Ca_{2+}$ or calmodulin, phosphorylates three serine residues (sites-3a, 3c and 3c) all located within nine amino acids on the polypeptide chain (Table 1).

Phosphorylation by each of the three glycogen synthase kinases decreases the activity of glycogen synthase in the absence (but not in the presence) of glucose-6P, and increases the $A_{0.5}$ for glucose-6P (Embi *et. al.* 1980b). Phosphorylation by glycogen synthase kinase-3 produces larger decreases in activity than cyclic AMP-dependent protein kinase or phosphorylase kinase for a given amount of phosphate incorporated. Phosphorylation at all six sites (1a, 1b, 2, 3a and 3c) is required to achieve an enzyme which is almost completely inactive in the absence of glucose-6P (Embi *et.al*.1980b).

Glycogen synthase is known to be highly phosphorylated *in vivo* and its degree of phosphorylation increases in response to adrenaline (Cohen 1978), but the state of phosphorylation of the individual sites *in vivo* is still under investigation.

Phosphorylase kinase and glycogen synthase were the first examples of enzyme regulation by 'multisite phosphorylation' and the phosphorylation of a protein at more than one site or by more than one kinase is turning out to be a very common phenomenon (reviewed in Cohen 1980a). A second phosphorylation may amplify or even antagonize the effects of the first phosphorylation, or influence the rate at which the first site is phosphorylated or dephosphorylated. Such interactions between phosphorylation sites may explain, at the molecular level, how the effects of different neural and hormonal stimuli can become integrated into the structures of key regulatory proteins. 'Multisite phosphorylations' may allow proteins to respond to different degrees of hormonal stimulation, and explain other effects, such as the transient nature of many neural and hormonal responses.

### Evidence for Involvement of the Regulatory Proteins of Glycogen Metabolism in other Metabolic Pathways

*Cyclic AMP-dependent Protein Kinase*

A variety of hormones with diverse physiological effects on a wide range of tissues can all elevate the intracellular concentration of cyclic AMP (Robinson *et.al.*1971), and yet cyclic AMP dependent protein kinase appears to be the only high affinity binding protein for cyclic AMP in mammalian tissues. Furthermore the concentration of this enzyme is as high or even higher in tissues where glycogen metabolism is of very minor importance (Kuo and Greengard 1969). These findings have given rise to the idea shown in figure 7 (Krebs 1972). According to this hypothesis the specificity of a hormone is determined by whether the receptor for that hormone is present on the outer membrane of the target cells and which physiological substrates for cyclic AMP-dependent protein kinase happen to be present within those cells. If the receptor is present, then the hormone-receptor interaction leads to the activation of adenylate cyclase, elevation of cyclic AMP and activation of cyclic AMP-dependent protein kinase. The protein kinase then phosphorylates whatever substrate proteins happen to be present within those cells. As a result the biological properties of the substrate may become modified, although the magnitude of the effect will depend on the metabolic state of the cell. Phosphorylation of the enzyme often changes the Km for a substrate, the Ka for an activator or the Ki for an inhibitor. Allosteric effectors may also affect the rate at which an enzyme is phosphorylated or dephosphorylated. Phosphorylation-dephosphorylation should not therefore be regarded as a mechanism for switching an enzyme on or off, but rather as a mechanism for interconverting an enzyme between two forms (or very many more than two in the case of enzymes with complex subunit structures which exhibit 'multisite phosphorylation') which respond differently to substrates and allosteric effectors (Cohen 1980a). Therefore whether the phosphorylation of an enzyme *in vivo* actually changes its activity, depends on the concentration of substrates and regulatory metabolites which have the power to amplify or suppress the effects of phosphorylation. The interplay between phosphorylation and allosteric effectors represents the means by which extra cellular (neural and hormonal) and intracellular information become inte grated to determine the precise activity of a metabolic pathway *in vivo*. However, should the metabolic state of the cell allow the activity of a protein to be altered

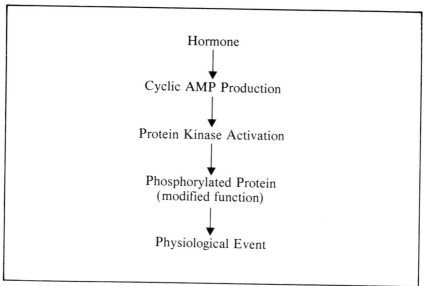

**Figure 7**
Hypothesis for the hormonal regulation of cellular functions working through cyclic AMP (38).

by phosphorylation, some change in the physiology of the cell will occur (figure 7).

One obvious prediction of this model is that a very large number of substrates for cyclic AMP-dependent protein kinase must exist in different cells to explain the great diversity of action of many hormones, and it has become increasinly clear that this is the case. Nine enzymes that are likely to be physiological substrates for cyclic AMP-dependent protein kinase are listed in Table 2. The activation of triglyceride lipase (Steinberg 1976) and inactivation of glycerol phosphate acyl transferase (Nimmo 1980) in adipose tissue are likely to provide co-ordinated control of triglyceride breakdown and synthesis in adipose tissue in response to adrenaline, in the same way that the activation of phosphorylase kinase and inhibition of glycogen synthase co-ordinate glycogen breakdown and synthesis in skeletal muscle and liver (figure 2). The phosphorylation of acetyl-CoA carboxylase decreases its activity and raises the $A_{0.5}$ for the allosteric activator, citrate (Hardie and Guy 1980). This underlies the inhibition of fatty acid synthesis which occurs in adipose tissue in response to adrenaline, and in liver in response to glucagon (Brownsey and Hardie 1980). The phosphorylation of L-type pyruvate kinase increases the $K_m$ for phosphenol-pyruvate and is an important mechanism for stimulating gluconeogenesis in liver in response to glucagon (Engstram 1980). The activation of cholesterol esterase increases the pool of cholesterol for steroidogenesis in the adrenal cortex in response to ACTH (Boyd and Gorban

1980). The inactivation of myosin light chain kinase is likely to be a key event in the relaxation of smooth muscle by adrenaline (Adelstein *et.al.*1980). The activation of tryosine hydroxylase stimulates the synthesis of catecholamines (Joh *et.al.*1978; Yamauchi and Fujisawa 1979a, Vulliet *et.al.*1980).

However, perhaps the majority of hormonal effects influence processes where the protein components are not enzymes. These include effects on muscle contractility, secretion, membrane permeability and transport, protein induction and protein degradation. Although it is likely that the hormonal regulation of many of these processes involves protein phosphorylation, progress is hampered by the lack of understanding of the molecular nature of the processes themselves. However the importance of cyclic AMP-dependent protein kinase has been established in several cases. For example the phosphorylation of troponin-I in cardiac muscle by cyclic AMP-dependent protein kinases reduced the affinity of tropinin-C for $Ca^{2+}$, which may be important in stimulating the rate of relaxation of heart muscle by adrenaline (reviewed in England 1980). The phosphorylation of a protein in cardiac sarcoplasmic reticulum, termed phospholamban, is associated with increased rates of calcium uptake into the sarcoplasmic reticulum, and may also promote the decrease in relaxation time of the heart by adrenaline (reviewed in England 1980). The growth of a number of mammalian cells in culture is inhibited by cyclic AMP, and this has allowed the isolation of mutant cells in which this phenomenon no longer occurs. Many of these mutant cells have been shown to lack cyclic AMP-dependent protein kinase (Gottesman *et.al.*1980) Thus even

**Table 2**
List of enzymes that are regulated by cyclic AMP-dependent protein kinase*

| Enzyme | Tissue | Activated (A) or Inhibited (I) |
|---|---|---|
| Phosphorylase kinase | Muscle, liver | A |
| Glycogen synthase | Muscle, liver | I |
| Triglyceride lipase | Adipose tissue | A |
| Glycerol phosphate acyl transferase | Adipose tissue | I |
| Acetyl-CoA carboxylase | Adipose tissue, liver, mammary gland | I |
| L-pyruvate kinase | Liver | I |
| Cholesterol esterase | Adrenal cortex | A |
| Myosin light chain kinase | Smooth muscle | I |
| Tyrosine hydroxylase | Adrenal gland and brain | A |

*Steinberg 1976; Nimmo 1980; Hardie and Guy 1980; Brownsey and Hardie 1980; Engstram 1980; Boyd and Gorban 1980; Adelstein *et.al.*1978; Joh *et.al.*1978; Yamauchi and Fujisawa 1979; Vulliet *et.al.*1980.

the long-term effects of cyclic AMP on cell growth are clearly mediated by cyclic AMP-dependent protein kinase, and must involve the phosphorylation of as yet unidentified proteins.

It is, however, important to stress that cyclic AMP-dependent protein kinase is a very specific enzyme which phosphorylates very few proteins at signficant rates (Nimmo and Cohen 1977). Even among substrate proteins only one or two out of a large number of potentially available serine or threonine residues become phosphorylated. The determination of the amino acid sequences around some of the phosphorylation sites in recent years has demonstrated that two adjacent basic amino acids, at least one of which is arginine, just N-terminal to the residue that is phosphorylated, is a feature common to all the

**Table 3**
Amino acid sequences at the phosphorylation sites of substrates for cAMP-dependent protein kinase

| Substrate | Sequence[a] |
|---|---|
| Phosphorylase kinase ($\beta$-subunit) | 100<br>ala-arg-thr-lys-arg-ser-gly-ser(P)-val-tyr-glu-pro-leu-lys |
| Glycogen synthase (site-1a) | 80<br>pro-gln-trp-pro-arg-arg-ala-ser(P)-cys-thr-ser-ser-ser-gly |
| Pyruvate kinase, rat liver | 35<br>gly-val-leu-arg-arg-ala-ser(P)-val-ala-glx-leu |
| Pyruvate kinase, pig liver | ?<br>leu-arg-arg-ala-ser(P)-leu-gly |
| Inhibitor-1 | 30<br>ile-arg-arg-arg-arg-pro-thr(P)-pro-ala-thr |
| Phosphorylase kinase ($\alpha$-subunit) | 20<br>phe-arg-arg-leu-ser(P)-ile-ser-thr-glu-ser-gln-pro |
| Glycogen synthase (site-1b) | 10<br>ser-ser-gly-gly-ser-lys-arg-ser-asn-ser(P)-val-asp-thr-ser-ser-leu-ser |
| Troponin 1, rabbit heart | ?<br>val-arg-arg-ser(P)-asp-arg-ala-tyr-ala |
| Histone H1, calf thymus | 8<br>ala-lys-arg-lys-ala-ser(P)-gly-pro-pro-val-ser |
| Type 2 regulatory subunit of cAMP-dependent protein kinase | asp-arg-arg-val-ser(P)-val |

[a]The numbers above the phosphorylated residues refer to the rates at which the sites are phosphorylated relative to the $\beta$-subunit of phophorylase kinase (100%) at a $6\mu M$ substrate concentration under a defined set of assay conditions.
Each protein was from rabbit skeletal muscle unless otherwise stated.

*Cohen 1978; Yeaman et. al. 1977; Parker et. al. 1981; Cohen et. al. 1977; Engstram 1980; Moir and Perry 1977; Huang et. al. 1979.

best substrates for cyclic AMP-dependent protein kinase (Table 3). Work with synthetic peptides corresponding to some of these sites has confirmed that this feature is critical for specific substrate recognition (reviewed in Engstram 1980). The finding that the specificity of cyclic AMP-dependent protein kinase largely resides in the primary structure (or secondary structure determined by local primary structure) in the immediate vicinity of the phosphorylation site suggests a simple mechanism whereby proteins have evolved sensitivity to hormones. If, by mutation, a protein acquires two adjacent basic amino acids N-terminal to a serine (or occasionally a threonine) residue located on an accessible region on the surface of a protein, then that protein will become phosphorylated by cyclic AMP-dependent protein kinase *in vivo*. Should that phosphorylation affect the function of the protein in a biologically useful way, the mutation will be selected for and eventually spread through the population. It seems likely that the specificity of other protein kinases, such as phosphorylase kinase (table 1), will also be found to reside in primary structures surrounding particular phosphorylation sites.

*Calmodulin*
Although the importance of calcium ions in cellular regulation has been recognised for many years, the concept of an intracellular calcium receptor which mediates the actions of this divalent cation, in a manner analogous to the regulatory subunit of cyclic AMP-dependent protein kinase, is a very recent development. It is only since the discovery of calmodulin and the identification of its multiple actions that this idea has started to gain widespread acceptance (Klee *et.al.* 1980; Wolff and Brostrom 1979; Cheung 1980).

   Calmodulin, formerly termed the 'modular protein' or 'calcium dependent regulator protein' was originally discovered as a small thermostable calcium binding protein which stimulated the activity of one of the cyclic nucleotide phosphodiesterases in brain. This protein was subsequently found to be present in very large amounts in brain and other tissues (50-500 mg per 1,000 g tissue), a huge excess over the concentration of cyclic nucleotide phosphodiesterase. The amino acid sequence of calmodulin, which demonstrated its considerable similarity to troponin-C (Cheung 1970) was really the stimulus which started the search for other proteins whose activities might be affected by calmodulin. Seven enzymes which are known to be activated by or completely dependent on calmodulin are given in table 3. In all these cases calmodulin is only an activator in the presence of calcium ions. This list includes three protein kinases, myosin light chain kinase, phosphorylase kinase, and tryptophan hydroxylase kinase. In addition membranes isolated from a variety of tissues have been shown to contain endogenous calmodulin-dependent protein kinases which phosphorylate membrane proteins whose identity and function are unknown (Schulman and Greengard 1978). Calmodulin has been shown to become associated with the mitotic spindles during

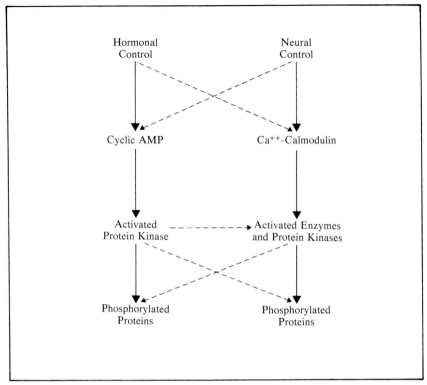

**Figure 8**
Interrelationships between cyclic AMP and calmodulin in the neural and hormonal control of intermediary metabolism.

cell division (Welsh *et. al.* 1978; Dedman *et. al.* 1979) and to stimulate the depolymerisation of microtubules (Dedman *et. al.* 1979). It seems likely that many more calmodulin-dependent enzymes will be identified over the next few years, and that its involvement in other cellular processes, such as secretion, will become recognised.

It seems, however, already justified to describe this protein as a major intra cellular calcium receptor, and the calcium-calmodulin and cyclic AMP-cyclic AMP-dependent protein kinase systems are closely analogous as illustrated in Figure 8.

A major difference between the two systems is that mammalian cells contain just one catalytic subunit of cyclic AMP-dependent protein kinase which phosphorylates a variety of proteins. On the other hand, the current evidence suggests that there is a large number of different calmodulin-dependent protein kinases, each of which has a very restricted substrate specificity. Nevertheless, both mechanisms produce the same end result, namely the phos phorylation of a number of proteins in response to either cyclic AMP or calcium ions.

Another important point illustrated by the broken lines in figure 8 is that the cyclic AMP and calcium-calmodulin pathways are closely interlinked and may often be interchangeable in different tissues. Thus the stimulation of glycogenolysis in skeletal muscle is a $\beta$-adrenergic effect mediated by cyclic AMP, whereas in rat liver it appears to be largely an $\alpha$-adrenergic effect mediated, at least in part, by calcium ions (Exton and Harper 1975). Similarly, electrical stimulation of skeletal muscle leads to an elevation in the concentration of calcium ions in the muscle sarcoplasm, whereas electrical activity of the brain elevates the intracellular level of cyclic AMP. The latter effect could be due to the activation of the calmodulin sensitive adenylate cyclase, which is present in brain but not apparently in most other tissues.

A second point at which the cyclic AMP and calcium-calmodulin pathways may interconnect is at the level of the protein kinases. Figure 8 suggests that cyclic AMP-dependent protein kinase may often phosphorylate calmodulin sensitive enzymes. There are already two well documented examples of this phenomenon, namely the activation of phosphorylase kinase in skeletal muscle and the inactivation of myosin kinase in smooth muscle (table 2).

Further interconnection may also occur at the level of the phosphorylated substrates. Figure 8 suggests that cyclic AMP-dependent and calmodulin-dependent protein kinases may often phosphorylate the same proteins, although at different sites, due to the high specificity of protein kinases. Three examples of this phenomenon have already been described; glycogen synthase, phospholamban (the protein in cardiac sarcoplasmic reticulum believed to regulate the uptake of calcium ions from the sarcoplasm (Lepeuch *et.al*.1979), and a brain membrane protein, termed protein-1, which is believed to be involved in synaptic transmission (Huttner and Greengard 1979).

*Protein phosphatase-1*

As the number of enzymes reported to be regulated by phosphorylation-dephosphorylation has increased, an important generality that is emerging is that enzymes in biodegradative pathways are activated by phosphorylation, whereas enzymes in biosynthetic pathways are inactivated by phosphorylation (Cohen 1980a; Cohen *et.al*.1979 table 5). Two implications of this finding are that different enzymes may be regulated by the same protein kinases and protein phosphatases, or that different protein kinases and protein phosphatases may be controlled by the same regulator proteins. Both these concepts are already established in the case of protein kinases. Cyclic AMP-dependent protein kinase regulates enzymes involved in both degradative and synthetic pathways (table 4), while a number of protein kinases are controlled by the same regulator protein, namely calmodulin (tables 4,5).

Protein phosphatase-1 catalyses a number of functionally related dephos phorylation reactions involved in the control of glycogen metabolism (table 1, figure 3), and it dephosphorylates serine and threonine residues phosphorylated by cyclic AMP-dependent protein kinase, phosphorylase kinase and glycogen synthase kinase-3 (Cohen 1978; Stewart $et.al.$1981). This raises the question of whether its specificity is even broader, and whether it may dephosphorylate enzymes involved in cellular processes other than glycogen metabolism. The tissue distribution of protein phosphatase-1 is consistent with the idea that this enzyme has a wider role in metabolism (Burchell $et,al.$1978). Its concentration only varies by about 2-fold from tissue to tissue, and its concentration is therefore high in adipose tissue, brain and mammary gland where the glycogen metabolising enzymes are present in extremely low concentrations. The tissue distribution of protein phosphatase-1 is consistent with the idea that this enzyme has a wider role in metabolism (Burchell $et.al$ 1978). Its concentration only varies by about 2-fold from tissue to tissue, and its concentration is therefore high in adipose tissue, brain and mammary gland where the glycogen metabolising enzymes are present in extremely low concentrations. The tissue distribution of protein phosphatase-1, therefore resembles that of cyclic AMP-dependent protein kinase. Protein phosphatase-1 has now been shown to dephosphorylate all of the enzymes listed in Table 5 (Stewart $et.al.$1981; Nimmo 1980; Boyd and Gorban 1980; Ingebritsen and Gibson 1980; Stewart $et. al.$1980; Hardie 1980; unpublished), except for triglyceride lipase which has not yet been tested. The enzymes involved in biodegradative pathways are inactivated and those involved in biosynthetic pathways are activated by this enzyme. These experiments do not however prove that protein phosphatase-1 is a *major* protein phosphatase acting on these enzymes *in vivo*. There is currently only evidence for this in the case of acetyl-CoA carboxylase in lactating mammary gland (Hardie 1980) and

**Table 4**
List of enzymes that are activated by or completely dependent on calmodulin[*]

| Enzyme | Tissue |
| --- | --- |
| High Km cyclic nucleotide phosphodiesterase | Brain, heart |
| Adenylate cyclase | Brain |
| Calcium-magnesium ATPase | Erthrocyte membrane |
| NAD-kinase | Higher plants |
| Phosphorylase kinase | Skeletal muscle |
| Myosin kinase | Skeletal musle and smooth muscle |
| Tryptophan hydroxylase kinase | Brain |

[*]Cohen $et.al.$1978; Shenlikar $et.al.$1979; England 1980; Cheung 1970; Kakuichi $et.al.$1970; brostrom $et.al.$1975; Gopinath and Vicenzi 1977; Jarrett and Penniston 1977; Anderson and Cormier 1978; Yamauichi and Fujisawa 1979b; Kuhn $et.al.$1980.

hydroxymethylglutaryl-CoA reductase in liver (Ingebritsen and Gibson 1980). However the results so far are suggestive and indicate that protein phosphatase-1 (and also perhaps inhibitor-1), like cyclic AMP-dependent protein kinase and calmodulin, has a widespread role in cellular regulation. The finding that several of the proteins involved in the regulation of glycogen metabolism also participate in the control of other metabolic pathways, indicates that a relatively simple network of phospho rylation-dephosphorylation reactions may underlie the regulation of a variety of cellular processes by neural and hormonal stimuli.

## The Mechanism of Action of Insulin - An Hypothesis

Although it has been known for over 50 years that insulin lowers the concentration of glucose in the blood, the molecular mechanism by which this hormone acts has so far defied solution. Insulin not only stimulates glucose uptake, but a range of biosynthetic processes including glycogen, fatty acid, triglyceride, cholesterol and protein synthesis. Inspection of table 5 indicates that most, if not all, of the actions of insulin could be explained by a net decrease in the extent of phosphorylation of the key rate limiting enzymes of these pathways. Evidence in favour of this idea was first obtained in the field of glycogen metabolism. Joseph Larner and co-workers found that when rat hemidiaphragms were incubated with insulin, the activity of glycogen synthase measured in the absence (but not in the presence) of glucose-6P was increased

**Table 5**

Enzyme found in the cytoplasm of mammalian cells that are regulated by phosphorylation (see Cohen 1980a; Burchell *et al* 1978)

| | Types of protein kinase involved | | | |
|---|---|---|---|---|
| | cAMP | Ca$^2$+-calmodulin | Other | |
| *Activation by phosphorylation* | | | | *Biodegradative pathway* |
| Glycogen phosphorylase | — | + | — | Glycogenolysis |
| Phosphorylase kinase | + | + | — | Glycogenolysis |
| Myosin | — | + | — | ATP hydrolysis |
| Triglyceride lipase | + | — | — | Triglyceride breakdown |
| Cholesterol esterase | + | — | — | Cholesterol ester hydrolysis |
| *Inactivation by phosphorylation* | | | | *Biosynthetic pathway* |
| Glycogen synthase | + | + | + | Glycogen synthesis |
| Acetyl-CoA carboxylase | + | — | — | Fatty acid synthesis |
| L-pyruvate kinase | + | — | — | ATP synthesis |
| Glycerol phosphate acyl transferase | + | — | — | Triglyceride synthesis |
| HMG-CoA reductase | — | — | + | Cholesterol synthesis |
| Initiation factor e1F-2 | — | — | + | Protein synthesis |

(Villar-Palasi and Larner 1960; Craig and Larner 1964). These results indicated that insulin had either decreased the activity of glycogen synthase kinase or increased the activity of glycogen synthase phosphatase. The interpretation of these results has been complicated by the realization that glycogen synthase can be phosphorylated and inactivated by a number of different protein kinases *in vitro*. The recent finding that insulin activates glycogen synthase in the soleus muscle of I-strain mice which lack phosphorylase kinase (LeMarchand Brustel *et. al.* 1979), does however appear to exclude the possibility that insulin activates glycogen synthase by decreasing the activity of phosphorylase kinase. It also implies that the action of insulin on glycogen synthesis is unrelated to decreases in the intracelular concentration of $Ca^{2+}$, or to a direct effect on the $Ca^{2+}$-calmodulin pathway (figure 8).

In order to avoid the complication of multiple phosphorylations, the effect of insulin on the state of phosphorylation of inhibitor-1 was investigated, since this protein is phosphorylated on a single threonine residue by just one protein kinase (cyclic AMP-dependent protein kinase). Using a perfused hind limb system, insulin was found to produce a 2-fold decrease in the phosphorylation of inhibitor-1. This indicates that insulin must either inhibit cyclic AMP-dependent protein kinase or activate the protein phosphatase which dephosphorylates inhibitor-1 *in vivo*. The latter enzyme may be protein phosphatase-1 (see section 3). It should be stressed that insulin does not affect the concentration of cyclic AMP in skeletal muscle under conditions where glycogen synthase and inhibitor-1 are dephosphorylated (Goldberg *et.al.*1967; Craig *et.al.*1969). An inactivation of cyclic AMP-dependent protein kinase by insulin would therefore need to proceed through a different mechanism (Walkenbach *et.al.*1978).

Recent studies on the control of cholesterol synthesis appear to be of some significance to our understanding of insulin action. The rate limiting enzyme in this pathway - hydroxymethylglutaryl-CoA (HMG-CoA) reductase - is inactivated by phosphorylation and the enzyme which carries out this reaction - HMG-CoA reductase kinase - is also an interconvertible enzyme which is activated by an HMG-CoA reductase kinase kinase (figure 9). Ingebritsen and Gibson have shown that insulin promotes the dephosphorylation of both HMG-CoA reductase and HMG-CoA reductase kinase in isolated hepatocytes (Ingebritsen *et. al.* 1979), so that stimulation of cholesterol synthesis by insulin is highly analogous to the regulation of glycogen synthesis by this hormone. However, neither HMG-CoA reductase kinase nor HMG-CoA reductase kinase kinase is cyclic AMP-dependent protein kinase (Ingebritsen and Gibson 1980). The action of insulin in this system cannot therefore be explained by the inactivation of cyclic AMP-dependent protein kinase. On the other hand, protein phosphatase-1 has been implicated as a major HMG-cOA reductase phosphatase and HMG-CoA reductase kinase phosphatase (Ingebritsen and Gibson 1980), and the striking finding that emerges from the effects

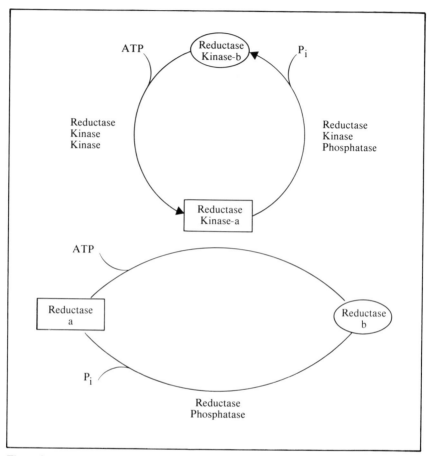

**Figure 9**
Bicyclic model for the regulation of HMG-CoA reductase (reductase) and cholesterol synthesis (72). *b*, inactive; *a*, active form.

of insulin on glycogen synthase, inhibitor-1, HMG-CoA reductase and HMG-CoA reductase kinase is that protein phosphatase-1 may be the inter-converting enzyme which is common to each of these systems. Many of the actions of insulin on intermediary metabolism could therefore be explained if protein phosphatase-1 became activated in response to insulin. It is therefore of considerable interest that a new mechanism for activating this enzyme appears to have been discovered.

Merlevede and co-workers reported some years ago that liver contained a phosphorylase phosphatase activity which was only active in the presence of ATP-Mg (Merlevede *et. al.* 1969). This ATP-Mg dependent phosphorylase phosphatase was recently resolved into two components termed FC and FA (Goris *et.al.*1979). FC was an inactive phosphorylase phosphatase, while FA was a factor which in the presence of ATP-Mg activated $F_C$ (Goris *et.al.*1980). This system has now been demonstrated to exist in skeletal muscle and cardiac muscle as well as liver, and accounts for a substantial proportion of the total phosphorylase phosphatase activity of these tissues (Yang *et.al.*1980).

It has recently been discovered that the ATP-Mg dependent phosphorylase phosphatase is not specific for the dephosphorylation of phosphorylase. Furthermore, this enzyme has been shown to have an identical specificity to protein phosphatase-1 and to be inhibited by the same concentrations of inhibitor-1 that inactivate protein phosphatase-1 (Stewart *et.al.*1981). These observations raise the possibility that the ATP-Mg dependent protein phosphatase may merely be an inactive form of protein phosphatase-1, and that its activation by $F_A$ may be the key event in the stimulation of biosynthetic pathways by insulin. The requirement for ATP-Mg suggests that $F_A$ is a protein kinase which phosphorylates $F_C$, but there is currently no evidence to support this idea (Goris *et.al.* 1980). Further analysis of this system must clearly concentrate on understanding how $F_C$ and protein phosphatase-1 differ at the molecular level, and on the characterisation of $F_A$ and the mechanisms by which its activity is regulated.

## Acknowledgements

This work was supported by a Programme Grant from the Medical Research Council, London, and by the British Diabetic Association, British Heart Foundation and Cancer Research Campaign.

## References

Adelstein, R.S., Conti, M.A., Hathaway, D.R. and Klee, C.B. (1978) J. Biol. Chem., *253*, 8347-8300.

Anderson, J.M. and Cormier, M.J. (1978) Biochem. Biophys. Res. Commun., *84*, 595-602.

Antoniw, J.F. and Cohen, P. (1976) Eur. J. Biochem., *68*, 45-54.

Boyd, G.S. and Gorban, A.M.S. (1980) *in Molecular Aspects of Cellular Regulation, 1*, 95-134 (Cohen, P. ed.) Elsevier/North Holland, Amsterdam.

Brostrom, C.O., Hunkeler, F.L. and Krebs, E.G. (1971) J. Biol. Chem., *246*, 1961-1967.

Brostrom, C.O., Huang, Y.C., Breckenridge, B.M. and Wolff, D.J. (1975) Proc. Natl. Acad. Sci. USA, *72*, 64-68.

Brownsey, R.W. and Hardie, D.G. (1980) FEBS Lett., *120*, 67-70.

Burchell, A., Foulkes, J.G., Cohen, P.T.W., Condon, G.D. and Cohen, P. (1978) FEBS Lett., *92*, 68-72.

Cheung, W.Y. (1970) Biochem. Biophys. Res. Commun., *38*, 533-538.

Cheung, W.Y. (1980) Science, *207*, 19-27.

Cohen, P. (1973) Eur. J. Biochem., *34*, 1-14.

Cohen, P. (1978) Curr. Top. Cell. Reg., *14*, 117-196.

Cohen, P. (1980a) *in Molecular Aspects of Cellular Regulation*, volume *1*, pp 1-276, *'Recently Discovered Systems of Enzyme Regulation by Reversible Phosphorylation'*, Elsevier/North Holland Biomedical Press, Amsterdam.

Cohen, P. (1980b) Eur. J. Biochem., *111*, 563-574.

Cohen, P. (1980c) FEBS Lett., *119*, 301-306.

Cohen, P., Burchell, A., Foulkes, J.G., Cohen, P.T.W., Vanaman, T.C. and Perry, S.V. (1978) FEBS Lett., *92*, 287-293.

Cohen, P., Embi, N., Foulkes, J.G., Hardie, D.G., Nimmo, G.A., Rylatt, D.B. and Shenolikar, S. (1979) Miami Wint. Symp., *16*, 463-481.

Cohen, P., Rylatt, D.B. and Nimmo, G.A. (1977) FEBS Lett., *76*, 182-186.

Corbin, J.D., Sugden, P.H., West, L., Flockhart, D.A., Lincoln, T.R. and McCarthy, D. (1978) J. Biol. Chem., *253*, 3997-4003.

Craig, J.W. and Larner, J. (1964) Nature (London), *202*, 971-973.

Craig,, J.W., Rall, T.W. and Larner, J. (1969) Biochim. Biophys. Acta, *177*, 213-219.

Dedman, J.R., Brinkley, B.R. and Means, A.R. (1979) Adv. Cyc. Nuc. Res., *11*, 131-174.

DePaoli-Roach, A.A., Roach, P.J. and Larner, J. (1979) J. Biol. Chem., *254*, 4212-4219.

Embi, N., Rylatt, D.B. and Cohen, P. (1979) Eur. J. Biochem., *100*, 339-347.

Embi, N., Parker, P.J. and Cohen, P. (1980a) Eur. J. Biochem., submitted for publication.

Embi, N., Rylatt, D.B. and Cohen, P. (1980b) Eur. J. Biochem., *107*, 519-527.

England, P.J. (1980) in Molec. Aspects of Cell. Reg., *1*, 153-173 (Cohen, P. ed.) Elsevier/North Holland, Amsterdam.

Engstram, L. (1980) *in Molecular Aspects of Cellular Regulation, 1*, 11-13 (Cohen, P. ed.) Elsevier/North Holland, Amsterdam.

Exton, J.H. and Harper, S.C. (1975) Adv. Cyc. Nuc. Res., 5, 519-532.

Foulkes, J.G. and Cohen, P. (1979) Eur. J. Biochem., *97*, 251-256.

Foulkes, J.G., Jefferson, L.S. and Cohen, P. (1980) FEBS Lett., *112*, 21-24.

Friedman, D.L. and Larner, J. (1963) *Biochemistry, 2*, 669-675.

Goldberg, N.D., Villar-Palasi, C., Sasko, H. and Larner, J. (1967) Biochim. Biophys. Acta, *148*, 665-672.

Gopinath, R.M. and Vicenzi, F.F. (1977) Biochem. Biophys. Res. Commun., *77*, 1203-1209.

Goris, J., Defreyn, G. and Merlevede, W. (1979) FEBS Lett., *99*, 279-282.

Goris, J., Dopere, F., Vandenheede, J.R. and Merlevede, W. (1980) FEBS Lett., *117*, 117-121.

Gottesman, M.M., LeCam, A., Bukowski, M. and Pastan, I. (1980) Somatic Cell Genet.

Grand, R.J., Shenolikar, S. and Cohen, P. (1980) Eur. J. Biochem., in press.

Hardie, D.G. (1980) Molec. Aspects of Bell. Reg., *1*, 33-62 (Cohen, P. ed.) Elsevier/North Holland, Amsterdam.

Hardie, D.G. and Guy, P.S. (1980) Eur. J. Biochem., *110*, 167-177.

Huang, T.S., Feramisco, J.R., Glass, D.B. and Krebs, E.G. (1979) Miami Winter Symp., *16*, 449-461.

Huttner, W.B. and Greengard, P. (1979) Proc. Natl. Acad. Sci. USA, *76*, 5402-5406.

Ingebritsen, T.S., Geelen, M.J.H., Parker, R.A., Evenson, K.J. and Gibson, D.M. (1979) J. Biol. Chem., *254*, 9986-9989.

Ingebritsen, T.S. and Gibson, D.M. (1980) in Molec. Aspects of Cell. Reg., *1*, 63-93 (Cohen, P. ed.) Elsevier/North Holland, Amsterdam.

Jarrett, H.W. and Penniston, J.J. (1977) Biochem. Biophys. Res. Commun. 77, 1210-1216.

Joh, T.H., Park, D.M. and Reis, D.J. (1978) Proc. Natl. Acad. Sci., *75*, 4744-4748.

Kakuichi, S., Yamazaki, R. and Nakajima, H. (1970) Proc. Jap. Acad., *46*, 589-592.

Klee, C.B., Crouch, T.H. and Richman, P.G. (1980) Ann. Rev. Biochem. *49*, 489-515.

Krebs, E.G. (1972) Curr. Top. Cell. Reg., 5, 99-133.

Krebs, E.G. and Fischer, E.H. (1956) Biochim. Biophys. Acta, *20*, 150-157.

Krebs, E.G., Graves, D.J. and Fischer, E.H. (1959) J. Biol. Chem., *234*, 2867-

Kuhn, D.M., O'Callaghan, J.P., Juskerich, J. and Lovenberg, W. (1980) Proc. Natl. Acad. Sci., *77*, 4688-4691.

Kuo, J.F. and Greengard, P. (1969) Proc. Natl. Acad. Sci., *64*, 1349-1355.

LeMarchand-Brustel, Y., Cohen, P.T.W. and Cohen, P. (1979) FEBS Lett., *105*, 235-238.

Lepeuch, C.J., Haiech, J. and Demaille, J.G. (1979) Biochemistry, *18*, 5150-5157.

Merlevede, W., Goris, J. and DeBrandt, C. (1969) Eur. J. Biochem., *11*, 499-502.

Moir, A.J.G. and Perry, S.V. (1977) Biochem. J., *167*, 333-343.

Nimmo, H.G. (1980) *in Molecular Aspects of Cellular Regulation, 1*, 135-152 (Cohen, P. ed.) Elsevier/North Holland, Amsterdam.

Nimmo, H.G. and Cohen, P. (1977) Adv. Cyc. Nuc. Res., *8*, 145-266.

Nimmo, G.A. and Cohen, P. (1978) Eur. J. Biochem., *87*, 353-365.

Ogreid, D. and Dosekeland, S.O. (1980) FEBS Lett., *121*, 340-344.

Parker, P.J., Aitken, A., Bilham, T., Embi, N. and Cohen, P. (1981) FEBS Lett., in press.

Picton, C., Klee, C.B. and Cohen, P. (1980) Eur. J. Biochem., *111*, 553-561.

Roach, P.J., DePaoli-Roach, A.A. and Larner, J. (1978) J. Cyc. Nuc. Res., *4*, 245-257.

Robison, G.A., Butcher, R.W. and Sutherland, E.W. (1971) *'Cyclic AMP'*, Academic Press, New York.

Rylatt, D.B., Aitken, A., Bilham, T., Condon, G.D., Embi, N. and Cohen, P. (1980) Eur. J. Biochem., *107*, 529-537.

Schulman, H. and Greengard, P. (1978) Proc. Natl. Acad. Sci. USA, *75*, 5432-5436.

Shenolikar, S., Cohen, P.T.W., Cohen, P., Nairn, A.C. and Perry, S.V. (1979) Eur. J. Biochem., *100*, 329-337.

Skuster, J.R., Jesse Chan, K.F. and Graves, D.J. (1980) J. Biol. Chem., *255*, 2203-2216.

Soderling, T.R., Srivastava, A.K., Bass, M.A. and Khatra, B.S. (1979) Proc. Natl. Acad. Sci. USA, *76*, 2536-2540.

Steinberg, D. (1976) Adv. Cyc. Nuc. Res., *7*, 157-198.

Stewart, A.A., Crouch, D., Cohen, P. and Safer, B. (1980) FEBS Lett., *11*, 16-19.

Stewart, A.A., Hemmings, B.A., Cohen, P., Goris, J. and Merlevede, W. (1981) Eur. J. Biochem., in press.

Villar-Palasi, C. and Larner, J. (1960) Arch. Biochem. Biophys., *94*, 436-442.

Vulliet, P.R., Langan, T.A. and Weiner, N. (1980) Proc. Natl. Acad. Sci., *77*, 92-96.

Walkenbach, R.J., Hazen, R. and Larner, J. (1978) Mol. Cell. Biochem., *19*, 31-

Walsh, D.A., Perkins, J.P. and Krebs, E.G. (1968) J. Biol. Chem., *243*, 3763-3765.

Walsh, K.Y., Millikin, D.M., Schlender, K.K. and Reimann, E.M. (1979) J. Biol. Chem., *254*, 6611-6616.

Watterson, D.M., Sharief, F. and Vanaman, T.C. (1980) J. Biol. Chem., *255*, 962-975.

Welsh, A.J., Dedman, J.R., Brinkley, B.R. and Means, A.R. (1978) Proc. Natl. Acad. Sci. USA, *75*, 1867-1871.

Wolff, D.J. and Brostrom, C.O. (1979) Adv. Cyc. Nuc. Res., *11*, 27-88.

Yamauchi, T. and Fujisawa, H. (1979a) J. Biol. Chem., *254*, 6408-6413.

Yamauchi, T. and Fujisawa, H. (1979b) Biochem. Biophys. Res. Commun., *90*, 28-35.

Yang, S.D., Vandenheede, J.R., Goris, J. and Merlevede, W. (1980) FEBS Lett., *111*, 201-204.

Yeaman, S.J. and Cohen, P. (1975) Eur. J. Biochem., *51*, 93-104.

Yeaman, S.J., Cohen, P., Watson, D.C. and Dixon, G.H. (1977) Biochem. J., *162*, 411-421.

## Questions

*Hahlbrock*

Calmodulin is involved in calcium storage in transport processes, does that also involve these interactions with ATP and cyclic AMP levels?

*Cohen*

You are referring to the effects of calmodulin on the calcium ATPases which are really the calcium pump of a number of cells. To my knowledge, there are no connections with cAMP at the present time in those systems although that does not rule out the possibility that these will be discovered.

*Critchley*

You are proposing that insulin somehow modifies the activity of Glycogen Synthase Kinase 3. If GSK 3 is located in the cytoplasmic compartment how do you envisage that the interaction of insulin with its cell surface receptor might modify the activity of the enzyme?

*Cohen*

We isolate as a soluble enzyme, that does not say anything of its distribution. The one thing one has to say is that concentration of insulin in the blood is $10^{-9}$ or $10^{-10}$ molar. This enzyme and other interconverting enzymes are at levels of $10^{-6}$ or $10^{-7}$ molar and therfore you are always looking for an amplification factor that would give that 100 to 1,000-fold amplification that one needs. Of course, this is where the second messengers like cAMP and calcium come in and so what one is looking for is some analogous regulator of the glycogen synthase kinase 3 enzyme. But I am afraid I cannot give you any more information that that.

*Lodish*

Could you comment on the possible role of any of the other phos phatases or protein kinases such as the *src* protein. Is there any possible interconversion here with - cyclic AMP?

*Cohen*

Well I suppose the only connection would really come when you start to talk not just about the *src* kinase which labels tyrosine residues but, of course, the epidermal growth factor system which when that interacts with its receptor, the receptor appears to be a protein kinase which also phosphorylates tyrosine residues. So this is, of course, in the membrane and that actually gives you an idea of how you could have an amplification without the need for a second messenger. So if EGF interacts with its receptor which is itself a protein kinase, and that activates it, you can go straight into a phosphory lation cascade without need of a second messenger. Of course, the effects of EGF on stimulating growth you might say were somewhat analogous to insulin's effects on protein synthesis and that perhaps somewhere in the system there is the phosphorylation of some tyrosine kinase that starts off a cascade. One alternative possibility for the model presented at the end is that the conversion of this inactive phosphatase to the activated phosphatase - the difference between them might be, for example, a tyrosine phosphorylation that started everything off. This is not impossible so I think it is something one obviously has to look for, that those tyrosine phosphorylating systems do somehow plug into these normal systems and in the case of *src* and other protein kinases they plug in an abnormal way and that the phosphorylation of certain target proteins is the cause of the transformed state.

*Crumpton*

Could I just expand that by saying that the indications from the latest work from Racker's laboratory would suggest that perhaps the point at which they have an effect is ATPase.

*Cohen*

Right. Ephraim Racker has shown that in the tumour cells -it has been known for a long time they have a low sodium, potassium ATPase activity, and that this now appears to be due to the phosphorylation of a tyrosine residue and I understand along the grape-vine that this is a rather complex system now in which they have four tyrosine kinases acting one on top of another in a cascade finally coming through to the modification of the Na+, K+ ATPases or membrane-bound tyrosine kinases. Although one should not get carried away with tyrosine kinases because only 0.03% of all phosphorylated amino acid in cells is phosphotyrosine and greater than 99% are serine or threonine. However, of course, when cells are transformed by any range of viruses, the phosphotyrosine content goes up five to ten-fold but that is still only up to levels of something like 0.2% of the total phosphorylated amino acid.

*Crumpton*
A number of people would subscribe to the view that EGF acts via the same potassium ATPase with an increase in sodium level so, in fact, one could tie the whole of that sort of system around that particular enzyme.

*Cohen*
Yes. What is known about the systems I have been describing is that there are multiple interactions and therefore it would not at all be surprising that these interconnecting reactions would also occur at the level of this different class of protein kinases.

*Hunt*
You raised an interesting point when you

mentioned 99% - how much of the phosphate in cells is actually of regulatory significance?

*Cohen*
This is a difficult question to answer in a short time. A lot of proteins that are household names have got phosphate attached to them, like fibrogen has two (three?) phosphoserines, ovalbumin has two phosphoserines, pepsin has a phosphoserine and these appear to be stable phosphoserines that do not turn over at all. Their role is not known, they may be involved in controlling turnover or secretion or they may have metal ion-binding properties 99.7% of the serine or threonines is a difficult one - O.K., I will guess a half.

*Willingham*
There was an interesting tie-in between Racker's reports about cAMP resistance and tyrosine sensitivity. Each of these kinases, has a second serine site on it which is phosphorylated by cAMP-dependent protein kinase and that inhibits the activity, but the tyrosine site activates the activity. The serine site seems to be dominant for both phosphorylated protein kinases.

*Cohen*
Well again this comes into the significance of these multi-site phosphorylations where one phosphorylation can either amplify or antagonise a second phosphorylation - that is quite right.

# Genetic and Biochemical Analysis of Regulation by Cyclic AMP

*Philip Coffino*

## Mutants and Cyclic AMP

Cells recognise certain molecules as regulatory. Some of these, including hormones, behave in the following ways: they have effects on multiple processes that are not necessarily directly related to each other biochemically and their structure gives no direct clues as to what these effects will be (Tomkins 1975). In general, several distinct steps intervene between the initial effects of these molecules and the biological results of their presence. Cyclic AMP (cAMP) is an example of such a signal molecule.

Much is known from biochemical studies about how cAMP acts. Most amine and peptide hormones work by binding to membrane associated receptors and thus stimulating the activity of adenyl cyclase in the membrane. This results in an increased rate of conversion of ATP to cyclic AMP and thereby to an increase in the intracellular level of the latter. The target molecule of cAMP is a kinase, a holoenzyme composed of catalytic (C) and regulatory (R) subunits; the latter bind cAMP (Kuo and Greengard 1969; Nimmo and Cohen 1977). In the presence of cAMP, catalytic subunits become dissociated from the holoenzyme, and are thus converted from an inactive to an active form. They phosphorylate specific protein substrates, commonly enzymes, whose biochemical properties are altered. The panoply of modifications results in a change in the biological properties of the cell.

This scheme has been substantiated by two approaches: purification and characterisation of the individual biochemical constituents and pharmacologic manipulation of whole cells or cell fractions. My laboratory has supplemented these with a third approach, somatic cell genetics. By studying cells with mutations that produce defects in specific components of this system, I have attempted to understand the nature and degree of complexity of the response.

The use of animal cell mutants to study regulation is not widespread. A respect for the technical problems associated with mutant isolation rather than a failure to appreciate their utility accounts for this. Isolation of cells genetically deficient in cAMP associated functions is greatly facilitated by exploiting a property of cultured mouse T cell lymphomas: cAMP causes them to commit suicide. This response is specific for cAMP and occurs regardless of whether the cells are made to generate and accumulate endogenous cAMP or are exposed to biologically active congeners such as dibutyryl cAMP (Bt₂cAMP) or 8-bromo cAMP.

In most of these studies I have used S49, a permanent line derived from a Balb/c mouse T cell lymphoma. These cells grow in suspension culture with a 17 hour generation time and also grow and form colonies in soft agar. Because cAMP specifically and efficiently kills these cells, it is straightforward to isolate a variety of resistant mutants, even when these are present at low incidence, by cloning large numbers of cells under selective conditions.

The series of events described above, triggered in S49 by hormone-receptor interaction, is illustrated in Figure 1. Also shown are the sites of alterations in different mutant classes. Their properties can be summarised as follows:

1) Receptor mutants, deficient in beta-adrenergic receptors (R). These cells have a quantitative deficiency (about 50% to 90% in independent clones) in the membrane receptors for one of the classes of hormones that activate cyclase in S49 (Johnson *et.al.* 1979).

2) Deficient or altered in a cyclase subunit (N). Some mutant cells lack a functional subunit that in wild-type cells mediates coupling of receptor-hormone (RH) interaction to adenyl cyclase (AC) activation. In other mutants, the subunit is present, but is functionally and structurally altered (Bourne *et.al.* 1975a; Johnson *et.al.* 1979).

3) Kinase mutants, deficient or altered in cAMP-dependent protein kinase. Some of these have structural changes in the R subunit. Others appear to have little or no functional kinase (Coffino *et.al.* 1975a; Bourne *et.al.* 1975b; Insel *et al.* 1975).

4) Deathless mutants, deficient in a function, not yet biochemically defined, required for cAMP-induced suicide (Lemaire *et.al.* 1975).

5) Transport mutants, with excess efficiency in cAMP transport. These mutants remove cAMP from cells more rapidly than do wild-type cells (Steinberg *et.al.* 1979).

6) Phosphodiesterase mutants. Excess activity of cAMP phosphodiesterase (PDE). These mutants degrade cAMP to 5′AMP more rapidly than do wild-type cells (Salomon and Bourne, in press).

I will here confine my discussion to the properties and uses of the kinase and deathless mutants. Receptor and cyclase mutants have been extensively exploited to elucidate the biochemical mechanisms of adenyl cyclase activation by beta-adrenergic hormones, notably in independent work from the laboratories of Dr H Bourne and Dr A Gilman. Recent reviews have described this work (Johnson *et.al.* 1980; Ross and Gilman 1980). The mutants with

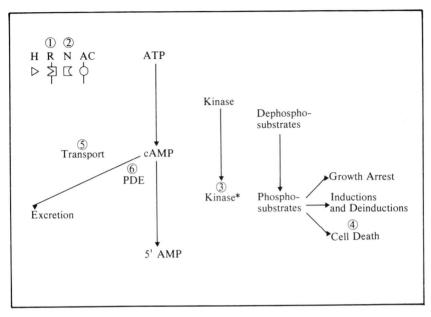

**Figure 1**
The sequence of cyclic AMP mediated events in S49 cells. The functions altered in different mutant cells are indicated by numbers that correspond to those used in the text. H, hormone; R,N and AC, respectively, receptor, coupling component and catalytic subunit of the membrane associated adenyl cyclase complex; PDE, cAMP phosphodiesterase; kinase and kinase*, inactive and active forms of cAMP dependent protein kinase.

alterations in cAMP transport and degradation have been little exploited, but may provide useful tools in investigating the metabolism of cAMP.

Mutants with altered kinase activity are isolated by cloning cells in medium containing Bt₂cAMP. They arise spontaneously at a rate of $2 \times 10^{-7}$ per cell per generation (Coffino *et.al.* 1975a); their frequency is greatly augmented by treating cultures with chemical mutagens (Friedrich and Coffino 1977). Analysis of cAMP-stimulated protein kinase activity in extracts from wild-type and mutant cells reveals that the mutants differ from wild-type and are heterogeneous (Figure 2). Three general mutant classes can be distinguished.

Type A have kinase with reduced apparent affinity for cAMP compared to that of wild-type cells. Independently selected mutants of this kind vary in the degree of alteration of the enzyme's sensitivity to cAMP; a five-to twenty-fold reduction in sensitivity is typical. In all cases examined, the defect results from a structural alteration in the R subunit in the kinase. This can be demonstrated by studying the kinetic properties of holoenzyme reconstituted from separated R and C subunits derived from wild type or mutant cells (Hochman *et.al.* 1977). In addition, analysis on two-dimensional gels, which fractionate proteins on the basis of charge as well as size, reveals that most Type A mutants contain R

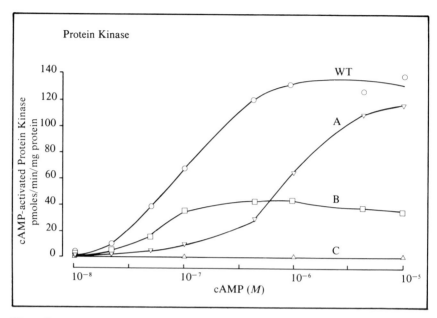

**Figure 2**

Cyclic AMP-stimulated phosphotransferase activity in extracts of wild-type and type A, B, and C kinase mutants of S49 cells. From Insel *et.al.*1975

subunits whose charge is altered, but whose molecular weight is not significantly changed (Steinberg *et. al.* 1977). Interestingly, mutant cells invariably contain R subunits of wild-type mobility as well. It is likely that wild-type cells are homozygous at a diploid locus coding for the R subunit. In a mutant, one locus has undergone a mutation that results in an amino acid substitution, or perhaps in a small carboxy-terminal deletion.

Type B cells have a kinase with apparently normal kinetic properties, but extracts express less activity than is found in wildtype cells, generally half or less. These mutants have not been extensively studied, but may be due to a structural mutation in one of two alleles coding for the R or C subunit.

Type C mutants have no detectable cAMP-stimulated kinase activity. This is the case when extracts are assayed *in vitro* using an exogenous substrate. It is true also of endogenous activity. In wild-type cells, phosphorylation of endogenous substrates can be demonstrated as follows (Steinberg and Coffino 1979). Cells are labelled with $^{35}$S-methionine in the presence or absence of Bt₂cAMP and the cell lysates analyzed on two-dimensional gels. Proteins whose phosphorylation is stimulated by addition of Bt₂cAMP become more acidic,and that change is seen as an alteration in their position of the protein in the gel. About sixteen proteins are seen to be modified in this way when wild-

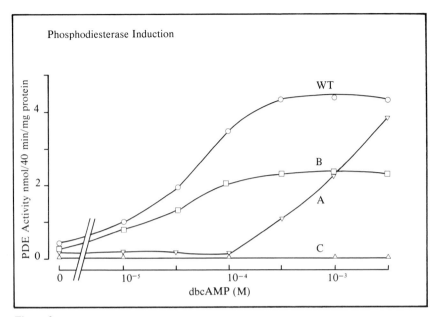

**Figure 3**
Induction of cAMP phosphodiesterase in wild-type and mutant S49 cells.   The cells are designated as in Figure 2.
  Cells were treated with the indicated concentrations of Bt₂cAMP and the cAMP phosphodiesterase activity of cell lysates determined. From Insel *et.al.*1975.

type cells are treated with Bt₂cAMP.  No changes are seen in response to that treatment in Type C mutants.

  The genetic change that results in Type C mutants is not clear. The mutation is trans-dominant: hybrid tetraploid cels formed by fusing wild-type cells with mutant cells of this type also express no detectable cAMP-dependent kinase activity (Steinberg *et.al.*1978). This is not due to the presence of a soluble inhibitor, for lysates from mutant and wild-type cells mixed in various proportions show strict additivity of activity. It is likely that a genetic change in a regulatory gene, one coding for neither the R nor C subunit, causes this phenotype.

  The availability of these different mutant cells makes it possible to design critical experiments testing the function of cAMP-dependent kinase in the biological responses of a cell to cAMP. If kinase plays a central role, the responses of the different types of mutants to cAMP should be altered in different and characteristic ways. This is the case (Insel *et.al.*1975). Among the responses of S49 cells to cAMP is induction of the enzyme cAMP phosphodiesterase. Figure 3 shows the effect of different concentrations of Bt₂cAMP on the induction of that enzyme in wild-type S49 cells and in the same three mutant clones whose kinase activities were previously depicted in

Figure 2. Comparison of Figures 2 and 3 reveals that in each case the response of kinase to cAMP in cell lysates correlates well with the induction of phosphodiesterase by Bt₂cAMP in the whole cell. Sensitivity is reduced in Type A, response is attenuated in Type B, and response is abolished in Type C. These same characteristic changes in the dose-dependent response to Bt₂cAMP holds regardless of which biological change is examined in S49 cells. These include cell killing, growth arrest, and extinction of the activities of ornithine decarboxylase and S-adenosylmethionine decarboxylase (Insel *et.al.* 1975; Insel and Fenno 1978).

Some general conclusions can be made. Perhaps most surprising is that cAMP's regulatory function is not essential for cell life. S49 cells deficient in adenyl cyclase or in cAMP dependent kinase or even in both enzymes, for mutants with the double defect can be selected, are not readily distinguishable from wild-type cells in morphology or growth. Mutants with altered or deficient cAMP-dependent kinase have now been described in a variety of cell lines (Schimmer *et.al.* 1977; Evain *et.al.* 1979; Rosen *et.al.* 1979), suggesting that cAMP-mediated control is generally gratuitous in animal cells. The analogy with *E coli* mutants with defects of cyclase or of CRP protein, the bacteria's cAMP receptor, is striking (Pastan and Perlman 1972). Both S49 cells and *E coli* survive the ablation of cAMP mediated regulation, despite the loss of some adaptive regulation.

All measured responses to cAMP are similarly affected by genetic changes in kinase. All responses, including those detected using two-dimensional gels, occur in wild-type cells regardless of the source of cAMP, whether presented as an exogenous analog or generated endogenously. This implies that active kinase is the central parameter relevant to the activity of the system. Lastly, in S49 cells, the amount of kinase present is rate-limiting for the response, because Type B mutants having a two-fold quantitative deficiency of enzyme show sub-optimal effects compared to wild-type cells.

The response of a cell to cAMP may be described as a one parameter control system, with active protein kinase as the relevant parameter. For a given cell, inputs at the level of hormone receptors may be multiple and outputs in the form of biochemical effects are invariably so, but these complexities are individual properties of particular cells. This view (Langan 1973), supported by the work presented here, provides a reassuring sense of simplicity when confronting a literature that describes scores of stimuli that change cAMP and hundreds of effects produced by that molecule. It must, however, be qualified as follows.

Regulation by cAMP does not occur in isolation; it is interactive with other control systems, eg. kinase inhibitors, phosphatases, and multiple calcium-responsive enzymes (Ashby and Walsh 1972; Cohen *et. al.* 1978). The temporal pattern of kinase stimulation may be significant. The differential biological role of iso-enzymes of cAMP-dependent kinase is poorly under-

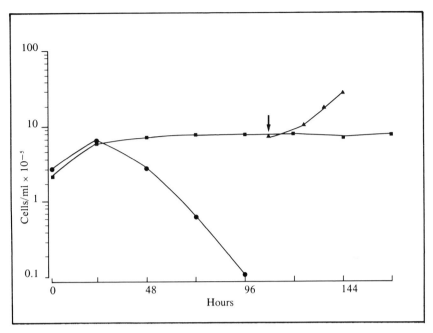

**Figure 4**
Effect of Bt₂cAMP on S49 cell growth. Wild type ( ● ) and deathless  ( ■ ) S49 cell cultures were
treated with Bt₂cAmp 1.0mM and the cell concentration sequentially determined thereafter. At
the indicated time ( arrow ) Bt₂cAmp was removed from an aliquot of the deathless culture ( ▲ ).

stood. The R subunit of protein kinase may have significant interactions with
macromolecules other than the C subunit.

## Growth Regulation and Cyclic AMP

One consequence of protein kinase activation in S49 cells is inhibition of cell
growth (Coffino et.al. 1975b). The biochemical mechanisms that cells use to
regulate their rate of growth are poorly understood. Because at least the initial
events in cAMP's action are known, it seemed reasonable to explore this
phenomenon in S49 to determine the nature of the growth inhibition, and
ultimately its mechanism.

Figure 4 shows the effect of Bt₂cAMP on S49 cell growth. There is a period of
somewhat less than a day before proliferation stops, followed by a fall in cell
number over the next several days as killing takes place. The killing facilitates
isolation of mutants, but complicates the analysis of growth inhibition per se.
The deathless (D-) mutant was isolated to solve this problem (Lemaire and
Coffino 1977). It is not killed by cAMP, but its other  responses remain
unaffected. The protein kinase of D- is like that of wild-type S49 cells.

The proliferation cycle of animal cells is divisible into four periods. One of

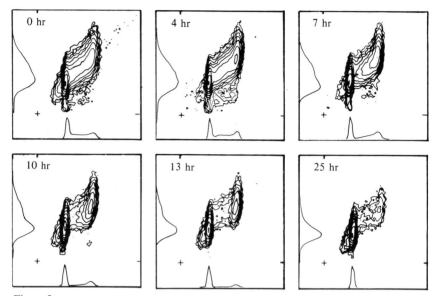

**Figure 5**
Effect of Bt$_2$cAMP on the relationship between cell size and DNA content. S49 cAMP deathless cells growing exponentially at a concentration of 0.5 x 10 6 ml were treated with 1 mM Bt$_2$cAMP, and samples were removed at the indicated times for dual mode analysis. The density distribution of cells is represented as a series of contour lines on a coordinate system that represents fluorescence per cell (as a measure of DNA content) on the abscissa and 90 light scattering per cell (as a measure of size) on the ordinate. The distribution of cell number as a function of fluorescence alone or of light scattering alone is projected on the appropriate axis. At each time point the G 1 cells are responsible for the most prominent feature of the density map.

these, mitosis (M), is distinguishable morphologically. The period of DNA synthesis (S) was originally observed as the discrete phase of the cycle during which radioactive precursors to DNA are incorporated. There is a gap period (G$_1$) free of DNA synthesis preceding S and a second gap period (G$_2$) that follows S. A convenient way to monitor progression of a cell population through the cycle and to observe perturbations in that progression is flow cytometry (Gray and Coffino 1979; Gray *et.al.* 1979). This can be used to measure DNA content per cell. On an arbitrary scale G$_1$ cells have 1 unit or DNA, G$_2$ or M cells 2 units, and S phase cells between 1 and 2 units. By flow cytometry one finds that the 17 hours generation time of S49 cells in exponential growth is composed of G$_1$, S, and G$_2$ + M periods having modal durations of 1, 12, and 3 hours respectively.

Flow cytometry can be used to obtain, simultaneously, information on the size as well as DNA content of each cell in a population (Gray and Coffino 1979). S49 cells in exponential growth were examined using this dual analysis mode at various times after treatment with Bt$_2$cAMP (Coffino and Gray 1978;

Figure 5). The data is displayed as a topographic density map in a coordinate system whose axes represent DNA content per cell (horizontal) and cell size (vertical).

Cells in exponential growth (O time) have about 30% of their population in $G_1$ these are the smallest class of cells. After addition of $Bt_2cAMP$, there is a progressive depletion, first of the early S phase cells and eventually of the $G_2$ and M cells. The result is a population of cells about 90% of which are arrested in $G_1$.

These data support the following conclusions. Cyclic AMP produces a block in cell cycle progression whose onset is rapid and which drastically slows progression through $G_1$. The block is not absolute. Under steady-state conditions of maximally effective $Bt_2cAMP$ treatment, the $G_1$ population never reaches 100% and those cells that do escape the block progress through the remainder of the cycle. The size of arrested $G_1$ cells is the same as that of exponentially growing $G_1$ cells, as can be seen by superimposing the density distributions for the first and last time points of Figure 5. Cyclic AMP does not, therefore, dissociate the DNA replicative cycle from the growth cycle that achieves, on average, the net doubling once per division of other cellular constituents. Rather, it slows both cycles coordinately.

Related experiments show that the arrested cells re-enter the cycle when $Bt_2cAMP$ is removed. The kinetics of emergence from $G_1$ are the same, regardless of the duration of the arrest (Coffino and Gray submitted for publication). Growth arrest is therefore $G_1$ specific, probabilistic rather than absolute, coordinate with respect to growth and replication, and reversible. These characteristics together suggest that in S49 cells cAMP regulates growth by triggering a coordinated endogenous physiologic change.

## Proteins and Growth Regulation

Because the pre-eminent effect of cAMP on cell growth is arrest in $G_1$, I sought next to determine whether there were biochemical correlates of that event specific to $G_1$ cells. Populations of exponentially growing cells were fractionated according to size to yield rather pure populations of cycling $G_1$ cells and less pure populations of cells in early or late S. Each of these populations was treated as described above to determine what proteins were present and which were phosphorylated in a cAMP-dependent manner. Cells were incubated with $^{35}$S-methionine in the presence or absence of $Bt_2cAMP$ and the labelled proteins analysed on two-dimensional gels. The results were not encouraging. There was little significant difference in pattern that depended in cell cycle position (Coffino and Groppi, in press). This was true both for the rate of synthesis of about 800 proteins seen when cells were labelled without $Bt_2cAMP$ and for the small group of proteins, previously examined in unsynchronised cells, whose mobility is modified by the addition of Bt₂cAMP. The cells do not seem to make or modify protein in a manner dependent on cell cycle position.

A naive approach had thus produced a genuine but distinctly negative result. To bolster this finding, it seemed important to show, as a positive control, that events known to depend on cell cycle position could be reproduced in synchronised S49 cells. Histone synthesis was chosen for that purpose, because an extensive literature documented the finding that histone synthesis was confined to S phase (Borun 1975).

Histones are among the most basic proteins and therefore are not visualised in the two-dimensional gel system used in the studies described above, which best resolves proteins whose isoelectric points lie between 5 and 7.5. However, a different two-dimensional gel system, one designed for the resolutiion of basic proteins, had been recently developed and shown capable of visualising the histones present in whole cell lysates (O'Farrell *et.al.*1977; Sanders *et.al.*1980). Again cells were synchronised, labelled, and analysed on this gel system.

The result was surprising. The rates of H₁ and nucleosomal histone synthesis did not differ in G₁ and S phase S49 cells (Groppi and Coffino 1980). Analysis of histone synthesis in Chinese hamster ovary cells produced the same result, despite the fact that previous studies on these cells had found histones to be made only in S phase (Gurley *et.al.*1972). Subcellular fractionation revealed the basis of the discrepancy. In S phase cells, histones were found in the nuclear fraction within minutes after their synthesis in the cytoplasm. Under the same experimental conditions, the histones made in G₁ cells were found in the cytoplasmic fraction. In the past, the preferred methods of analysis of histones began with the isolation of nuclei or nuclear fractions. It is reasonable to infer that in many cases synthesis of histones in G₁ was not recognised because the cell fraction containing them was discarded. Because the two dimensional gels have sufficient resolution, it was possible instead to discard nothing and to analyse whole cell lysates.

## Anticipations

Genetics and biochemistry provide complementary approaches to the understanding of biological questions. The application of genetics to the study of complex regulation in animal cells has been limited. It has largely depended on fortuitous circumstances, such as the availability of patients with genetic diseases or the existence of a readily selectable phenotype in mutant cells. This situation has begun to change. We can expect that it will soon be possible to isolate any gene, modify it at will, replace it in a cell and ask how it then behaves. We will, in a few years, be in a position to assess just how primitive is our present understanding of biology. The prospect is both intimidating and exciting.

## References

Ashby Cd. Walsh, DA. *Characterisation of the interaction of a protein inhibitor with adenosine 3', 5'-monophosphate protein kinases,* J Biol Chem *247,* 6637-6642, 1972.

Borun, T.W. *Histones, differentiation, and the cell cycle. IN Results and Problems in Cell Differentiation* (J. Reinert, H. Holtzer, eds). New York, Springer Verlag, 1975, pp 249-290.

Bourne, H.R., Coffino, P., Tomkins, G.M. *Selection of variant lymphoma cell deficient in adenyl cyclase.* Science, *187,* 750-752, 1975a.

Bourne, H.R., Coffino, L.P., Tomkins, G.M. *Somatic genetic analysis of cyclic AMP action: Characterization of unresponsive mutants.* J. Cell Physiol. *85,* 611-620, 1975b.

Coffino, P., Bourne, H.R., Tomkins, G.M. *Somatic genetic analysis of cyclic AMP action: Selection of unresponsive mutants.* J. Cell Physiol. *85,* 603-610, 1975a.

Coffino, P., Gray, J.W. *Regulation of S49 lymphoma cell growth by cyclic AMP.* Cancer Res., *38,* 4285-4288, 1978.

Coffino, P., Gray, J.W., Tomkins, G.M. *Cyclic AMP, a nonessential regulator of the cell cycle.* Proc. Nat. Acad. Sci. USA. *72,* 878-882, 1975b.

Cohen, P., Nimmo, G.A., Burchell, A., Antoniw, J.F. *The substrate specificity and regulation of the protein phosphatases involved in the control of glycogen metabolism in mammalian skeletal muscle. IN advances of Enzyme Regulation, V 16* (G. Weber, ed). Pergamon Press, New York, 1978, pp 97-119.

Evain, D. Gottesman, M., Pastan, I., Anderson, W.B. *A mutation affecting the catalytic subunit of cyclic AMP-dependent protein kinase in CHO cells.* J. Biol. Chem. *254,* 6931-6937, 1979.

Friedrich, U., Coffino, P. *Mutagenesis in S49 mouse lymphoma cells: Induction of resistance to ouabain, 6-thioguanine, and dibutyryl cyclic AMP.* Proc. Nat. Acad. Sci. USA. *74,* 679-683, 1977.

Gray, J.W., Coffino, P. *Cell cycle analysis by flow cytometry. IN Methods in Enzymology* (W.B. Jakoby, I.H. Pastan, eds). Academic Press, New York, 1979, pp 233-248.

Gray, J.W., Dean, P.N., Mendelsohn, M.L. *Quantitative cell-cycle analysis. IN Flow Cytometry and Sorting* (M.R. Melamed, P.P. Mullaney, M.L. Mendelsohn, eds) Wiley, New York, 1979, pp 383-407.

Groppi, V., Coffino, P. *G₁ and S-phase mammalian cells synthesise histones at equivalent rates.* Cell, *21,* 195-204, 1980.

Gurley, L.R., Walters, R.A., Tobey, R.A. *The metabolism of histone fractions: IV. Synthesis of histone during the G₁ phase.* Arch. Biochem. Biophys. *148,* 633-644, 1972.

Hochman, J., Bourne, H.R., Coffino, P., Insel, P.A. Krasny, L., Melmon, K.L. *Subunit interaction in cyclic AMP-dependent protein kinase of mouse lymphoma cells.* Proc. Nat. Acad. Sci. USA, *74,* 1167-11771, 1977.

Insel, P.A., Bourne, H.R., Coffino, P., Tomkins, G.M. *Cyclic AMP-dependent protein kinase: Pivotal role in regulation of enzyme induction and growth.* Science, *190,* 896-898, 1975.

Insel, P.A., Fenno, J. *Cyclic AMP-dependent protein kinase mediates a cyclic AMP-stimulated decrease in ornithine and S-adenosyl-methionine decarboxylase activities.* Proc. Nat. Acad. Sci. USA, 75, 862-865, 1978.

Johnson, G.L., Bourne, H.R., Gleason, M.K., Coffino, P., Insel, P.A., Melmon, K.L. *Isolation and characterisation of S49 lymphoma cells deficient in beta-adrenergic receptors. Relation of receptor number to activation of adenylate cyclase.* Molec. Pharmacol. *15,* 16-27, 1979.

Johnson, G.L., Kaslow, H.R., Farfel, Z., Bourne, H.R. *Genetic analysis of hormone-sensitive adenylate cyclase.* Adv. in Cyclic Nucleotide Res. *13,* 1-37, 1980.

Kuo, J.F., Greengard, P. *Cyclic nucleotide protein kinases. IV. Widespread occurrence of adenosine 3':5' monophosphate dependent protein kinase in various tissues and phyla of the animal kingdom.* Proc. Nat. Acad. Sci. USA. *64,* 1349-1355, 1969.

Langan, T.A. *Protein kinases and protein kinase substrates. IN Advances in Cyclic Nucleotide Research, V1.* (P. Greengard, G.AM Robison, eds). Raven Press, New York, 1973, pp 99-153.

Lemaire, I., Coffino, P. *Cyclic AMP-induced cytolysis in S49 cells: selection of an unresponsive 'deathless' mutant.* Cell, *11*, 149-155, 1977.

Nimmo, H.G., Cohen, P. *Hormonal control of protein phosphorylation. IN: Advances in Cyclic Nucleotide Research, V8* (P. Greengard and G.A. Robison, eds). Raven Press, New York, 1977, pp 145-266.

O'Farrell, P.Z., Goodman, H.M., O'Farrell, P.H. *High resolution two- dimensional electrophoresis of basic as well as acidic proteins.* Cell, *12*, 1133-1142, 1977.

Pastan, I., Perlman, R.L. *Regulation of gene transcription in Escherichia coli by cyclic AMP. IN Advances in Cyclic Nucleotide Research, V1,* (P. Greengard, R. Paoletti, G.A. Robison, eds). Raven Press, New York, 1972, pp 11-16.

Rosen, N., Piscitello, J., Schneck, J., Muschel, R., Bloom, B.R., Rosen, O.M. *Properties of protein kinase and adenylate cyclase-deficient varients of a macrophage-like cell line.* J. Cell Physiol. *98*, 125-136, 1979.

Ross, E.M., Gilman, A.G. *Hormone sensitive adenylate cyclase.* Ann. Rev. Biochem. *49*, 533, 1980.

Salomon, M.R., Bourne, H.R. *Novel S49 lymphoma variants with aberrant cyclic AMP metabolism.* Mol. Pharm. in press.

Sanders, M.M., Groppi, V.E., Browning, E.T. *Resolution of basic cellular proteins including histone variants by two-dimensional gel electro-phoresis:* Analytic Biochem. *103*, 157-165, 1980.

Schimmer, B.P., Tsao, J., Knapp, M. *Isolation of mutant adrenocortical tumour cells resistant to cyclic nucleotides.* Molec and Cell Endocrinol,: 135-145, 1977.

Steinberg, R.A., Coffino, P. *Two-dimensional gel analysis of cyclic AMP effects in cultured S49 mouse lymphoma cells: protein modifications, inductions, and repressions.* Cell, *18*, 719-733, 1979.

Steinberg, R.A., van Daalen Wetters, T., Coffino, P. *Kinase-negative mutants of S49 mouse lymphoma cells carry a trans-dominant mutation affecting expression of cAMP-dependent protein kinase.* Cell, *15*, 1351-1361, 1978.

Steinberg, R.A., O'Farrell, P.H., Friedrich, U., Coffino, P. *Mutations causing charge alterations in regulatory subunits of the cyclic AMP-dependent protein kinase of cultured S49 mouse lymphoma cells.* Cell, *10*, 381-391, 1977.

Steinberg, R.A., Steinberg, M.G., van Daalen Wetters, T. *A varient of S49 mouse lymphoma cells with enhanced secretion of cyclic AMP.* J. Cell Phsiol. *100*, 579-588, 1979.

Tomkins, G.M. *The metabolic code.* Science, *189*, 760-763, 1975.

## Questions

*Yoeman*

It is interesting that when you release the cells they do not come out synchronously, they come out slowly - does this suggest that they actually lengthen the $G_1$ period and that the cells are actually moving very slowly and continuously through $G_1$?

*Coffino*

Yes. I think the data under steady-state conditions before cAMP, is consistent with that. By putting in a secondary block, using colcemid for instance, it allows quantitation of the accumulation in mitosis. One can show that the cells which have come out of the block are continuing to cycle. There are several components to the kinetics when dibutyryl cyclic AMP is removed - there is a delay during which nothing happens in terms of $G_1$ exit. Following this delay there is an emergence with kinetics quite different from that of exponentially-growing cells. It is not until the cells have completed successfully one cycle that they resume kinetic characteristics of exponential growth. There appear to be 3 stages, then, to the process: one is a delay in which one sees no emergence, the second in which the emergence is characterised by kinetics different from those seen in exponential growth and there is a third which requires a cycle to occur in which kinetics become restored.

*Questioner*

You have measured the lenght of $G_1$?

*Coffino*

We have measured the lenght of $G_1$ using a synchronised cell populations aid flow microfluorimetry and we find that in exponential growth that the $G_1$-exit kinetics are characterised by a half-life of about 1½ hours.

*Wolpert*

What happens if you mix your cells with other cells. I would be curious to know if they form gap junctions with the other cells.

*Coffino*

Yes, these are suspension cultures; they are non-adherent cells so I doubt very much that they would form gap junctions. I think that offers some interesting advantages as well as some disadvantages. The cells are essentially monads, they do not speak to each other and so one is asking questions about what happens to a single cell. Of course one cannot ask about interactions but it does give a simpler system to work with.

*Pardee*

The appearance of histones in $G_1$ in the cytoplasm and then their appearance in the nucleus in S is very reminiscent of results we have obtained with about 8 enzymes that are involved in DNA metabolism. These are also found synthesised in $G_1$ in the cytoplasm and in the nucleus in S phase so it sounds like there is a similar movement to the one you describe for histones. On the other hand we have over the years done some experiments looking for histone synthesis in the cell cycle and I do not remember which cells they were (either CHO or 3T3, back in 1970) but we looked for histones that bind to a DNA column in the total cell extract and did not find any histones or proteins that bind to DNA until S phase - none in $G_1$. Secondly, taking 3T3 cells out of $G_0$, looking both in the cytoplasm and in the nucleus for histone, the peak didn't appear until S phase, so there is a discrepancy that I do not really understand.

*Coffino*

Yes, I will comment on what I take to be a two-part question. I agree that there may be some similarities with respect to cytoplasmic to nuclear transport. I do not know either the kinetics or the mechanism with respect to histone transport in the cells we have worked with. If the mechanism that you are suggesting is one that triggers DNA synthesis then one has to presume that migration would precede the onset of DNA synthesis. If I had to make a guess at why histones position differently in $G_1$ and S phase, my guess would be that in S phase there is naked DNA that is being synthesised and that is acting as a kind of affinity sink for histones. If that is the case, then DNA synthesis would be a pre-requisite for the change in the positioning rather than an event that follows it. With respect to the experiments that you have done on histone synthesis in the cell cycle: without knowing that work in detail I cannot really comment on it but I think that one of the problems in working with histones is that they are slippery, elusive, sticky beasts. If one starts doing fractionation, one may miss them and this has certainly been shown in yeasts and probably in other contexts as well. So, I think it is important to check results against a system in which one throws away as little as possible and it is that that this two-dimensional gel system can do for you.

*Lodish*
A related question concerning the way in which you fractionate the cells to give you a population of what you call $G_1$. Do you really know that these cells are *not* synthesising DNA?

*Coffino*
Yes, we know that by doing thymidine labelling. Essentially, we have taken an exponentially-growing population and label it simultaneously with thymidine and $S^{35}$ methionine using different labels and then we sorted the cells by DNA content and asked how much of each label was in each fraction with respect to DNA content and the result was as you would expect. The cells that were in $G_1$ by other criteria did not incorporate thymidine; if one looked at amino acid synthesis then there is a smooth gradient - the cells made protein in proportion to their size. This bears upon a potential artefact that we are

worried about, namely that there might be a great burst of protein synthesis in early S phase that could account by virtue of a very tiny contamination of early S phase in the $G_1$ population for the apparent inequality of the rate of histone synthesis, but that was not the case. The protein synthesis is a smooth function of DNA content per cell.

*Bradbury*
Can you comment on the state of acetylation of histones in $G_1$ compared to S?

*Coffino*
I am afraid I cannot because this gel system is not one that resolves such charge changes very well, so we do not know much about phosphorylation or acetylation.

*Hahlbrock*
We have used cultured plant cells and their growth and division is retarded under UV light and with respect to your sink hypothesis, histone synthesis is also retarded, not completely inhibited but reduced 50% or so and histone messenger RNA activity *in vitro* is reduced to the same extent within a few hours of irradiation of these cells. So the sink cannot, in this system, be the only explanation.

*Coffino*
I think it is important to point out that all of the experiments we have done have been done with exponentially growing cells. I do not mean to suggest that if a cell were arrested in $G_1$ or A phase or whatever terminology you prefer that it would behave similarly to a cycling $G_1$ cell, nor do I mean to imply necessarily that all $G_1$ cells will make histones at a great rate. The two cells with which we are dealing here have relatively short $G_1$ periods - of the order of 2 hours - and it may be that cells that have a longer $G_1$ would have different properties. So we are planning to look at He La cells and a variety of other cells as well.

*Questioner*
Have you tried gene complementation analysis of your protein kinase mutant?

*Coffino*
Yes. We have made hybrids between a variety of these mutants. The finding with the mutants that are completely deficient in cAMP dependent protein kinase is that this mutation is fully dominant. That is, if one makes a hybrid between a wild-type cell and a kinase-deficient mutant, the resultant mutant is as kinase- deficient as the apparent mutant cell. This is one of our bases for inferring that the mutation is a regulatory one.

*Questioner*
What happens if you use your deathless mutants - treat them with dbcAMP and look for $H_1$ synthesis. Then you can keep them in $G_1$, or whatever it is, for a long time?

*Coffino*
Preliminary experiments suggest that the effect of dbcAMP treatment on protein synthesis is to greatly reduce the rate of protein synthesis but not to greatly alter the pattern that one sees using either the equilibrium gels or the gels for basic proteins. I think we will have to do some more work before I am really sure of all that. It does seem to be the case that protein synthesis may be a critical factor in the growth arrest. Once again, preliminary experiments with synchronised populations suggest that the inhibition of protein synthesis, insofar as one can infer that from a reduction in incorporation of amino acids, that the event is specific for $G_1$. Cells in $G_1$ are sensitive to inhibition of protein synthesis; cells in other phases of the cycle are not.

*Garcia-Bellido*
You have heard about the work in *Drosophila* where you remove the gene for phosphodiesterase and not only do the cells live but they fly.

*Coffino*
Yes, but they are stupid aren't they?

# 5
# Differentiation versus Proliferation

An important strategy in development is to divide or to differentiate at the right place, at the right time and this is a theme explored in the present section.

Taking the formation of blood cells as his model, Dr Metcalf evaluates possible roles of glycoprotein regulator molecules in directing multipotential stem cells towards a particular differentiation pathway. The decision as to whether to continue growth or go into the differentiation pathway occurs in the post mitotic phase and Dr Pardee has been eminent in evaluating ideas concerning the role of the decision point in cell cycle control. In the present paper, however, the central argument put forward by Pardee & Sager is that the de-regulated differentiation of tumours is due to cells undergoing genomic re-arrangements.

This finds parallels in Dr Natalie Teich's work who like Dr Metcalf, uses an *in vitro* haemopoietic system for studying differentiation with the exception that RNA tumour viruses (retroviruses) are employed here to affect differentiation and proliferation. It is known that incorporation of viral RNA (as a reverse copy) into the host genome produces a variety of neoplastic states and this serves to emphasise the relationship between the organisation of DNA and its function. Indeed, in the field in general there is great interest in the possibility that controlled re-arrangements ('jumping') of genes may be a feature of normal development.

# Control of Granulocyte-Macrophage Differentiation by the Glycoprotein GM-CSF

*Donald Metcalf*

## Introduction

*Haemopoiesis*

Haemopoiesis (blood cell formation) presents a fascinating opportunity for analysis of the mechanisms controlling cell proliferation and differentiation, not only because dispersed viable cells are readily accessible for analysis but because haemopoiesis occurs continuously throughout foetal and adult life.

Haemopoiesis is initiated by a population of multipotential haemopoietic stem cells that arises in the yolk sac, then migrates to the foetal liver. Populations of differentiating haemopoietic cells subsequently develop in the liver and later in the spleen and bone marrow. Following birth, haemopoiesis continues throughout life in the marrow and to a lesser degree in the spleen. These events have been described in full elsewhere (Metcalf and Morre 1971).

This haemopoiesis is sustained entirely by the extended capacity for self-replication of the initial stem cells and their capacity also to generate more differentiated progenitor cells that are the specific committed precursor cells for the various differentiated haemopoietic families the erythroid, granulocytic, macrophage, eosinophil, megakaryocyte and lymphoid populations. The remarkable feature of this massive daily haemopoiesis is the fact that at no stage following the initial events in the yolk sac are new haemopoietic stem cells generated from cells of some other type. This curious biology of haemopoietic stem cells is shared by two other stem cell populations the primordial germ cells and primordial melanoblasts. All three populations arise outside the body and, after a brief interval, migrate into the embryo proper. It seems likely that the initial residence outside the body may protect these stem cells from differentiation events occurring within the embryo early in development but this has yet to be investigated.

Because fully differentiated haemopoietic cells exhibit highly characteristic nuclear and cytoplasmic structures, simple morphological studies performed early in this century on the more mature haemopoietic populations were able to delineate the final sequential maturation steps within the various haemopoietic families. In more recent years this descriptive work has been supplemented by kinetic studies using tritiated thymidine and by studies on specialised biochemical components and membrane markers in such populations.

However it has only been in the past 15 years that techniques have become available that have permitted the earliest cellular events in haemopoiesis to be analysed with precision and use of these techniques has led to the identifi cation and characterisation of a family of specific regulatory factors controlling haemopoietic cell proliferation and differentiation. These recent advances have depended almost entirely on the introduction of semi-solid culture techniques that support the clonal proliferation and differentiation of individual stem and progenitor cells. The first of these techniques permitted the clonal proliferation of neutrophilic granulocytes and/or macrophage progenitors (granulocyte-macrophage colony-forming cells or GM-CFC) (Bradley and Metcalf 1966; Ichikawa et. al. 1966) but comparable cloning techniques subsequently have been developed for all other haemopoietic progenitor and stem cells (see review Metcalf 1977).

The present discussion will concern some aspects of the control of granulocyte-macrophage (GM) populations and some of the general principles raised by these studies that are likely to apply to other haemopoietic populations and may well apply to other cell populations within the body. In restricting discussion to the control of GM populations, it should be emphasised that comparable specific glycoprotein regulators exist for each distinct haemopoietic family e.g. erythroid, eosinophil, megakaryocytic and that essentially the same phenomena are demonstrable in each system.

## Proliferation and Differentiation

In the mouse bone marrow, approximately 1 cell in 400 is a progenitor cell apparently committed irreversibly to the formation of granulocyte and/or macrophage progeny. Such GM-CFC have been shown to be the progeny of multipotential haemopoietic stem cells (CFU-S), to have essentially no capacity for genuine self-replication, to be unable to become progenitor cells of any other cell lineage or to revert to multipotential, self-replicative, CFU-S. In the normal adult marrow, GM-CFC are in active cell cycle and thus represent a transitional population of cells, continually being generated by CFU-S and continually being expended by generating more differentiated G and M progeny. These relationships are indicated diagrammatically in Figure 1. The transition CFU-S - GM-CFC may possibly be achieved by a single commitment event, with or without an accompanying cell division, but it is more likely to involve a progressive sequence both of differentiative and proliferative events since there is evidence that the CFU-S compartment is itself stratified at least on the basis of previous mitotic history (Rosendaal et.al. 1979).

Each GM-CFC can generate up to 10,000 granulocytic or macrophage end

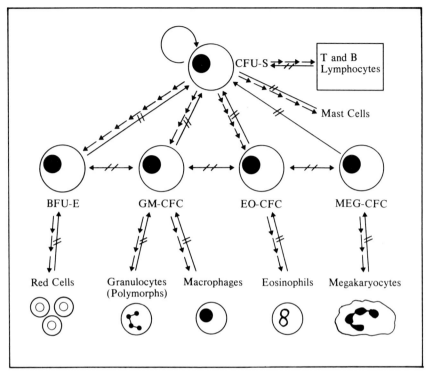

**Figure 1**
Schematic diagram of the early events in the production of blood cells. Multipotential haemopoietic stem cells (CFU-S) are capable both of self-replication and the generation of a variety of specific progenitor cells by a sequence of proliferative and differentiative events. Progenitor cells cannot dedifferentiate or transform to other progenitors but are able to generate clones of maturing progeny cells, the most mature of which appear in the blood. Note that many granulocyte-macrophage progenitors (GM-CFC) are bipotential and able to form both granulocytes and macrophages.

cell progency and this process also necessitates a sequence of differentiative and proliferative events. It is important to emphasise that considerable flexibility exists in the system with respect to the final number of progeny produced, their type and the time lag required for differentiation to mature end cells.

Pure populations of haemopoietic progenitor cells have now been obtained from mouse marrow and foetal liver using separative procedures combining density separation and separation using the fluorescence-activated cell sorter with fluorescein-conjugated pokeweed mitogen and rhodamine-conjugated antineutrophil/monocyte serum (Nicola *et.al.* 1980; Nicola, NA, Burgess, AW and Metcalf, D, unpublished data). These cells have the morphology of undifferentiated blast cells, 11-13 $\mu$m in diameter, with basophilic cytoplasm

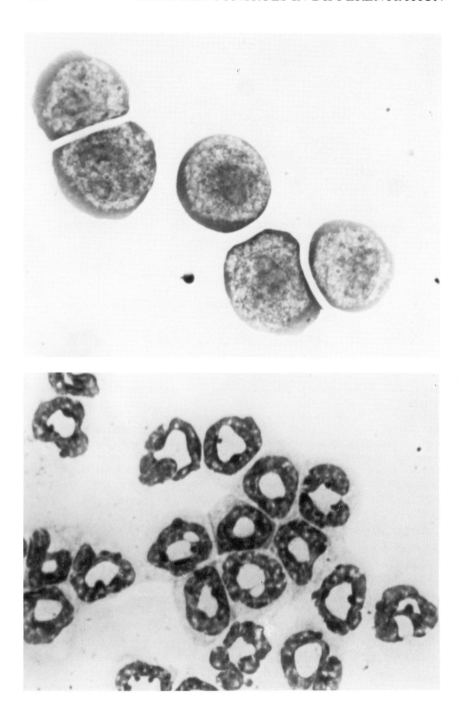

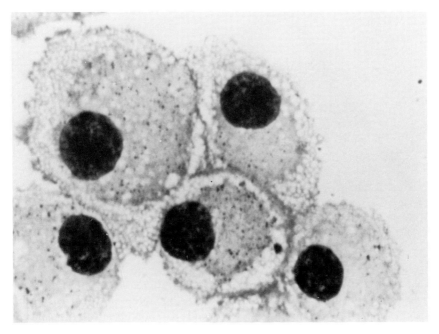

**Figure 2**
Progenitor cells purified from mouse foetal liver populations by density separation and fluorescence-activated cell sorting
Top left: and the mature cell ends, granulocytes (polymorphs)
Bottom left: and macrophages
Above: generated *in vitro* by purified progenitor cells after stimulation by GM-CSF

but no cytoplasmic granules and a somewhat variable size due to their active cell cycle status (Figure 2). However these separative procedures co-purify the progenitor cells of all haemopoietic families and a pure population consisting solely of GM-CFC has yet to be achieved. CFU-S have been purified from rat bone marrow using somewhat similar techniques (Goldschneider *et.al.* 1980) and have essentially the same morphology as that of progenitor cells although they are slightly smaller in size. From this it can be concluded that the critical differentiative events involved in the commitment step from CFU-S to GM-CFC are not associated with any distinctive changes in morphology.

   While GM-CFC have yet to be obtained in pure form, it is relatively simple to analyse the proliferation and differentiation of individual GM-CFC using culture of unfractionated marrow cells because of one important general property of semi-solid cultures. In the absence of a specific stimulating factor, no proliferation is possible and few progenitor cells can even survive for more

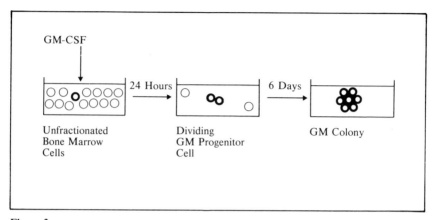

**Figure 3**
When mouse bone marrow cells are cultured in agar-medium in the presence of GM-CSF, granulocyte-macrophage progenitor cells selectively survive and proliferate to form colonies of mature granulocytes and/or macrophages.

than 24 hours. For this reason, in marrow cultures containing only the regulator for GM proliferation (GM-CSF), the only proliferating cells present are those that will subsequently progress to form granulocytic and/or macrophage colonies (Figure 3). Such cultures after 24 hours of incubation are remarkably free of all the other cells initially present in the culture and permit a wide range of micromanipulative procedures to be performed on GM-CFC and their progeny even though such cells cannot be formally identified as being GM progenitor cells.

The successful culture of colonies from micromanipulated single GM-CFC has formally proved that GM colonies are clones and that, while some GM-CFC appear to be unipotential (capable of forming only G or M progeny), many are bipotential since single cultured cells are able to form colonies containing both G and M progeny (Moore *et. al.* 1972; Metcalf *et. al.* 1980; Metcalf 1980).

GM colony formation has been achieved in semi-solid methylcellulose cultures using serum-free, fully-defined, medium and purified GM-CSF (Guilbert and Iscove 1976; Guilbert, LJ, Iscove, NN, Burgess, AW and Metcalf, D, unpublished data) so this system is unique in presenting an opportunity for analysis of the mechanisms controlling the formation of two very different end cells - polymorphs and macrophages (Figure 2) - from single progenitor cells under fully definable conditions in the complete absence of any interactions with other cells.

*Granulocyte-Macrophage Colony Stimulating Factor (GM-CSF)*
Analysis of the growth of GM colonies *in vitro* revealed that the proliferation

of these populations required continuous stimulation by a specific macro-molecule, now termed 'granulocyte-macrophage colony stimulating factor' (GM-CSF) (see review Metcalf 1980a). GM-CSF has been purified to homogeneity from mouse lung conditioned medium and is a neuraminic acid-containing glycoprotein of molecular weight 23,000, the carbohydrate portion of which is not required for biological activity *in vitro* (Burgess *et.al.* 1977). The molecule is active at molar concentrations as low as $10^{-11}$ and is required continuously for every cell division during colony formation. If target GM-CFC's are not in cycle, they enter S phase within 3 hours of exposure to GM-CSF (Moore and Williams 1973) and there is a concentration-dependent shortening by GM-CSF of mean cell cycle times of GM colony cells (Metcalf and Moore 1973; Metcalf 1980).

Since purified GM-CSF is able to stimulate GM colony formation by GM-CSF in serum-free cultures, it can be concluded that the molecule interacts directly with GM-CFC. Although various cyclic nucleotides can modify GM colony formation *in vitro*, the molecular events following interaction of GM-CSF with GM-CFC have yet to be determined and it is not known for example whether the molecule enters the nucleus or activates the cyclic AMP system in the cytoplasm.

GM-CSF is known to be synthesised by a number of cell types including macrophages, mitogen-stimulated lymphocytes, L-cells and endothelial cells. Furthermore, all organs are able to synthesise GM-CSF either because of their content of these cells or because many types of cells also are able to synthesise the molecule (see review Metcalf 1980a).

Although most of the GM-CSF's generated by mouse tissues are of the same type as that purified from mouse lung conditioned medium (Nicola *et al.* 1979), the situation is complex since other forms of GM-CSF have been documented. A major-variant produced by L-cells and mouse yolk sac cells has a preferential (but not exclusive) capacity to stimulate macrophage formation (M-CSF). M-CSF has been purified to homogeneity from L-cell conditioned medium (Stanley and Heard 1977) and while also being a neuraminic acid-containing glycoprotein, M-CSF has a molecular weight of 70,000, the molecule appearing to have two subunits of molecular weight 35,000. M-CSF shares antigenic cross-reactivity with GM-CSF from many, but not all, mouse-derived sources (Shadduck and Metcalf 1975; Stanley 1979). Recent evidence indicates the existence of another major variant molecule, preferentially stimulating granulocyte colony formation (G-CSF) (Horiuchi and Ichikawa 1977; Lotem *et.al.* 1980; Burgess and Metcalf 1980).

*GM Progenitor Cell Heterogeneity*

The heterogeneity of GM-CSF's is matched by a corresponding heterogeneity in the GM-CFC target cell population. From cell separation studies on GM-CFC's it is clear that subpopulations of GM-CFC's exist that are prefer-

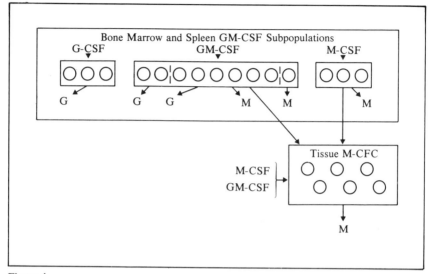

**Figure 4**

Schematic representation of the subpopulations of granulocyte- macrophage progenitor cells (GM-CFC) in the mouse bone marrow and spleen and the macrophage progenitors (M-CFC) in non-haemopoietic tissues. Subsets exist that respond only to G-CSF or M-CSF but the major progenitor cell population responding to GM-CSF contains unipotential cells generating granulocytes (G) or macrophages (M) and a large bipotential group of cells, each of which can form both granulocyte and macrophage progeny.

entially (or only) stimulated by M-CSF. The progenitor population able to form exclusively M progeny includes a much larger population of slightly more mature cells that are possibly the progeny of GM-CFC. These latter cells are present not only in the haemopoietic tissues but also in nonhaemopoietic tissues such as the liver, lung, lymph nodes, etc. When stimulated by GM-CSF or M-CSF, these cells are capable of generating small numbers of macrophage progeny (Lin and Stewart 1974; Stanley *et. al.* 1978).

It is likely that a similar subset of GM-CFC's responds preferentially to G-CSF and is capable only of forming G progeny. Within the major subset responding to the prototype GM-CSF molecule, it is also likely that minor subsets exist that are preprogrammed only to generate G or M progeny. The remaining major group of GM-CFC's are bipotential and able to form both G and M progeny. These interrelationships are illustrated diagrammatically in Figure 4.

Although it has been suggested that these various subsets of GM-CFC may be interrelated and represent a maturational sequence (Bol and Williams 1980) there is no clear evidence supporting this suggestion and it may equally be that each subset is a distinct differentiation stream derived independently from CFU-S. Recent experiments using M-CSF and GM-CSF on paired daughter cells of individual GM-CFC indicate that the subsets may overlap and that many cells can respond to either M-CSF or GM-CSF. This suggests that on some occasions the two molecules may compete for, or act in collaboration on, the same target cells (Metcalf, D and Burgess, AW, unpublished data).

From the viewpoint of cell division and differentiation, the most instructive situation of GM formation involves the production by single bipotential GM precursor cells of both G and M progeny. Studies using purified GM-CSF confirmed earlier observations that, in the presence of high GM-CSF concentrations, there is a preferential formation of G colonies whilst with low GM-CSF concentrations the only colonies formed are composed of macrophages. This appeared to document a situation in which a single regulator molecule was able to control the formation of two quite different end cells simply on the basis of the concentration of the molecule impinging on the target cells.

However the demonstration that GM-CFC's were heterogeneous offered an alternative explanation for the concentration-related effects of GM-CSF. GM-CFC's forming M progeny were shown to be able to respond to relatively low concentrations of GM-CSF whereas cells forming G progeny required high concentrations of GM-CSF before being able to proliferate (Metcalf and MacDonald 1975). The effects of varying GM-CSF concentrations might therefore be explained simply on the basis of selective activation of preprogrammed GM-CFC's, the GM-CSF having no capacity to modify the pathway of differentiation.

This problem has recently been approached in a manner designed to avoid the problems of heterogeneity by making paired studies on the daughter cells of individual GM-CFC's. Individual GM-CFC's were stimulated to proliferate with GM-CSF then the pair of daughter cells separated by micromanipulation and cultured separately, one in a culture with a high GM-CSF concentration, the other in a culture with a low GM-CSF concentration. This study showed that some GM-CFC's could generate pure populations of G or M progeny regardless of the GM-CSF concentration used. However it was shown that for many daughter cell pairs, one daughter could be stimulated to form a granulocytic colony by high GM-CSF concentrations whilst the other formed a macrophage colony if stimulated by low GM-CSF concentrations (Metcalf 1980) (Figure 5). The results of this experiment appear to document clearly that the regulator GM-CSF is able to dictate the pathway of differentiation entered by the progeny of individual GM-CFC's, provided the cell involved is bipotential.

One surprising finding on the action of GM-CSF was the demonstration that purified GM-CSF is able to stimulate the *initial* proliferation of multipotential haemopoietic cells. In cultures of micromanipulated single cells it was shown that GM-CSF was able to stimulate at least 5 divisions in such cells without suppressing their capacity to generate progeny of some other lineage. For

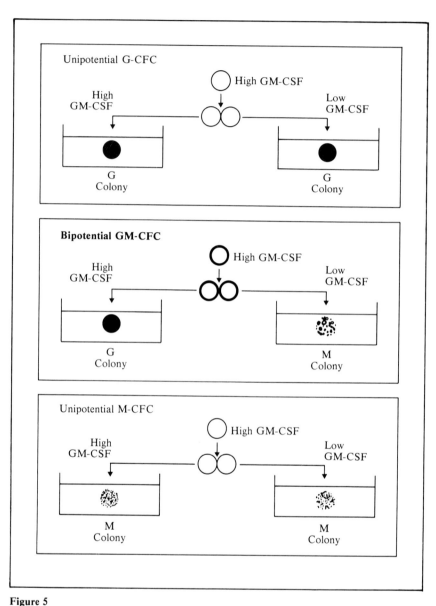

**Figure 5**

Demonstration that GM-CSF concentration can directly determine the differentiation pathway entered by bipotential GM-CFC. Individual GM-CFC are stimulated to divide then one daughter cell placed in a culture dish containing high GM-CSF concentrations, the other in a culture with low GM- CSF concentrations. Some CFC appear to be unipotential regardless of GM- CSF concentration but most GM-CFC are bipotential and, as shown in the centre panel, one daughter cell will form a granulocyte (G) colony if stimulated by a high GM-CSF concentration while the other daughter forms a macrophage (M) colony if stimulated by a low GM-CSF concentration.

example, a cell could be stimulated to generate 64 progeny under the action of GM-CSF. If pokeweed mitogen-stimulated spleen conditioned medium (SCM) was then added, (SCM contains glycoprotein factors for erythroid, eosinophil and megakaryocyte proliferation) such a developing colony could form a large colony composed only of erythroid cells (Metcalf *et.al.* 1980). In a similar manner, other proliferating cells could generate eosinophil, mega-karyocyte or mixed colonies following the delayed addition of SCM. In the absence of added SCM, only those colonies capable of forming GM progeny were able to continue proliferation and the formation of colonies of maturing GM cells. In contrast to these effects of GM-CSF, M-CSF had no capacity to stimulate the initial proliferation of multipotential cells (Metcalf *et.al.* 1980a).

There are two unusual aspects of these observations:

a) It was unexpected that the highly specific GM regulator, GM-CSF, would be able to stimulate the initial proliferation of precursors of erythroid, eosinophil or megakaryocytic cells, and;
b) Equally unexpected was the ability of GM-CSF, with its obvious capacity to stimulate the differentiated functions of GM cells, to be able to stimulate repeated cell divisions over a 48 hour period without irreversibly committing the responding cells to the GM pathway of differentiation.

**Differentiation**
Although differentiation to mature end cells is the inevitable accompaniment of cellular proliferation in a GM colony stimulated by GM-CSF, it is unclear whether all facets of the cellular differentiation are under the *direct* control of GM-CSF. For example, it might be postulated that GM cells are programmed to go through a developmental sequence if triggered by a certain number of previous mitotic divisions. If this were so, differentiation would occur as a secondary effect of GM-CSF-stimulated proliferation. However, there are several observations that make it probable that GM-CSF acts directly to enforce differentiation:

a) Differentiation seems not to be related to the number of divisions the cell has undergone. Indeed, high GM-CSF concentrations result in the formation of larger GM colonies apparently by *delaying* maturation to post-mitotic end cells,
b) GM-CSF has a direct effect on G verus M differentiation in bipotential cells and
c) GM-CSF stimulates obvious increases in the functional activity of end cells, e.g. RNA and protein synthesis of polymorphs (Burgess and Metcalf 1977), phagocytosis and killing activity of macrophages (Handman and Burgess 1979), and plasminogen-activator synthesis by macro-phages (Lin and Gordon 1979). To the degree that this latter type of action on end cells can

be regarded as 'enhancement' of differentiation, GM-CSF has to be a differentiation-enforcing factor, with actions not linked to mitotic activity.

While recent results strongly indicate that GM-CSF is a genuine differentiation factor, it is not clear what factor 'commits' a multipotential cell to become a GM progenitor cell. The general question of what factors commit the progeny of multipotential cells to the various pathways of differentiation remains a tantalising and unresolved problem. Single multipotential cells can form mixed colonies in clonal cultures *in vitro* in the course of which they generate committed progenitor cells of the various cell classes. Thus the whole process can be monitored *in vitro* and it would be reasonable to expect that the events would be relatively easy to analyse. The proliferation and commitment of the multipotential cells requires addition to the medium of SCM, known to contain a mixture of regulatory glycoproteins - GM, erythroid, eosinophil, megakaryocytic and possibly many others. However, attempts to purify these various regulators by separative protein chemistry have been frustrated by the close physical similarities of the active molecules - all are glycoproteins of molecular weight 23,000 with similar hydrophobic binding properties and heterogeneous surface change.

One obvious possibility is that GM-CSF itself might commit a multipotential stem cell to the GM pathway of differentiation. However, excess levels of GM-CSF do not commit all precursors to this pathway (Metcalf and Johnson 1979). Again the problem is compounded by the likely heterogeneity of multipotential stem cells which renders simple competition experiments difficult to interpret.

*Speculations on the Mechanism of Action of GM-CSF*
There are four key aspects of the action of GM-CSF that must be taken into account in any model constructed to explain the mechanism of action of this regulator. These are:

a) GM-CSF stimulates the proliferation of multi potential stem cells without preventing differentiation of some of their subsequent progeny to other haemopoietic pathways,
b) GM-CSF is required continuously for all cell divisions in the GM-pathway,
c) GM-CSF has a concentration-dependent capacity to determine whether some progeny of GM precursors differentiate to G cells whilst others differentiate to M cells and
d) GM-CSF has a concentration-dependent influence on mean cell cycle times of dividing GM cells.

Recent binding and metabolic studies using comparable polypeptide hormones tend to indicate

a) That specific cytoplasmic membrane receptors for such polypeptides exist on target cells and
b) That intact or minimally modified hormone molecules are internalised into the cells (see Kolata 1978). The most logical conclusion from these observations is that, if such hormones are to influence the differentiation of the target cells, the hormones are likely to actually enter the nucleus and there interact directly with one or more appropriate genes within thenucleus of the target cell.

Despite recent evidence from lymphoid cells that gene deletion occurs during differentiation (Cory and Adams 1980) it is still likely that most nuclei in a mammalian organism contain most of the genes appropriate for that organism. This has led to the conclusion that many genes controlling potential specialised cell functions must be repressed in most cells. Consideration of the known facts regarding haemopoietic cells requires an elaboration of this conclusion by defining two types of repression. Because, even under most extreme conditions of experimental manipulation, there has been no suggestion that haemopoietic stem cells can generate skin, liver or gut cells, the genetic information in the haemopoietic stem cell nucleus coding for the formation of such specialised cells can be regarded as permanently repressed. On the other hand, while a haemopoietic stem cell synthesises no haemoglobin or neutrophil granules, it clearly contains the genetic information for such functions since they will be exhibited by at least some of the progeny of these cells. Genes for such information could be regarded as either incompletely repressed (if in fact miniscule amounts of the gene products *are* produced in stem cells) or potentially derepressible.
The process by which a stem cell or one of its progeny is 'committed' to become a GM progenitor cell would therefore represent a selective derepression of the gene or gene complex required to transform a stem cell to a GM progenitor cell. Present data strongly suggest

a) That this commitment is irreversible in the sense that such a committed cell can never revert to a multipotential cell and
b) That commitment to the GM pathway irreversibly blocks any future possibility that the cell or any of its progeny may activate any of the other 'haemopoietic' genes that were potentially derepressible in the stem cell. Thus a granulocytic cell can never synthesise haemoglobin, eosinophil granules or platelets.

In view of the example of gene deletion occurring during lymphoid cell differentiation, the possibility needs to be raised that 'mono-commitment' of a multipotential cell involves deletion of other haemopoietic genes, e.g. commit ment to the GM pathway involves deletion of E, EO, MEG genes etc. This would certainly achieve irreversibility of the commitment process but at the present time insufficient evidence exists for such a radical process and other processes could achieve the same end results.

Permanent gene repression in a non-dividing cell could be visualised as resulting either from binding of a repressor molecule to the gene or from the insertion of a blocking sequence preventing transcription of that region of DNA. In a dividing cell it is a little difficult to envisage how a binding repressor could remain in place. During the production of two daughter cells the repressed genes must be derepressed to permit duplication and what process then ensures 'rerepression' of the two consequent gene regions? A simpler system is to envisage that repressor binding to genes is a dynamic equilibrium process, there being a sufficiently high intranuclear concentration of the repressor to ensure at all times that a repressor molecule is bound to the appropriate gene segment.

Commitment of a stem cell to a defined pathway of differentiation would then represent a process resulting in derepression of one particular haemopoietic gene or gene complex, either by removing a bound repressor molecule or by so reducing the intranuclear concentration of repressor molecules that the gene complex was effectively derepressed.

The intriguing problem posed by the haemopoietic stem cell is why this commit ment process irreversibly represses other related gene sequences in the cell. Consider the case of the cell potentially able to form erythroid (E), granulocyte-macrophage (GM), eosinophil (EO) and megakaryocytic (M-EG) progeny. How does GM commitment irreversibly repress E, EO and MEG gene sequences? A consideration of phylogenetic ontogeny of these cells may provide an answer to this problem. In more primitive organisms, the functions of E, GM, EO and MEG cells are likely to have been fulfilled by the same cell. With the increasing specialisation associated with mammalian development these individual functions were delegated to distinct families of monofunctional cells. Since the various haemopoietic cells presumably share more in common with each other than they do with any other cells it is not inconceivable that the genes or gene complexes programming the specialised functions of various haemopoietic cells are derived ontologically from a common ancestral gene and exhibit significant regions of sequence homology.

If these considerations are valid, then a rather simple mechanism can be envisaged to ensure simultaneous permanent repression of related genes following activation of one member of the family. It may be that the initial trans cription product (RNA) of the activated gene, when present in high enough concentrations, is able to bind to, and thereby repress, transcription or related genes. While binding of RNA to gene DNA has been searched for un-successfully in past years, it seems improbable that the methods used would have been capable of detecting the binding of a single RNA molecule such as is postulated here. Furthermore, if binding was dependent on maintenance of a sufficiently high intranuclear concentration of the blocking RNA, the extraction process to obtain the DNA for examination would, by disrupting the nucleus, simultaneously remove the RNA from the milieu of the DNA in question and allow dissociation and loss of the RNA being sought.

On this hypothesis, commitment to the GM pathway of differentiation would lead to the generation of GM-RNA as a transcription product which binds to gene sequences for E, EO and MEG. The virtue of this proposition is that such RNA would have the correct configuration to bind to these DNA's if they exhibited significant sequence homology with the GM gene. If RNA is unacceptable as the binding molecule, a more complex model could be constructed using some protein product coded for by the GM gene sequence.

This hypothesis is shown diagrammatically in Figure 6. For simplicity, the genes are illustrated as being present and adjacent on a single chromosome although this is not essential. If the process depends on maintenance of an adequate intranuclear concentration of the activated gene product, the related genes could be located anywhere on the various chromosomes.

The key feature of the proposition is that the act of activation is also the mechanism generating the molecules needed to repress *related* genetic information, thus ensuring irreversible monocommitment of the multipotential cell.

Unfortunately no obvious examples are available for analysis in other cell systems to determine whether commitment to one pathway of differentiation also irreversibly blocks other options for multipotential cells. Since mesenchymal cells appear to have the capacity to form various specialised end cells these might be promising candidates for further investigation.

In the model illustrated in Figure 6, GM-CSF is shown as the molecule derepressing the GM genome by competing with or inactivating a cell product that was partially or reversibly suppressing the gene. Commitment might be a stochastic event not requiring the intervention of a regulatory molecule or some quite different molecule might function as the commitment factor. While there is no clear indication from the present data that GM-CSF is the actual molecule that commits a multipotential stem cell to the restricted GM pathway, conversely there is no example of commitment occurring in the certified absence of GM-CSF. Since other actions of GM-CSF on committed GM cells are most readily explained if GM-CSF penetrates the nucleus and interacts directly with GM genes it is assumed for the purposes of the present discussion that one molecule (GM-CSF) mediates both commitment and the subsequent events occurring in the GM cells. The model would require that the haemopoietic stem cell possesses receptors for GM-CSF, permitting entry of this molecule or a product of the molecule to the nucleus. Since GM-CSF has been shown to stimulate at the division of multipotential stem cells (Metcalf *et al.* 1980; Metcalf 1980), it is reasonable to conclude that such receptors must exist on the multipotential cell. Since neither M-CSF nor erythropoietin has a

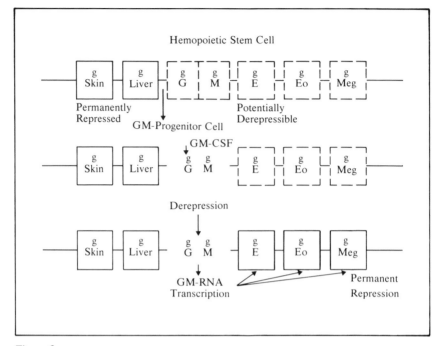

**Figure 6**

Schematic representation of a possible mechanism by which a multipotential haemopoietic stem cell is committed to one pathway of differentiation with subsequent permanent loss of capacity to form other types of haemopoietic cells. Many gene complexes are permanently repressed in the haemopoietic stem cell e.g. for skin (g skin) liver (g liver). Activation of the gene complex for granulocyte-macrophage differentiation (gG,gM), e.g. by the action of GM-CSF, leads to the synthesis of transcribed GM-RNA that binds to the gene complexes for erythroid (E), eosinophil (Eo) and megakaryocyte (Meg) differentiation because these genes share sequence homology with the GM gene. Binding of the transcribed GM products to these other gene complexes causes permanent repression of these genes.

similar capacity to stimulate the proliferation of multipotential cells, these cells may lack receptors for these molecules or for some other reason be in an unresponsive state to their intranuclear action.

Since GM-CSF can stimulate up to five divisions of a multipotential cell without blocking the capacity of the progeny to subsequently enter some other pathway of haemopoiesis, e.g. erythropoiesis, it needs to be postulated that the accumula tion of sufficiently high intranuclear concentrations of the GM-RNA product to block any other haemopoietic gene complexes is a slow process requiring several days. The process might well be made slower by the fact that the cells are dividing continuously and thus continuously reducing the accumulated intra nuclear concentrations of this transcribed GM-RNA.

If maintenance of a critical intranuclear concentration of GM-CSF is essential for the continued derepression of the GM gene complex, this could account for the observation that GM-CSF is required continuously in the culture medium throughout the process of proliferation and differentiation of GM cells.

Can the above model be used to explain the action of GM-CSF on the differentiation of the progeny of bipotential GM progenitor cells? It could be envisaged that a bipotential GM progenitor cell contains two related genes or gene complexes, one coding for the formation of G. cells, the other for M cells. Both gene complexes would be derepressible by GM-CSF. The observed facts would then suggest that the M gene complex was more readily able to be derepressed than the G gene complex and thus in the presence of low GM-CSF concentrations, only M progeny would be produced.

In the presence of high concentrations of GM-CSF leading to activation of the G gene complex, it would need to be postulated that the G gene product had some capacity to block the M gene complex, thus permitting bipotential cells to form pure G populations. Removal of such cells to low GM-CSF concentrations would again allow expression of the M gene complex and the formation of M progeny.

The mechanism of action of M-CSF raises some problems. Transfer of paired daughter cells of bipotential cells responsive to both GM-CSF and M-CSF has shown that if the cells are cultured for more than 48 hours in the presence of GM-CSF, many are no longer responsive to stimulation by M-CSF (Johnson and Burgess, 1978; Metcalf, D, unpublished data).

This implies that M-CSF is not equivalent in its action to that of a low concentration of GM-CSF but it is difficult to explain what process might result in unresponsiveness to M-CSF since many of the progeny produced by continuing GM-CSF stimulation will be macrophages, a process requiring continuing function of the M-gene complex.

The present model also will not explain why some progenitor cells form M colonies in the presence of high GM-CSF concentrations. It may be however that within the heterogeneous group of GM progenitor cells, some cells exist whose M gene complexes are not suppressible by G gene products, thus permitting the production of M cells. Since, on continued colony growth, G cells tend to mature and disintegrate, this process would transform a previously mixed GM colony to a colony containing only M cells and be a second method by which pure M colonies could form.

A major problem presented by haemopoietic regulators is the fact that they can simultaneously exert two quite different biological effects - stimulation of cell division and initiation or amplification of specialised cell functions. For example, how can one molecule simultaneously stimulate a myeloblast to divide and at the same time direct the synthesis of specific granules? Resolution of this problem clearly depends on a better understanding of what functions are encoded in the postulated G gene complex. Nothing is known of the mechanism controlling cell division if indeed a single mechanism exists. It does seem improbable that the genetic information controlling cell division in a myeloblast should happen to reside in the same region as that coding for granule synthesis - or if in different regions to be derepressible by the same specific molecule. Such a situation would then require that genes regulating erythroid cell proliferation be also linked physically or functionally to genes controlling haemoglobin synthesis, etc.

As discussed earlier the acquisition and expression of specialised functional activity seems not to be linked passively to cell division. This requires a mechanism whereby one highly specialised molecule can have diverse sites of action within an appropriate target cell. This possibility seems rarely to have been considered by cell biologists working with regulatory factors but the recent work with haemopoietic cells forces such a concept to be seriously investigated. The use of somatic cell hybrids with deletions of all but one or two chromosomes of one partner may be a method for approaching this problem. In view of the availability of purified haemopoietic regulatory factors for GM and E cells it is urgent that fusions be attempted of GM or E cells with CHO or other cells to generate target cell populations for the exploration of possible sites of regulator action on the chromosomes.

What is puzzling about GM-CSF action is that high concentrations of GM-CSF shorten mean cell cycle times. Does this imply a dynamic equilibrium between repressor and activating GM-CSF, with graded transcription of the RNA products controlling cell division, the presence of multiple gene copies with varying thresholds for derepression or some extremely indirect action of GM-CSF in controlling the rate of cell division? Furthermore, what happends when a G cell passes from the dividing myelocyte - to the post-mitotic metamyelocyte or polymorph stage? Clearly the latter cells do not lack GM-CSF receptors since they respond rapidly to added GM-CSF by major changes in RNA and protein synthesis. But what event makes it now impossible for this cell to divide? Does GM-CSF no longer enter into the nucleus? Is the gene complex controlling cell division permanently repressed in a polymorph and, if so, by what gene product? Again, cell fusion studies using polymorphs may provide some insight into this problem as may studies on the intracellular fate and localisation of labelled GM-CSF.

## References

Bols, S. and Williams, N. *The maturation state of three types of granulocyte-macrophage progenitor cells from mouse bone marrow.* J. Cell. Physiol. *102*, 233-244 (1980).

Bradley, T.R. and Metcalf, D. *The growth of mouse bone marrow cells in vitro.* Aust. J. Exp. Biol. Med. Sci. *44*, 287-300 (1966).

Burgess, A.W. and Metcalf, D. *The effect of colony stimulating factor on the synthesis of ribonucleic acid by mouse bone marrow cells in vitro.* J. Cell. Physiol. *90*, 471-484 (1977).

Burgess, A.W. and Metcalf, D. *Characterisation of a serum factor stimulating the differentiation of myelomonocytic leukemic cells.* Int. J. Cancer (in press) (1980).

Burgess, A.W., Camakaris, J. and Metcalf, D. *The purification and properties of colony stimulating factor from mouse lung conditioned medium.* J. Biol. Chem. *252*, 1998-2003 (1977).

Cory, S. and Adams, J.M. *Deletions are associated with somatic rearrangement of immunoglobulin heavy genes.* Cell. *19*, 37-51 (1980).

Goldschneider, I., Metcalf, D., Battye, F. and Mandel, T. *Analysis of rat hemopoietic cells on the fluorescence-activated cell sorter. I. Isolation of pluripotent hemopoietic stem cells and granulocyte-macrophage progenitor cells.* J. Exp. Med. *152*, 419-437 (1980).

Guilbert, L.J. and Iscove, N.N. *Partial replacement of serum by selenite, transferrin, albumin and lecithin in haemopoietic cell cultures.* Nature *263*, 594-595 (1976).

Handman, E. and Burgess, A.W. *Stimulation by granulocyte-macrophage colony stimulating factor of Leishmania tropica killing by macrophages.* J. Immunol. *122*, 1134-1137 (1979).

Horiuchi, M. and Ichikawa, Y. *Control of macrophage and granulocyte colony formation by two distinct factors.* Exp. Cell. Res. *110*, 79-85 (1977).

Ichikawa, Y., Pluznik, D.H. and Sachs, L. *In vitro control of the development of macrophage and granulocyte colonies.* Proc. Natl. Acad. Sci. (USA) *56*, 488-495 (1966).

Johnson, G.R. and Burgess, A.W. *Molecular and biological properties of a macrophage colony-stimulating factor from mouse yolk sacs.* J. Cell. Biol. *77*, 35-47 (1978).

Kolata, G.B. *Polypeptide hormones: What are they doing in cells?* Science *201*, 895-897 (1978).

Lin, H.S. and Gordon, S. *Secretion of plasminogen activator by bone marrow-derived mononuclear phagocytes and its enhancement by colony-stimulating factor.* J. Exp. Med. *150*, 231-245 (1979).

Lin, H.S. and Stewart, C.C. *Peritoneal exudate cells. I. Growth requirement of cells capable of forming colonies in soft agar.* J. Cell. Physiol. *83*, 369-378 (1974).

Lotem, J., Lipton, J.H. and Sachs, L. *Separation of different molecular forms of macrophage- and granulocyte-inducing proteins for normal and leukemic myeloid cells.* Int. J. Cancer *25*, 763-771 (1980).

Metcalf, D. *Hemopoietic Colonies. In vitro Cloning of Normal and Leukemic Cells.* Springer-Verlag. Heidelberg-New York (1977).

Metcalf, D. *Clonal analysis of the proliferation and differentiation of paired daughter cells: Action of GM-CSF on granulocyte-macrophage precursors.* Proc. Natl. Acad. Sci. (USA) (in press) (1980).

Metcalf, D. *Hemopoietic Colony Stimulating Factors. In: 'Tissue Growth Factors'* Ed. R. Baserga. Springer - New York (in press) (1980a).

Metcalf, D. and Johnson, G.R. *Interaction between purified GM-CSF, purified erythropoietin and spleen conditioned medium on hemopoietic colony formation in vitro.* J. Cell. Physiol. *99*, 159- 174 (1979).

Metcalf, D. and MacDonald, H.R. *Heterogeneity of in vitro colony- and cluster-forming cells in the mouse marrow. Segregation by velocity sedimentation.* J. Cell. Physiol. *85*, 643-654 (1975).

Metcalf, D. and Moore, M.A.S. *Haemopoietic Cells.* North-Holland. Amsterdam (1971).

Metcalf, D. and Moore, M.A.S. *Regulation of growth and differentiation in haemopoietic colonies growing in agar. In: 'Haemopoietic Stem Cells'* Eds E.W. Wolstenholme and M. O'Connor. Elsevier-Excerpta Medica - North Holland, Amsterdam, pp 157-175 (1973).

Metcalf, D., Burgess, A.W. and Johnson, G.R. *Stimulation of multipotential and erythroid precursor cells by GM-CSF. In: 'Experimental Hematology 1979'* Ed. S.J. Baum. Springer - Berlin-New York (in press) (1980a).

Metcalf, D., Johnson, G.R. and Burgess, A.W. *Direct stimulation by purified GM-CSF of the proliferation of multipotential and erythroid precursor cells.* Blood 55, 138-147 (1980).

Moore, M.A.S. and Williams, N. *Functional, morphologic and kinetic analysis of the granulocyte-macrophage progenitor cell. In: 'Hemopoiesis in Culture'* Ed. W.A. Robinson. DHEW Publication No. (NIH) 74-205, Washington pp 16-26 (1973).

Moore, M.A.S., Williams, N. and Metcalf, D. *Purification and characterisation of the in vitro colony forming cell in monkey hemopoietic tissue.* J. Cell. Physiol. *79*, 283-292 (1972).

Nicola, N.A., Burgess, A.W. and Metcalf, D. *Similar molecular properties of granulocyte-macrophage colony stimulating factors produced by different mouse organs in vitro and in vivo.* J. Biol. Chem. *254*, 5290-5299 (1979).

Nicola, N.A., Burgess, A.W., Staber, F.G., Johnson, G.R., Metcalf, D. and Battye, F.L. *Differential expression of lectin receptors during hemopoietic differentiation: Enrichment for granulocyte-macrophage progenitor cells.* J. Cell. Physiol. *103*, 217-237 (1980).

Rosendaal, M., Hodgson, G.S. and Bradley, T.R. *Organisation of haemo-poietic stem cells: the generation-age hypothesis.* Cell Tissue Kinet. *12*, 17-29 (1979).

Shadduck, R.K. and Metcalf, D. *Preparation and neutralisation characteristics of an anti-CSF antibody.* J. Cell. Physiol. *86*, 247-252 (1975).

Stanley, E.R. *Colony-stimulating factor (CSF) radioimmunoassay: Detection of a CSF subclass stimulating macrophage production.* Proc. Natl. Acad. Sci. (USA) *76*, 2969-2973 (1979).

Stanley, E.R. and Heard, P.M. *Factors regulating macrophage production and growth.* J. Biol. Chem. *252*, 4305-4312 (1977).

Stanley, E.R., Chen, D-M and Lin, H-S. *Induction of macrophage production and proliferation by a purified colony stimulating factor.* Nature *274*, 168-170 (1978).

## Questions

*Teich*

If the cell you initiate to proliferate is multipotential, couldn't you determine the pattern with which that property was transmitted in the same way that Dr Brenner was showing for his worms this morning.

*Metcalf*

Yes, you can. We have only just recently learned how to exaggerate the self-proliferation as opposed to the end-cell differentiation - to make it feasible to do - but those experiments are in progress. I cannot tell you what the answer will be but I suspect that the two systems have a lot in common. We have certainly already had examples but are exactly the same: one grand-daughter remaining multipotential, the other three grand-daughters differentiating - one into one pathway, two into another. Yes, it is possible and it is fun to do the experiments because in the haemopoietic cells you have got nice markers at the other end; there is a lot of difference between a red cell and a megakaryocyte. So the markers are there, the regulator molecules are there and the techniques are available.

*Questioner*

What are the targets of the regulator molecules?

*Metcalf*

The targets are the haemopoietic cells themselves. So far as we know, GMCSF has no action on any other cell type other than the ones we are talking about: the granulocytes; the macrophages and the ancestors of those cells. So if you check them out on fibroblasts there is no measurable activity, no activity on endothelial cells, epithelial cells. These are a new group of regulatory molecules that are the exact converse of the classical hormones. If you think of something like insulin coming from one defined cell, but with actions on almost every cell in the body,

the haemo poietic regulators are the opposite. They are possibly generated by every cell in the body but have an exquisite target cell specificity. The same also seems to be true of things like nerve growth factor; a multiplicity of cells able to produce the factor and a very specific target-cell activity. One of the puzzles is how can you affect cell proliferation and differentiation at the same time. Surely those targets within a cell must be separate and one would imagine the genes controlling replication are up here and those controlling granular-synthesis are somewhere else. I am only giving facts; the explanation is for somebody who likes model-building like Dr Raff.

*Gardner*

Can I ask what the percentage of cases is in which both daughters surive and what happens if both daughters are put in the same conditions. In other words, have you completely ruled out the possibility of selection.

*Metcalf*

The answer is, whether we had luck or good technique, that the number of failures was quite low - of the order of 10%. When you do the control experiment and put both daughters in the same culture there is an extraordinary similarity in the colonies produced. Culture dishes are mixed up on a tray at the end of a day and you can sort them out (when you are scoring them just for fun) into parts because no two colonies are exactly the same in shape or size and you can just line them up in pairs. There is also a lot of synchrony and symmetry in early divisions.

*Brenner*

So it is not the cells that diffentiate, it is their progeny.

*Metcalf*

Ah, but I am using your Brenner defination of what differentiation is.

*Brenner*
No, that was a definition of a difference, not differentiation.

*Metcalf*
It is a definition of behaviour by end-cell function which I think is fine. You cannot stain a cell and have it keep growing so we never know what the cells look like that we have been manipulating and we are judging them by their subsequent behaviour, that is true. But there is this intriguing time interval. If you do everything in the first 24 hours, the options seem to be open for the cells and few of those fail to grow. You might have noticed if you looked closely at the 2 day and 3 day experiments that there was a very high percentage of failures particularly cells initiated by GMCSF that MCSF could not support, and that is true, that a sub-set of cells that are uni-responsive but this first 24 hour period is quite intriguing.

*Raff*
I cannot understand how these factors might operate physiologically, can you demonstrate any of these molecules *in vivo*?

*Metcalf*
I hate to challenge you out of my area but the salivary gland has 5% of its dry weight as nerve growth factor.

*Metcalf* (in response to a question)
Are these things circulating in the body? Yes. It is very easy to measure directly the levels of CSF present in the serum or urine of all you people. The minute you get an infection, the levels will rise 20-50 fold, the minute the infection resolves, they pull back. There is a disease called cyclic neutropaenia where the production of granulocytes fluctuates in a cyclic fashion and there are inverse cycles of monocyte production. When you measure the CSF levels you find that they cycle with the same periodicity and exhibit that relationship between concentration and whether or not you make the

granulocytic or macrophage progeny. There is no reason to believe that they are *in vitro* artifact and if all else failed and they were - it is the only way we know to make such cells proliferate and it is a very predictable system. But the evidence is quite good that this is essentially what is going on *in vivo*. It is complicated because there are multiple sites of production and because most of the target cells are in the bone marrow you might wonder about local production of these regulators in the bone marrow and this does seem to be very important and the behaviour of local production can differ quite a lot from the behaviour of production sites elsewhere. So it is not easy to get some of the answers.

*Questioner*
You have shown that the concentration of GMCS will influence the relative proportions of granulocyte versus macrophage colonies, but you have also illustrated an effect of factors on proliferation rate. I wondered if you have ever done the experiment of using excess amounts of GMCSF and varying proliferation rate in some other way. Do you alter the relative proportion of the types of colony you see?

*Metcalf*
How would you suggest we alter the rate of proliferation of the cells?

*Questioner*
By amino acid limitation.

*Metcalf*
We have such trouble in getting them growing that we have not tried to stop them.

*Questioner*
No, slow them down.

*Metcalf*
But I take the point. It is true that when the culture conditions are sub-optimal you tend to end up with a high proportion

of macrophage colonies for whatever reason - whether everything reduces a responsiveness and only the macrophage ones which are highly responsive are still responsive - whether macrophages are tougher (which they are) - there is a number of other explanations.

*Questioner*

But you could say that the probability of differentiating into granulocytes or macrophages is in some way to rate of proliferation?

*Metcalf*

It is possible that that could be resolved. There are some systems - if you start with foetal liver cells which proliferate more rapidly than adult marrow-derived cells, I think I could prove your suggestion wrong, but, it is a possibility.

*Lodish*

Is there any indication that these factors influence the differen tiation of the so-called CFUs along the macrophage line as opposed to other erythropoietic lines?

*Metcalf*

I cannot answer that. I would have said there was absolutely no chance until about a year ago when I did that last experiment with the multipotential cell and was horrified it find that it would act on the multi- potential cell and none of the other regulators will but GMC SF does give a problem and the experiment in which you expose a multipotential cell to a massive excess concentration of GMC SF and ask the question, have I now a significantly higher proportion of GM progenitor cells is one that we have not yet done but it is obviously possible to ask

that question. Things like erythropoietin have been claimed as commitment factors but this is obviously not true because the site of action is quite distal in the differentiation pathway. Now, one of our richest sources of regulatory molecules is actually mitogen-stimulated lymphocytes and if you use either concanavalin A or pokeweed mitogen and stimulate your T cells to synthesise these factors there are at least two other factors produced that are active on multipotential cells. Now, the difficulty has been in purifying those and separating them clearly from the other regulators because all of them have a molecular weight of 23,000 and it is their very similarity that raises the possibility that they are analogous molecules with maybe significant regions of homology so, we would like to do the experiment - we can do it with one molecule but need something else to match it against.

*Rees*

Has any chemistry been done on these factors and if so, do they show any relationships with other families of proteins?

*Metcalf*

You mean, have they been sequenced? No, the one that we spent so much time purifying has a blocked N-terminus, this has held us up. These molecules are not like nerve growth factor, they are available in miniscule amounts. The GMC SF that we purify from mouse lung conditioned medium - if we take batches of 1,000 mice and generate conditioned medium from that - we get something of the order of 80 micrograms of material and this is pretty tough going for sequencing.

# Retrovirus Infection of Murine Bone Marrow Cultures as a System for Studying Differentiation

*Natalie M Teich   Janice Rowe   Nydia G Testa and T Michael Dexter*

## Introduction

Model systems to study leukaemogenesis *in vitro* require differentiating haematopoietic cell cultures to provide the necessary targets for neoplastic events. In the past few years, such a system using mouse bone marrow cells has been developed (Dexter and Testa 1976). In these cultures, the pluripotential haematopoietic stem cell, CFU-S, is maintained in a proliferative phase for about 12 weeks, and normal granulopoiesis, resulting in the production of mature granulocytes, continues for a similar period. In addition, the committed granulocyte-macrophage precursor cell, CFU-GM, and the committed erythroid precursor cell, BFU-E, are detected for at least 10 weeks (Dexter and Testa 1976; Testa and Dexter 1977), whereas megakaryocyte (Williams *et.al.* 1978) and lymphocyte (Schrader and Schrader 1978) precursors are present for at least 5 weeks. The cultures, however, do not maintain these proliferative properties indefinitely and the end result is often the terminal differentiation of the haematopoietic progenitor cells. Given these limitations, the bone marrow cultures still provide a suitable milieu for studies on the effects of murine retroviruses on proliferation, differentiation, and leukaemogenicity of haematopoietic cells *in vitro*.

We have studied infection of bone marrow cultures with several pathognomonic variants of murine retroviruses. One of the rationales for this approach derives from the findings that these viruses generally induce leukaemias or sarcomas of one particular cell type (i.e. exhibit target cell specificity) and, therefore, such manifestations might also occur *in vitro* if the appropriate cell types and microenvironmental conditions were provided. The heterogeneous cell populations and long-term survival of the bone marrow constituents in these cultures and the availability of viruses with different target tropisms afforded the opportunity for oncogenicity studies *in vitro*. The results described below concentrate on our findings with three murine retrovirus complexes. With one complex, Abelson virus (Abelson and Rabstein 1970) which induces early B-cell leukaemias, the cells transformed in bone marrow cultures *in vitro* precisely mimic the phenotype of the tumours arising from infections *in vivo* (Teich and Dexter 1978; Boss *et.al.* 1979; Teich *et.al.* 1979). On the other hand, infection with the Friend leukaemia virus complex, which induces erythroleukaemia *in vivo* (Friend 1957), elicits a diverse spectrum of effects (Dexter *et.al.* 1977; Teich and Dexter 1978). A third murine retrovirus complex, FBJ osteogenic sarcoma virus (Finkel *et al.* 1966), which manifests no changes on the haematological picture *in vivo*, also affected the differentiation of the murine bone marrow cultures *in vitro*. In the retrovirus examples described above, each virus complex consists of two components, a replication competent helper virus which may itself be leukaemogenic and a replication defective virus which is generally considered to induce the acute changes characteristic of the disease. Therefore, the effects observed in bone marrow cultures may be attributable to one or both virus components. Our findings indicate that there are profound effects on the proliferation and differentiation of particular cells of haematopoietic origin; some of these phenomena were anticipated from the pathological process observed *in vivo*, whereas others were unexpected. In several cases, the *in vitro* infections resulted in the establishment of cell lines; characterisation of a few of these lines is described below. A number of cell lines are leukaemogenic, whereas others are not, and the cells exhibit varying capacities to differentiate *in vivo* and *in vitro*.

**Procedures**
The procedures for establishing long-term bone marrow cultures have been reported in detail elsewhere (Dexter and Testa 1976; Dexter *et.al.* 1977). Replication competent murine leukaemia viruses (MLV) were titrated by the XC syncytial plaque assay (Rowe *et. al.* 1970), whereas the defective components of Abelson and FBJ virus complexes were assayed by the induction of morphologically transformed foci on monolayers of embryo fibroblasts (Hartley and Rowe 1966). The replication defective component of the Friend virus complex was measured by the macroscopic spleen colony assay (Axelrad and Steeves 1964). CFU-GM were enumerated in agar using mouse heart conditioned medium as an exogenous source of colony stimulating activity (CSA) (Bradley and Metcalf 1966). CFU-S, BFU-E and the later committed erythroid precursor cell, CFU-E, were assayed by standard procedures (Till and McCulloch 1961; McLeod *et. al.* 1974; Guilbert and Iscove 1976).

*Effects of Friend Virus on Differentiation and Proliferation*
In these experiments, (C57BL/6 × DBA/2)F₁ (BDF₁) mouse marrow cultures were infected with an NB-tropic polycythemia variant of Friend erythroleukaemia virus (FV) complex. The complex consists of a helper virus (Fr-MLV) capable of inducing erythroblastosis and anaemia in neonates of

certain mouse strains (Troxler and Scolnick 1978) and a replication defective spleen focus forming virus (SFFV) which induces acute erythroleukaemia in adult mice. As we have reported previously (Dexter *et.al.* 1977; Teich and Dexter 1978), these infections generally produced the following effects:

1) Sustained replication of Fr-MLV and a more limited production of SFFV, as measured by the ability of cell-free supernatants to induce erythroleukaemia in susceptible mice;
2) Increased numbers and prolonged proliferation of CFU-S which, although they could form spleen colonies, did not protect mice from the mortality of lethal irradiation doses and thus can be considered a typical or restricted CFU-S;
3) Increased numbers and prolonged proliferation of CFU-GM; and
4) Sustained granulopoietic differentiation in the marrow cultures *in vitro* with a pre dominant increase in early granulocytes (promyelocytes and myelocytes). In addition, there was an increase in the numbers and proliferation of BFU-E in FV- infected cultures, although there was no apparent further differentiation to CFU-E (NG Testa *et.al.* unpublished observations) using the standard culture conditions. In most cases, however, it was difficult to provide evidence that virus infection caused the cells to become leukaemogenically transformed per se, because the chronic production of both Fr-MLV and SFFV caused the rapid appearance of neoplastic changes in recipient mice after transplantation of the cultured cells. However, in some experiments, we were able to establish feeder-independent cell lines from FV-infected bone marrow cultures. These cell lines are apparently immortalised and display varying extents of differen tiation *in vivo* and *in vitro* as present below.

## a) Properties of a Myelomonocytic Cell Line
One cell line, designated 427E, described briefly elsewhere (Testa *et. al.* 1980), was isolated two weeks post-infection with FV. Large compact colonies arose in methylcellulose and cells from these subsequently proliferated in suspension without a feeder layer. Approximately 20-40% of the cells were undifferentiated blasts with an equivalent proportion of promyelocytes; a few late granulocytes and mononuclear cells were also observed. Karyotype analysis revealed that most of the cells had 78 chromosomes including two large metacentrics. The latter may have arisen from Robertsonian translocations between acrocentrics, in which case the cells could be regarded as having a tetraploid constitution.

When plated in soft agar, colony formation was independent of the addition of exogenous CSA, suggesting that the cells produced CSA endogenously. This was confirmed by showing that conditioned medium harvested from 427E cell cultures stimulated the formation of granulocyte-macrophage colonies of normal bone marrow cells. The 427E agar colonies exhibited little evidence of differentiation; 90% of the cells were blasts and early granulocytes with a very low proportion of mature granulocytes and mononuclear cells. This finding contrasted with the extent of differentiation observed when the cells were grown in liquid culture.

Injection of 427E cells into neonatal or adult syngeneic mice rapidly induced development of myelomonocytic leukaemia with an incidence approaching 100%. Infiltration of haematopoietic organs and liver by leukaemic cells was always observed. Histological examination of tumour sections showed that, in addition to undifferentiated cells, a large proportion of the cells were metamyelocytes and segmented granulocytes. Thus *in vivo* the cells showed a pronounced enhancement of differentiation compared to any culture conditions *in vitro*, indicating that the host provides either an environment necessary for maturation or physiological factors that modulate haematopoiesis. In one case, a karyotype analysis of the tumour cells was performed; 90% of the cells were hypotetraploid with the same two metacentric marker chromosomes seen in the cultured 427E cells. In addition, cells from bone marrow, spleen or tumour from leukaemic mice were able to form CSA-independent colonies in soft agar. These findings provided evidence that 427E cells are truly leukaemogenically transformed.

The cells chronically produce Fr-MLV, but no SFFV, and this property suggests that early loss of the SFFV component may be a critical factor in establishing the pattern of differentiation for the leukaemically transformed cells. Preliminary studies demonstrate that there are no detectable levels of gp55 (the 55,000 dalton glycoprotein encoded by the SFFV genome) (Racevskis and Koch 1977; Ruscetti *et.al.* 1979) in these cells, as measured by immunoprecipitation of cell extracts with anti-FV serum followed by sodium dodecyl sulfate polyacrylamide gel electrophoresis (N Teich and J Rowe, unpublished observations). It is of obvious interest to elucidate whether the SFFV genome is maintained in the 427E cell genome in a proviral integrated state.

Thus, the 427E cell line represents the immortalisation and neoplastic transformation of cells of the granulocytic lineage in bone marrow cultures infected with FV.

*b) Properties of Myeloid Cell Lines*
Two clonal cell lines, called 427F and 458E, arose from $BDF_1$ or $BDF_1$ + C57BL/6 bone marrow cultures, respectively, infected with FV and, as has been emerging in recent experiments, represents the major type of immortalised feeder-independent cell lines recoverable from such cultures. Although detailed characterisation of many of these lines await further analysis, they have several features in common with each other. Firstly, the predominant cell type is an undifferentiated blast cell, with a low level of spontaneous

differentiation along the granulocytic pathway. Secondly, growth of the cells *in vitro* is generally characterised by the maintenance of both adherent and nonadherent cell populations. However, neither gross morphological examination nor functional analysis has yet revealed distinct segregation of cell types between the two populations. Thirdly, the cells chronically produce Fr-MLV but no biologically functional SFFV and there is no detectable expression of SFFV gp55 (N Teich and J Rowe, unpublished observations). Finally, inoculation of the cells into syngeneic recipients causes granulocytic leukaemias of either acute or chronic forms. Therefore, in many ways, these cell lines resemble the 427E cell line described above. On the other hand, differences in the rate and extent of spontaneous differentiation and in the type of disease produced suggest that the lines manifest unique phenotypes.

*c) Derivation of a Nonleukaemic CFU-GM Cell Line*
Yet another type of haematopoietic cell line has been isolated from an FV-infected BDF₁ bone marrow culture with properties different from the cell lines described above. Cell line 458C represents a clone derived about 6 moths post-infection. The cells grow independently of adherent marrow cells and consist of granulocytes at all stages of maturation. It is of interest that differentiation occurs spontaneously and that colony formation in soft agar also is independent of exogenous CSA. Morphological examination of the agar colonies revealed the presence of mature neutrophils, but no mature macrophages or other cells of the monocytic lineage were detected. Unlike the cell lines described above, however, these cells contain an apparently normal diploid chromosome complement, are not leukaemogenic *in vivo*, and cannot produce spleen colonies in irradiated mice. The fact that the cell line can be continuously propagated *in vitro* suggests that there is a stem cell which, in addition to being able to differentiate into mature granulocytes, is capable of self-renewal. In this regard, 458C cells can be considered 'restricted CFU-GM' or committed granulocyte progenitor cells. Obviously it is of interest to determine whether the cells produce CSA and whether they respond to treatment with physiological regulators of haematopoiesis, particularly those that influence the monocyte-macrophage pathway.

*d) Derivation of a Nonleukaemic Multipotential Stem Cell Line*
A preliminary characterisation of one cell line, 416B, derived from BDF₁ cultures infected with FV, has already been reported (Dexter *et.al.* 1979). For the first 5-6 weeks post-infection, the virus-infected cultures behaved similarly to uninfected controls. Subsequently, haematopoiesis declined in control cultures and eventually only phagocytic mononuclear cells remained. In FV-infected cultures, however, granulopoiesis was maintained with a predominant shift towards the immature forms (promyelocytes and myelocytes). In addition, there was a very marked increase in the number of CFU-S in the 12-

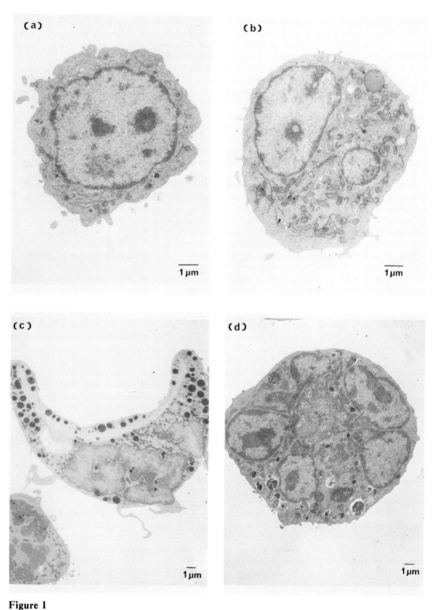

**Figure 1**
Electron micrographs of 416B cells.
a) Characteristic blast cell.
b) segmented nucleus and granulation noted; may represent a promyeloblast.
c) A more segmented nucleus and many granules; probably a relatively mature myelocyte.
d) Multi-lobed nucleus and large size, presumably a megakaryocyte; similar cells of up to 75$\mu$m diameter have also been observed. Scales are indicated on individual micrographs.

20 week post- infection period; these CFU-S showed limited differentiation capacity, producing spleen colonies containing only granulocytes and mega-karyocytes (such atypical CFU-S have sometimes been noted in our previous experiments) (Dexter *et.al.* 1977). The numbers of these restricted stem cells progressively increased such that at 18 weeks post-infection, approximately one cell in 100 was capable of forming a spleen colony. After 20 weeks, cells were transferred to fresh culture flasks and a proliferating nonadherent cell clone was established. Ultrastructurally, the majority of cells appear as undifferentiated blasts with a high nucleus:cytoplasm ratio, smooth nuclear profiles and condensed peripheral chromatin. A minor proportion (approx-imately 1%) of cells show nuclear segmentation characteristic of immature granulocytes and there are rare, large multi-lobed cells which resemble megakaryocytes. Electron microscopic examination confirmed this diversity, as illustrated in Figure 1. Intracellular and extracellular retrovirus particles are prominent in all cell types. An analysis of the karyotype revealed that approximately 95% of the cells possess a diploid chromosome number.

At high cell densities in soft agar, the cells formed colonies of loosely dispersed cells in the absence of CSA; thus the cells apparently produced growth-stimulating factors. However, there was no apparent differentiation to mature granulocytes or monocytes even in the presence of exogenous CSA, indicating a maturation block.

Measurements for CFU-S showed considerable variability with extended time of culture *in vitro*. Up to approximately 50 weeks, macroscopic colonies of granulocytes and megakaryocytes only were detected following inoculation of the cells into lethally irradiated syngeneic mice (Table 1); there was no evidence of erythropoiesis or lymphopoiesis. The same spectrum was obtained from smears of bone marrow from these mice. Thus in the *in vivo* environment, the cultured cells could undergo some apparently normal development and maturation. However, mice succumbed at 11-20 days post-irradiation,

**Table 1**
Characteristics of 416B Cultures

| Property | | | | | |
|---|---|---|---|---|---|
| Morphology* | EG+LG+MoEG+B | | B+M | B+EG+M | B |
| Karyotype | 40XX | 40XX | 40XX | 40XX | 41XX |
| CFU-S | G+M+E | G+M | G+M | G+M+E | Diffuse |
| Reconstitution ability | + | + | + | + | ? |
| Leukaemogenicity | − | − | − | − | ? |

*EG=early granulocytes (promyelocytes and myelocytes), LG=late granulocytes (metamyelocytes and polymorphonuclear neutophils), Mo=phagocytic mononuclear cells, B=blasts, M=megakaryocytes, G=gran-ulocytes, E=erythrocytes.

presumably due to defective erythropoiesis and/or thrombopoiesis. This suggestion prompted us to attempt to prolong survival by repeated inoculations of packed erythrocytes. Many of these reconstituted erythrocyte-hypertransfused mice have survived for periods greater than one year. One of the most interesting findings, however, was the ability to protect animals from lethal irradiation *without* hypertransfusion; this finding has been a reproducible phenomenon with 416B cells maintained *in vitro* for more than one year, without any passages *in vivo* (Table 1). In an attempt to rule out the possibility that the survival was due to the emergence of endogenous erythropoiesis, we increased the radiation dose substantially and were still able to protect the mice and to identify cells of erythroid, granulocytic and megakaryocytic lineages in the spleen colonies. Thus, the 416B cells had spontaneously become tripotential for differentiation *in vivo*. We are investigating the possibility that the tripotential stem cells may now respond to the inductive effects of erythropoiesis regulators *in vitro*. With further culture *in vitro*, the cells showed a diminished capacity for differen tiation *in vivo*; discrete spleen colonies were not formed although there was splenic enlargement due to a diffuse proliferation of erythroid cells. It is of interest to note that karyotype analysis of these late passage cells revealed an additional chromosome; identification of this chromosome is currently in progress (TM Dexter and D Scott, unpublished observations).

Throughout the culture period, high levels of Fr-MLV were produced; however, like the other cell lines described above, there was no evidence of SFFV replication or expression. More importantly, even though some of the 416B-reconstituted irradiated mice have survived for long periods, there is no evidence of leukaemia due to the inoculated cells or their chronically produced virus. Thus, despite immortalisation and chronic virus production, 416B cells are apparently normal nonleukaemic tripotential stem cells.

The occurrence of a continuous cell line as close to a normal haematopoietic stem cell as has been established to date provides a unique opportunity to characterise markers of pluripotential CFU-S *in vitro*. Preliminary characterisations for specific haematopoietic cell antigens indicate that there is no *Thy-1* (mature T cells), surface immunoglobulin (mature B cells), or Fc receptors (mature myelomonocytic cells). The 416B cells express the major histocompatibility antigen *H-2*, but are otherwise null with regard to surface markers tested to date (MF Greaves *et al.* unpublished observations).

Finally, as the cells have exhibited different spectra in their capacity to differentiate *in vivo* with continued propagation *in vitro* (Table 1), we are investigating whether variations in other biological properties occur with time.

*Effects of Abelson Virus on Differentiation and Proliferation*
Abelson murine leukaemia virus complex (AV) (Abelson and Rabstein 1970), consisting of a replication defective focus forming virus (Ab-MLV) and a

replication competent helper Moloney strain virus (Mo-MLV), causes a rapidly progressing pre-B-cell lymphosarcoma in BALB/c mice. Because of the haematopoietic nature of the target cell *in vivo*, it was of interest to investigate the effects of AV infection on the differentiation in BALB/c bone marrow cultures. Earlier experiments, using short-term cultures of bone marrow, spleen or foetal liver cells, showed that there were cells in these populations that could be successfully transformed by Abelson virus (Sklar *et al.* 1974; Rosenberg *et.al.* 1975). Although there are no detectable mature lymphocytes in the long-term cultures, it was possible that uncommitted stem cells or committed lymphoid precursors might be induced to proliferate if given an appropriate stimulus, such as a lymphotropic virus.

Within a few weeks post-infection, AV-infected cultures showed a dramatic shift toward undifferentiated blast cells and a decline in the proportion of granulocytes (of all stages). This contrasted with the control cultures in which the predominant population was composed of mononuclear phagocytic cells by week 7. On the other hand, the loss of CFU-S and CFU-GM occurred with approximately the same kinetics in uninfected and infected cultures. By week 15 post-infection, the infected cells demonstrated feeder-independent autonomy and were capable of forming colonies in agar in the absence of CSA. These colonies differed from normal CFU-GM in that they were tight clusters composed of undifferentiated blasts with no evidence of granulopoiesis. Such CSA-independent cells were also detected by 5 weeks post-infection; however, at this earlier time, mercaptoethanol was required for agar colony formation.

One cell line derived from these cultures, designated ABC-1, has been character ised in detail (Teich and Dexter 1978; Boss *et.al.* 1979; Teich *et.al.* 1979). Despite the absence of the mature lymphocyte surface markers, *Thy-1* antigen and surface immunoglobulin, a minor proportion (1-4%) of the cells contain intracytoplasmic IgM in the form of mu chains. A similar finding has been reported for Abelson virus transformed cells derived from short-term cultures (Siden *et.al.* 1979). Such observations provide substantial support to the hypothesis that Abelson tumour cells are early pre-B lymphocytes. Numerous rounds of single cell cloning have proven that the IgM-positive and IgM-negative cells are descendants from a single cell, as most clones have a low level of cells synthesising IgM constitutively. Attempts to increase the proportion of cells containing IgM with inducing agents have been successful; by far the best inducer is bacterial lipopolysaccharide (LPS), a B-cell mitogen (Boss *et. al.* 1979). In addition, butyric acid and interferon increase the percentage of IgM-positive cells. Interestingly, agents which effectively induce differentiation in other leukaemic haematopoietic cell lines (e.g., dimethyl sulfoxide or hexamethylene bisacetamide) do not act on ABC-1 cells. In testing different ABC-1 subclones with LPS, it was noted that clones with very low numbers of constitutively IgM-positive cells could be stimulated to virtually 100% IgM-positive cells, but clones containing no IgM-positive cells were not affected by LPS treatment. Another interesting finding is that no inducing compound has stimulated the cells to produce surface Ig; this suggests that there is an arrest in maturation that precludes the development of mature B-lymphocytes. Molecular analysis of cells transformed *in vitro* compared to those derived from virus inoculation *in vivo*, particularly the mature B-cell plasmacytomas that occur in animals receiving mineral oils as well (Sklar *et.al.* 1975), might shed some light on the nature of the maturation block.

*Effects of FBJ Osteosarcoma Virus on Differentiation and Proliferation*
The FBJ osteogenic sarcoma virus complex, consisting of a replication competent nonleukaemogenic helper virus (FBJ-MLV) and a replication defective fibroblast transforming component (FBJ-MSV), was isolated from a naturally occurring osteosarcoma (Finkel *et. al.* 1966). This complex is distinct from the more general class of oncogenic murine leukaemia viruses which have haematopoietic target cells and from the laboratory derived sarcoma viruses which transform cells of mesenchymal origin and produce undifferentiated fibrosarcomas only (or in a few cases to haematopoietic tumours as well). With these considerations in mind, we had no preconception about whether or not FBJ virus would have any effects on proliferation, differentiation or leukaemogenicity of long-term bone marrow cultures. For these experiments, DBA/2 strain mouse marrow aspirates were used.

Very soon after infection, the cultures showed a marked increase in blast cells, followed by a subsequent rise in the proportion of early granulocytes, pre dominantly promyelocytes. Apparently normal levels of CFU-S survived for periods analogous to those in uninfected cultures. However, in terms of CFU-GM production, there were marked changes. In agar colony assays for such progenitor cells, two distinct colony types were observed: those having loosely dispersed cells absolutely dependent on the presence of CSA and those forming tight clusters independent of exogenous CSA. Upon further examination, the former were identified to contain maturing granulocytes and macrophages, presumably reflecting the differentiation from a normal population of CFU-GM. The latter colonies, however, consisted predominantly of promyelocytes with about 5% metamyelocytes, thus indicating limited maturation potential. After several further weeks of continued culture, the latter colony types persisted and became the major cell type in the marrow population. From such cultures, clonal cell lines were established.

One such cell line, designated 426C, was further characterised. Following several rounds of single cell cloning, the cultures consistently contain both adherent and non-adherent cell types. Light and electron microscopy indicate that each population contains predominantly blast cells with some granulocytes and monocytes as well. A higher proportion of the monocytes occurs in the adherent cell layer. These results suggest that there is a self-renewing undifferentiated stem cell capable of maturing into both granulocytes and monocytes.

Virological analysis indicates that the cells continue to produce FBJ-MLV, but no detectable FBJ-MSV as measured by focus formation *in vitro* and tumouri genicity assays *in vivo*. Because the virus harvests were completely non-tumourigenic *in vivo* and some late passage clones produced no virus at all (T Curran and N Teich, unpublished observations), we could study unambiguously the neoplastic potential of the 426C cells *per se*.

Upon transplantation into syngeneic newborn mice, tumours arose in 100% of the recipients with a mean latency of 30-45 days. The disease was very similar to chronic myelogenous leukaemia and involved multiple sites including lymph nodes, marrow, spleen, and kidney, with frequent thymic metastases. Histologically, the tumours contained a predominance of promyelocytes and myelocytes, with the less frequent occurrence of metamyelocytes and band neutrophils. Thus, the 426C cell line is best characterised as a promyelocytic leukaemia. It is interesting that the tumours did not reveal large numbers of monocytes, as might be expected from the pattern of differentiation observed *in vitro*. This finding suggests that environmental factors provided in the host can markedly enhance or suppress particular pathways of haematopoietic differentiation into which a neoplastic cell is capable of maturing. Identification of these factors, whether they are due to micro environmental properties or specific hormonal regulators of haematopoiesis, would be extremely interesting.

## General Discussion

Interactions between retroviruses and haematopoietic cells form the basis of many recent studies on the importance of viral gene expression in leukaemo genesis *in vivo* and neoplastic transformation *in vitro*. It is generally felt that the target cell for neoplastic transformation is the same *in vitro* and *in vivo*; however, previous work by us and by others on Friend erythroleukaemia virus has shown that virus infection of haematopoietic cells *in vivo* (Golde *et.al.* 1976) and *in vitro* (Dexter *et.al.* 1977; Teich and Dexter 1978) can lead to the transformation of 'unusual' target cells, in this case, the malignant transformation of granulocytic rather than erythroid cells.

Our bone marrow culture system contains a heterogeneous cell population consisting of giant fat-containing cells, epithelioid cells, pluripotential stem cells, committed cells, maturing granulocytes and phagocytic mononuclear cells. This heterogeneity makes it difficult to assess the role of specific cell-cell and cell-virus interactions during the initial phases following virus infection which eventually lead to neoplastic transformation and/or immortalisation of specific cells. However, in the rare cases when a feeder-independent cell clone can be isolated, it is possible to identify those cells which have been either the target cells or, more likely, the descendants thereof, of 'transformation'.

## The Effects of Friend Virus Infection are Diverse

The data presented in this report demonstrate that infection of bone marrow cultures *in vitro* with Friend virus produces a diverse spectrum of biological effects. Initially normal haemopoiesis was followed by haematopoietic dysplasia. In some cases, the emergence of leukaemic cells resulted, whereas in others the process culminated in the extensive proliferation of apparently normal nonleukaemic 'stem cells' with restricted differentiation capacities. From some of these cultures, we established feeder-independent (i.e. autonomous with regard to the marrow microenvironment *in vitro*) cell lines which fall into several distinct categories.

By far the most prevalent class, at least using our culture techniques, comprises lines of myelocytic or myelomonocytic lineages (as exemplified by lines 427E, 427F, and 458E described above). In these cases, the majority of the cells within a clonal population are morphologically undifferentiated blast cells, with a minority of more differentiated cells, e.g. promyelocytes, identifiable at varying frequencies. Furthermore, in some instances, there is spontaneous differentiation into late granulocytes and mononuclear cells with the appropriate histochemical and immunological patterns associated with the myelomonocytic lineage. A further shared characteristic of these cells is their leukaemogenic potential *in vivo*, although the specific nature of the leukaemia (acute vs. chronic, myelocytic vs. myelomonocytic) varies with the particular cell line. In at least one case (line 427E), karyotype analysis and CSA-independence of tumour cells provided evidence that the cells are leukaemic transformants *per se*. Studies of this nature with the other cell lines are currently in progress. Because variants of retroviruses with potential for inducing different diseases arise, on occasion, following passage of virus *in vitro* (Rapp and Todaro 1978) or *in vivo* (for example, the derivation of the Abelson virus complex), it was conceivable that the cultured lines released viruses with the capacity to transform neoplastically cells of the myelomonocytic lineage. However, cell-free supernatants from these lines have not induced myeloid leukaemias *in vivo* and, furthermore, the pathological properties of the parental virus are usually unchanged, thus providing evidence that the cell lines are leukaemogenically transformed. An interesting feature of these cells is the absence of production and expression of the SFFV component of the Friend virus complex. If the immortalisation and neoplastic transformation processes are in fact direct effects of infection with Friend virus, it is possible that helper virus alone is sufficient. Elucidation of this issue will come from studies using Friend helper virus cloned free of SFFV biologically, or from experiments involving transfection with molecularly cloned Fr-MLV and SFFV.

The second category of cell line established from an FV infection of bone marrow is represented by the 458C line which is functionally characteristic of a committed granulocyte precursor cell, a restricted CFU-GM. The spontaneous differentiation to mature neutrophils suggests that

a) there is a self-renewing stem cell and
b) the cells produce granulopoietic stimulatory molecules, like CSA, and/or
the cells are independent of such signals. It is not yet known whether the cells
respond to regulators of monopoiesis or whether the stem cell of the clone
represents a stage of maturation beyond the commitment step of classical
CFU-GM for differentiation into distinct granulocytic and monocytic lineages. The additional observations that the cells have a diploid karyotype and
are nontumourigenic *in vivo* suggest that the cell line may be ideal for studying
differentiation-linked antigens of granulopoiesis, not only by using existing
antisera and monoclonal antibodies, but also by using the cells as immunogens
for producing monoclonal antibodies.

The last category of immortalised cell from FV-infected bone marrow
cultures is exemplified by the 416B cell line. This cell line has shown
phenotypic 'evolution' with continued passage *in vitro*. Initially the cells had a
high efficiency of spleen colony formation in irradiated mice, although the
animals were not protected from radiation death, presumably due to an
absence of erythropoietic differentiation. Thus, the cells were functionally
classified as bipotential stem cells (Dexter *et.al.* 1979). Later, the efficiency of
spleen colony formation diminished, but the cells made erythrocytic colonies
as well as granulocytic and megakaryocytic colonies and were able to
reconstitute irradiated mice; therefore, they were functionally tripotential. At
present, the cells appear to be evolving further with loss of distinct spleen
colonies and karyotypic instability. Whether these phenomena are auguries of
changes in differentiation capacity and tumourigenicity remains to be seen.

*Abelson Virus Infection In Vitro Mimics Infection In Vivo*
Whereas the experiments involving Friend virus led to the enhanced proliferation and establishment of cell lines of lineages not generally affected during
the oncogenic process *in vivo*, infection with Abelson virus gave the 'expected'
results, that is, derivation of transformed cells with a pre-B-cell phenotype.
The observed results corresponded to similar infections performed on freshly
isolated bone marrow cells, the only difference being that, in our system, the
requirement for 2-mercaptoethanol is abrogated. This difference could be
trivial or it could mean that the heterogeneous adherent cells in the marrow
population supply the critical factor(s) required during the early stages post-
infection before the transformed cells proliferate autonomously. A detailed
analysis might ascertain the nature of such factors. We have also detected a
rapid decline in stem cells, both CFU-S and CFU-GM in cultures infected
with Abelson virus or with the helper virus (Moloney MLV) alone. Therefore,
it would be interesting to monitor the early changes in differentiation induced
by Abelson virus stocks with a helper virus of another MLV strain.
  The ABC-1 cell line derived from infection *in vitro* phenotypically resembles
Abelson virus transformed haematopoietic cells from short-term cultures

(Siden *et.al.* 1979). A low proportion of cells synthesise intracellular immuno globulin mu chains spontaneously, although they are very responsive to the inductive stimulus of the B-cell mitogen lipopolysaccharide (Boss *et.al.* 1979; Teich *et.al.* 1979). This finding is very interesting in that leukaemic cells of other haematopoietic lineages can be induced to differentiate by a wide range of nonphysiological reagents, whereas all the Abelson transformed and tumour cell lines respond to B-cell mitogens primarily, suggesting that some semblance to normal growth control mechanisms is maintained. Another point in this regard is the finding that, although the inducers stimulate more cells to produce intracytoplasmic immunoglobulin, maturation to a B-cell with surface immunoglobulin is blocked. This phenomenon is consistent with the notion that leukaemogenesis in some instances may be due to abortive differentiation.

## Unexpected Effects of FBJ Osteosarcoma Virus Infection

Although FBJ osteogenic sarcoma virus complex can transform fibroblasts *in vitro*, the neoplastic process *in vivo* does not apparently affect haemato poiesis. Unlike other helper viruses isolated from mixtures containing a replication competent virus in conjunction with replication defective sarco magenic component, it is interesting that the helper virus of this naturally occurring complex, FBJ-MLV, is not leukaemogenic even for newborn animals.

The situation obtained following FBJ virus infection of DBA/2 bone marrow cultures *in vitro* reported here represents another example of the trans- formation of an 'unusual' target cell, in this case a myeloid cell. The transformed 426C cells could have arisen as a result of several possibilities.

1) For example, they could represent the consequences of a selection of a previously unidentified target which is not observed *in vivo* due to the presence of a target cell of greater affinity (presumably an osteoblast).
2) Selection of a new virus variant could have occurred by replication in unusual cells or by selection of a variant in the original virus stock due to the environmental milieu.
3) The bone marrow cultures are programmed predominantly for granulocyte- monocyte differentiation and virus infection may be a nonselective factor which triggers neoplastic mechanisms in this lineage. It is difficult to assess the first possibility due to the lack of suitable conditions for culturing osteoblasts *in vitro* at this time. The second consideration also seems unlikely because the virus produced by 426C cells does not induce myeloid leukaemia. Thus, the third possibility seems the most likely explanation at present. The 426C cells are truly neoplastically transformed as is evident from their ability to develop as myelocytic leukaemias *in vivo*, despite the absence of virus production in late passage cells.

The 426C cell line obviously contains a heterogeneous cell population as measured by morphological, biochemical and functional criteria. Presumably this is due to the presence of a self-renewing precursor cell, committed to the myelomonocytic lineage. The differentiation into predominantly atypical promyelocytes, but mature cells of granuolcytic and monocytic lineages as well, suggests that the cells produce a CSA-like factor. It will be interesting to test for this activity and to assess whether the differentiation process can be influenced by physiological and nonphysiological inducers.

## Overview

The experiments described here indicate that the long-term bone marrow culture system responds to retroviral infections in diverse and often unpredictable fashion. In the main, the results suggest that the cultures have a high propensity for granulocyte-macrophage differentiation. This pattern is observed in uninfected cultures as well. The use of conditioned medium from the murine myelomonocytic leukaemia cell line WEHI-3 leads to prolongation of the proliferation and survival of granulocytes and monocytes for indefinite periods of time, provided that the cultures are constantly supplemented with conditioned medium (Greenberger et. al. 1979). However, such WEHI-factor-dependent cells neither become established as permanent cell lines nor are they tumourigenic (TM Dexter, unpublished observations). Therefore, it seems that virus infection may directly or indirectly influence a factor-independent state, a characteristic which could be requisite for neoplastic conversion.

The spectrum of differentiation in marrow cultures can be enhanced for mature erythrocytic maturation or prolonged lymphocytic survival by using appropriate physiological factors, such as erythropoietin (Eliason et.al. 1979) or lymphocyte mitogens. In a similar fashion, the glucocorticoid hydrocortisone also stimulates haematopoiesis, presumably by increasing the levels of fat-containing cells in the adherent monolayer (Greenberger 1978) which represent a necessary population to the microenvironment. Therefore, alterations in the concentrations of these and other extrinsic factors may subtly alter the responses observed following virus infection and such variable conditions need to be assessed.

In the situation most closely analogous to leukaemogenesis in vivo, that of Abelson virus infection, the tumourigenic cell population is of the pre-B-lymphocyte class. Furthermore, in both virus production and response to inducing agents, the tumour cell lines derived in vivo and the transformed lines derived in vitro are apparently identical. Although there is no certainty in either case that the pre-B-cell is the primordial target for leukaemogenic transformation, the emergent tumour cell is phenotypically identifiable as this cell type. There has been one report of an Abelson virus transformed myelomonocytic cell line derived from a similar long-term bone marrow culture (Greenberger *et.al.* 1979); however, this may represent the granulocyte-monocyte propensity of the cultures in general, as described above.

The infections with the other two retrovirus systems described here, Friend erythroleukaemia and FBJ osteosarcoma virus complexes, led to transformation of cells that one might consider inappropriate target populations from what is known about the situation *in vivo.* If the culture conditions had been adjusted to augment differentiation along other pathways, as for example the erythropoietic lineage in the case of Friend virus infections, it is possible that cell-lines derived from the 'appropriate' lineage might have been established. Nevertheless, the cell lines that were recovered should prove useful in categorisation of cell lineage-specific determinants and in analysis of changes occurring during differentiation in response to various inducers. Interestingly, the nonleukaemic cell lines maintain an apparently normal karotype and generally respond to physiological inducers only.

The role of each of the retrovirus complexes of their individual components in the neoplastic transfromation and/or immortalisation of bone marrow cells culminating in the emergence of haematopoietic cell lines has yet to be determined. With the availability of molecularly cloned DNA copies of retrovirus genomes, it should be possible to analyse the distinct effects of both replication competent and replication defective viral components separately. In addition, such specific DNA molecules can be used to determine the status of retroviruses in the different cell types of the heterogeneous marrow population. Suffice it to say that virus infection has substantially increased the probability of obtaining cell lines from the bone marrow cultures and, therefore, we feel that virus infection has played a potentially vital role, directly or indirectly, in the establishment of these haematopoietic cell lines and we assume that this role is an event during the early stages post-infection.

## Acknowledgements

We would like to thank our colleagues Mike Boss, Mel Greaves and David Scott for allowing us to cite unpublished collaborative studies. We also thank Carol Upton and Richard Newman of the Electron Microscope Unit of ICRF. T.M.D. is a Fellow of the Cancer Research Campaign and is supported by the Medical Research Council and the Cancer Research Campaign.

## References

Abelson, H.T. and L.S. Rabstein. 1970. *Lymphosarcoma: virus-induced thymic-independent disease in mice.* Cancer Res. *30*, 2213-2222.

Axelrad, A.A. and R.A.Steeves. 1964. *Assay for Friend leukaemia virus : rapid quantitative method based on enumeration of macro scopic spleen foci in mice.* Virology, *24*, 513-518.

Boss, M., M. Greaves and N. Teich. 1979. *Abelson virus-transformed haematopoietic cell lines with pre-B-cell characteristics.* Nature, *278*, 551- 553.

Bradley, T.R. and D. Metcalf. 1966. *The growth of mouse bone marrow cells in vitro.* Austral. J. Exp. Biol. Med. *44*, 285-300.

Dexter, T.M. and N.G. Testa. 1976. *Differentiation and proliferation of haempoietic cells in culture.* Methods Cell Biol. *14*, 387-405.

Dexter, T.M., D. Scott and N.M. Teich. 1977. *Infection of bone marrow cells in vitro with FLV: effects on stem cell proliferation, differentiation and leukaemogenic capacity.* Cell, *12*, 355-364.

Dexter, T.M., T.D. Allen, D. Scott and N.M. Teich. 1979. *Isolation and characterisation of a bipotential haematopoietic cell line.* Nature, *277*, 471- 474.

Eliason, J.F., N.G. Testa and T.M. Dexter. 1979. *Erythropoietin-stimulated erythropoiesis in long-term bone marrow culture.* Nature, *281*, 382-384.

Finkel, M.P., B.O. Biskis and P.B. Jinkins. 1966. *Virus induction of osteosarcomas in mice.* Science, *151*, 698-701.

Friend, C. 1957. *Cell-free transmission in adult Swiss mice of a disease having the character of a leukaemia.* J. Exp. Med. *105*, 307-318.

Golde, D.W., A. Faille, A. Sullivan and C. Friend. 1976. *Granulocytic stem cells in Friend leukaemia.* Cancer Res. *36*, 115-119.

Greenberger, J.S. 1978. *Sensitivity of corticosteroid-dependent insulin-resistant lipogenesis in marrow preadipocytes of obese- diabetic (db/db) mice.* Nature, *275*, 752-754.

Greenberger, J.S., P.B. Davisson, P.J. Gans and W.C. Moloney. 1979. *In vitro induction of continuous acute pro myelocytic leukaemia cell lines by Friend or Abelson murine leukaemia virus.* Blood, *53*, 987-1001.

Guilbert, L.J. and N.N. Iscove. 1976. *Partial replacement of serum by selenite, transferrin, albumin and lecithin in haemopoietic cell cultures.* Nature, *263*, 594-598.

Hartley, J.W. and W.P. Rowe. 1966. *Production of altered cell foci in tissue culture by defective Moloney sarcoma virus particles.* Proc. Nat. Acad. Sci. USA. 55, 780-786.

McLeod, D.L., M.M. Shreeve and A.A. Axelrad. 1974. *Improved plasma culture system for production of erythrocytic colonies in vitro: quantitative assay method for CFU-E.* Blood, *44*, 517-534.

Racevskis, J. and G. Koch. 1977. *Viral protein synthesis in Friend erythroleukaemia cell lines.* J. Virol. *21*, 328-337.

Rapp, U.R. and G.J. Todaro. 1978. *Generation of new mouse sarcoma viruses in cell culture.* Science, *201*, 821-824.

Rosenberg, N., D. Baltimore and C.D. Scher. 1975. *In vitro transformation of lymphoid cells by Abelson murine leukaemia virus.* Proc. Nat. Acad. Sci. USA. *72*, 1932-1936.

Rowe, W.P., W.E. Pugh and J.W. Hartley. 1970. *Plaque assay techniques for murine leukaemia viruses.* Virology, *42*, 1136-1139.

Ruscetti, S.K., D. Linemeyer, J. Field, D. Troxler and E.M. Scolnick. 1979. *Characterisation of a protein found in cells infected with the spleen focus-forming virus that shares immunological cross-reactivity with the gp70 found in mink cell focus-inducing virus particles.* J. Virol. *30*, 787-798.

Schrader, J.W. and S. Schrader. 1978. *In vitro studies on lymphocyte differentiation. I. Long term in vitro culture of cells giving rise to functional lymphocytes in irradiated mice.* J. Exp. Med. *148*, 823-828.

Siden, E.J., D. Baltimore, D. Clark and N. Rosenberg. 1979. *Immunoglobulin synthesis by lymphoid cells transformed in vitro by Abelson murine leukaemia virus.* Cell 16, 389-396.

Sklar, M.D., B.J. White and W.P. Rowe. 1974. *Initiation of oncogenic transformation of mouse lymphocyte in vitro by Abelson leukaemia virus.* Proc. Nat. Acad. Sci. USA. *71*, 4077- 4081.

Sklar, M.D., E.M. Shevach, I. Green and M. Potter. 1975. *Transplantation and preliminary characterisation of lymphocyte surface markers of Abelson virus-induced lymphomas.* Nature, *253*, 550-552.

Teich, N.M. and T.M. Dexter. 1978. *Effects of murine leukaemia virus infection on differentiation of haematopoietic cells in vitro. In: Differentiation of Normal and Neoplastic Haematopoietic Cells,* (ed. B. Clarkson, P.A. Marks and J.E. Till), pp. 657-670. Cold Spring Harbor Laboratory, New York.

Teich, N.M., M. Boss and T.M. Dexter. 1979. *Infection of mouse bone marrow cells with Abelson murine leukaemia virus and establishment of producer cell lines. In: Modern Trends in Human Leukaemia III* (eds. R. Neth et al.,) pp. 487-490. Springer-Verlag, Berlin.

Testa, N.G. and T.M. Dexter. 1977. *Long-term production of erythroid precursor cells (BFU) in bone marrow cultures.* Differentiation, *9,* 193-195.

Testa, N.G., T.M. Dexter, D. Scott and N.M. Teich. 1980. *Isolation of malignant myelomonocytic cells after in vitro infection of bone marrow cells with Friend leukaemia virus.* Brit. J. Cancer, *41,* 33-39.

Till, J.E. and E.A. McCulloch. 1961. *A direct measurement of the radiation sensitivity of normal mouse bone marrow cells.* Radiat. Res. *14,* 213-222.

Troxler, D.H. and E.M. Scolnick. 1978. *Rapid leukaemia induction by cloned Friend strain of replicating murine type-C virus. Association with induction of xenotropic-related RNA sequences contained in spleen focus-forming virus.* Virology, *85,* 17-27.

Williams, N., H. Jackson, A.P.C. Sheridan, M.J. Murphy, Jr., A. Elste and M.A.S. Moore. 1978. *Regulation of megakaryopoiesis in long-term murine bone marrow cultures.* Blood, *51,* 245-255.

## Questions

*Lodish*

Are you implying that erythroprotein will cause Friend virus to replicate in otherwise resistant cells or that the effect is totally different?

*Teich*

No, what I was trying to say ther was that the cells were still there despite the fact that Friend virus shut off synthesis.

*Lodish*

...the stem cells?

*Teich*

The stem cells. They are still there and can be re-activated and respond normally. Leukaemic cells no longer respond to erythropoietin. The resistant cells in this case are there - are dormant until there is a natural or induced burst (as this was) of erythropoietin. There is no evidence in those animals that those cells ever became transformed. The way we did that was by trying to transplant the chimaeric cells into resistant mice and none of those ever took a transplantable tumour so we do not know if there is anything there. So we have not in any way been able to induce transformation in resistant cells. The only things we can say are what things do not cause transformation - we have no idea what would.

*Sager*

I am a little confused because earlier you said stem cells are refractory to infection by retroviruses.

*Teich*

The teratocarcimoma stem cells, are not in primitive stem cells.

*Sager*

But who reports that stem cells are not?

*Teich*

There is no evidence whatsoever, whether they are or are not sensitive to virus infection. No one can isolate a pure stem cell or population. Now, the one cell line I mention which was non-leukaemogenic and which during its life span was a pluri-potential (or at least a tri-potential) stem cell was obviously sensitive to at least the leukaemia virus although we had no evidence that the spleen focus forming virus was integrated in that cell.

*Sager*

In the last experiment, would the viral effects you were talking about, have to have been upon stem cells or did I miss that point?

*Teich*

Well it depends how far back the stem cell lineage can go One can say it infects /transforms a particular mate cell type and that the cell produces some factor which acts as a feed back inhibitor or in some positive sense to induce erythropoiesis. Now when one looks at the transplantable leukaemias they all contain virus. We do not know that those are the primary targets of the virus *in vivo*.

*Scholes*

It is only certain classes of the terato carcinoma cells that are susceptible to Friend virus or .

*Teich*

Yes, that is quite true in the sense that if you look at a total cell population and look at the proportion of cells which are injected by virus - it is quite small - it is under 5%. In no case that I know of has that particular cell type been identified. My personal feeling is that is is probably a fibroblastic type of cell because that would be one of the classical sensitive cells to these types of virus but I really have no idea on that.

*Pardee*

Is the transpositional activity of these viruses limited to moving the viral DNA around or are pieces of host DNA carried around on it also?

*Teich*
One can look at it in several ways in that there is really no good evidence that you are really getting transposition. The indirect evidence is the following: one, is that the viruses themselves pick-up cellular genetic material and, for example, the Kirsten or Harvey sarcoma viruses encode an oncogene which is not from a mouse (which the leukaemia virus is from), it is actually from a rat and in that sense, yes, there is a transduction of new material that is encoded now as an oncogenic virus. Also, if you pass viruses through heterologous cells you can show that they do pick up cellular DNA not only as oncogenic sequences but whether or not they move around any necessary functions or essential genes is not known yet.

*Borst*
If they move around, one could always argue that that is via an RNA transcript and what would be more convincing similarly with bacterial transposons would be if they also induce adjacent deletions or reversions - is there any evidence for that?

*Teich*
No, because very few of the flanking sequences have been sequenced so far.

*Borst*
How can you say that something is not a protein kinase because it might have a very narrow specificity for a protein expressed in very low concentrations?

*Teich*
I quite agree with you. I was once talking to someone who said that if you had to find an enzyme that a viral oncogene is coded for, protein kinase is one of the worst you could pick because of all the possible substrates. So what people have generally done is to stick with standard conditions used for looking at *src* or to examine as many ways as they know, and particularly looking for things like phosphotyrosines. There are several other

oncogenes of identifiable retroviruses that are kinases and by using those systems and looking at others you can find them. So, if you are quite right; a negative is not a good answer.

*Questioner*
Have people looked for increased phosphotyrosine levels in transformed cells of apparently non-kinase.

*Teich*
Yes. The trouble is that if you look, for example in Rous sarcoma virus transformed cells you see a rise in the amount of phosphotyrosine. If you look at something like Abelson which does have a phosphokinase activity within transformed cells you do not see an increase in the phosphotyrosine residues and in most of the others you do not see it.

*Sager*
Just to follow that point Art Pardee asked you, is there any evidence that transposition occurs in retroviruses?

*Teich*
In the sense of viral genes moving around, yes. For instance, in the AKP mouse, Steppen and Weinberg have shown that if you look at AKR mice either from different mouse colonies or even within their own mouse colony, you can see numerous copies of retroviruses but having different restriction enzyme patterns showing that they have moved. Certainly, if you look phylogentically in mouse strains, that have been derived from common progenitors you can see that restriction enzyme patterns have changed substantially. I should also mention, of course, what is learnt from the chicken is that they can be eliminated from the animal without changing the animal's lifespan or anything else, so you can have the reduction and loss (which you were suggesting before) of useless functions.

*Sager*
But has the actual process been seen in culture?

*Teich*
In tissue culture? Not that I know of.

# Cancer as Genetically Defective Differentiation

*Arthur B Pardee and Ruth Sager*

*It is at least arguable that the fundamental processes of neoplasia may be revealed most clearly in benign tumours which represent neoplasia in its simplest form, 'without frills' and uncomplicated by the numerous additional characteristics that complicate the study of malignant tumours. (Foulds 1964 see1969; 1975)*

## Cancer and Differentiation

Cancer is a cellular disease, characterised by the progressive loss of the organized properties of differentiated cells: growth control, karyotypic stability, particular morphological and biochemical traits, and the definite location of cells within the organism. Foulds (1969; 1975) recognized that cancer is progressive, dependent upon a sequence of phenotypic changes. He proposed that the earliest stages are the most instructive for understanding the origin of malignancy. The early changes can be considered as being in processes that control normal growth and development. Thus, a clearer understanding of the genetic and biochemical properties of benign cancer cells should provide insights into mechanisms of both growth and differentiation. Cellular growth control, which is defective in tumour cells and maintained with great stringency in normal cells, is the differentiated property on which we focus in this paper.

Growth of eukaryotic cells depends on external agents including protein growth factors, nutrients, and nearby cells. Our experiments to be described support the following hypothesis: that growth control is exerted before a specific point in the $G_1$ phase of the cell cycle, the R(restriction) point. Ability to pass this point and start DNA synthesis depends on production by the cell of a labile protein with a half-life of a few hours. Once the quantity of this protein is high enough the cells proceed into S phase and thence to cell division. We propose that this process is defective in tumour cells. We further propose that the same process of growth control is involved in regulation of terminal differentiation of stem cells. Selection operates on the heterogeneously changing cells of early tumours to favour fast-growing cells in which growth and differentiation controls are being lost. Thus, studies of the biochemistry of growth control are providing new understandings both of normal differentiation and of defective differentiation as expressed in tumour formation.

Our experiments on carcinogenesis show that acquisition of tumour forming ability requires karyotypic changes associated with alterations in growth regulation. The mechanism we propose to insure continuing genomic rearrangement is transposition, and experiments demonstrating the occurrence of transpositions in DNA tumour virus-transformed mouse cells will be described. We suggest that two different genetic alterations are required to initiate the progression of events that lead to malignancy. One change is decreased ability of cells to maintain a stable karyotype. The second is a diminution of growth control *in vivo*, thereby permitting many rounds of cell division during which the continually changing karyotype can arrive at a configuration that expresses characteristics of malignancy. Cancer cells thus are conceived to arise in a multistage process:

1) Creation of a kind of damage to DNA which initiates chromosome instability;
2) Cell proliferaton which together with genomic rearrangements, generates new phenotypes; and
3) Selection of those phenotypes conducive to decontrolled growth and metastasis.

*All constituents of living matter, whether functional or structural, of simple or complex constitution, are in a steady state of rapid flux.*
*(Schoenheimer R 1949).*

### Growth Control by Labile Protein

Cells *in vivo* become arrested in the $G_1$ part of the cell cycle, that is with an unduplicated DNA content. Some of these cells have achieved a quiescent state, as in the case with fibroblasts and various epithelial cells. They can be brought back into cycle and caused to divide, for example after wounding. Other cells terminally differentiate, eg. into nerve and muscle cells. Even those cells that have lost their nuclei, such as reticulocytes, terminally differentiated keratinocytes, or platelets, achieve an unduplicated DNA content before the nucleus is lost. All of these observations show that the terminal events of differentiation and of quiescence depend upon some process that occurs in the $G_1$ part of the cycle.

Cells established in tissue culture can reflect the *in vivo* growth controls. These cells, too, are generally arrested with a $G_1$ DNA content when growth conditions become suboptimal (Baserga 1976; Prescott 1976). We have

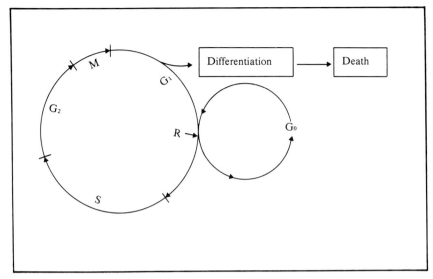

**Figure 1**
A cell cycle diagram. The conventional sequence of cell cycle phases $G_1$, S, $G_2$ and M are followed by cell division. Also included is a branch intended to indicate exit in $G_1$ of differentiating cells from the cycle. Non-differentiating cells exist into the quiescent ($G_0$) condition if they are unable to pass beyond the restriction point (R), also located in $G_1$.

normal cells with a DNA tumour virus were shown to lack the $G_1$ control totally. Under conditions that arrested growth of untransformed cells in $G_1$, the transformed cells continued slowly around the cell cycle and died (Pardee and James 1975).

More recently we have focused our studies on the biochemical nature of the event required for transit beyond the restriction point. We have shown that the progress of non-tumour forming cells through the early part of $G_1$, prior to the restriction point, is highly dependent upon rapid protein synthesis (Rossow *et al* 1979). By slowing the overall rate of protein synthesis with cycloheximide we were able to show that untransformed cells preferentially accumulate in the $G_1$ part of the cell cycle. Kinetic analysis of this lengthening of the $G_1$ part of the cycle led to formulation of a model which is adequate to explain our findings. According to this model, cells must produce a labile protein in a critical quantity in order to proceed to DNA synthesis and eventual cell division. We compute that the protein must have a half-life of a few hours in normal cells. Thus when conditions are inadequate for rapid synthesis of this protein its rapid degradation prevents its net accumulation. Only when conditions are optimal for protein synthesis can adequate amounts of the protein accumulate (Figure 2).

The great generalization of Schoenheimer (1949) that all molecules are in a steady state of rapid flux can now be extended to the regulatory molecules that

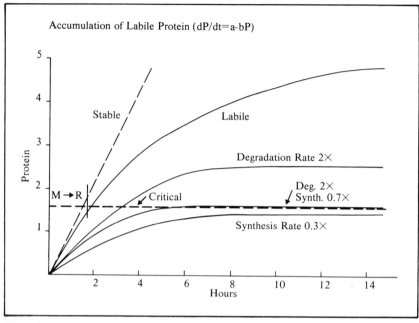

**Figure 2**

Kinetics of accumulation of a labile protein. Curves of quantity of a labile protein vs. time were calculated according to the equation shown. The curve marked 'Stable' represents accumulation of a protein with synthesis rate $a=1.0$ and zero degradation rate $b$. The curve marked 'Labile' is for a protein synthesised at rate 1.0 and degraded at rate $b=0.2$ (half-life 3.5 hr). Effects of increasing the degradation rate 2×, increasing degradation 2× and decreasing synthesis to 0.7, and of decreasing synthesis to 0.3 are shown in the three lower curves. Our model for transit past the R point proposes that a cell passes the R point when its labile protein exceeds a critical amount. Thus, the duration of M to R is given by the distance along the 'critical' line to the intersection. Note that this interval is greatly increased, and can easily become infinite as either synthetic or degradation rates or both are changed.

were discovered mainly since his time. Nature has taken advantage of this cells that have retained this control. Tumour cells, obtained by transforming earlier proposed that there is a crucial point in the cell cycle, the restriction (R) point in $G_1$, at which the decision is made as to whether a cell is to proliferate or not (Pardee 1974). We propose that cells pass this restriction point if they are able to carry out certain biochemical processes, and they are shifted into a quiescent state or differentiate if they cannot accomplish these processes (Figure 1).

Strong evidence that the restriction point is a physiologically significant signal was obtained by comparing cells that have lost their growth control with lability: responsiveness in eukaryotic cells of processes to physiological controls is rapid and flexible to the degree that regulatory molecules are labile (Schimke and Doyle 1970).

Once this protein has accumulated, and thus the restriction point has been passed, a period of several hours is required before the cells start to make DNA. Other recent experiments from our laboratory suggest that this interval is required so that the enzymes of DNA synthesis can move from the cytoplasm into the nucleus. There these enzymes assemble as a multienzyme complex called the replitase, required for DNA replication (Reddy and Pardee 1980).

How might this growth control mechanism be modified in transformed cells? Evidently, tumour cells could either produce the labile protein more readily or could degrade it more slowly under conditions that are inadequate for untransformed cells. In either case, the labile protein would accumulate more readily in transformed than in untransformed cells. Furthermore, transformed cells do not degrade their proteins as rapidly as untransformed cells in medium containing an inadequate supply of serum (Gunn et.al.1977). Rates of protein degradation in untransformed cells depend upon environmental conditions (Warburton and Poole 1979; Neff et.al.1977). Thus some transformed cells may continue to grow because their protein degradative systems are not responsive to external conditions. This possibility in no sense rules out the alternative of more rapid protein synthesis, or of a combination of these two factors, as suggested by our recent experiments. We have found that slower protein synthesis, in the presence of partially inhibitory concentrations of cyclo heximide, arrests untransformed cells readily in $G_1$, but does not arrest a variety of transformed and tumour forming cells (Medrano and Pardee 1980).

Growth of animal cells is controlled by external factors such as nearby cells (density dependent inhibition of growth), a surface for attachment, and availability of serum factors. Loss or decrease in these requirements is not sufficient for transformation to tumour forming ability in the animal, as discussed below. Apparently changes that facilitate growth in culture are not sufficient to permit these cells to grow into tumours in animals. But relaxed growth properties may be selected for, as cells in tumours evolve toward more successful growth. It is important also to appreciate that growth controls need not be lost entirely, but may only be partly relaxed in tumour cells; there need not be a complete absence of regulation. Cells transformed by DNA tumour viruses such as SV40 or polyoma largely lose growth control. However cells transformed by RNA tumour viruses or by chemicals such as benzopyrene only partly lose serum requirements and sensitivity to drugs that are capable of inhibiting growth of untransformed cells (Dubrow et.al.1978). Tumour cells are generally slowed down in their transit through $G_1$ by drugs or low serum, but are not completely arrested, thereby permitting a certain fraction of the cell population to continue growing under inadequate conditions. The SV40 transformed cells appear to continue proliferating because they synthesise a factor (T antigen) which permits the cell to bypass growth controls. The cells transformed by other means do not have this dominant factor, since (unlike

SV40 transformed cells) they are arrested when they are fused with quiescent untransformed cells (Yanishevsky and Stein 1981). These results are consistent with negative control through an inhibitor which becomes active when cells are made quiescent. Such an inhibitor could possibly be a protein degrading enzyme, according to the labile protein hypothesis.

Turning now to deregulated differentiation of tumour cells, the following recent experiments on cells in culture suggest a mechanism for differentiation very similar to the one just described for converting growing into quiescent cells. Myoblasts in culture continue to grow and divide if they are supplied with a complete medium, including chick embryo extract or fibroblast growth factor. After the growth factor is removed the cells rapidly differentiate, fusing and forming acetylcholine receptors. They do not divide again. Thus the terminal differentiation can be controlled by a growth factor. Furthermore the decision as to whether to continue growth or go into the differentiation pathway is accomplished within two hours in the early part of the $G_1$ phase, thus being very similar to the previously described entrance into quiescence of fibroblasts (Linkhart et. al. 1981).

Experiments with keratinocytes suggest a similar mechanism for differentiation. When supplied with complete medium including EGF, or agents that raise the intracellular cAMP level such as cholera toxin, these cells continue to grow and divide. However when growth is arrested, much as in the case of fibroblasts, by diminishing the EGF supply or by putting the cells into suspension, differentiation begins rapidly as exhibited by keratin formation and loss of nuclei (Rheinwald and Green 1975).

Head and neck tumour cells have recently been examined with regard to their terminal differentiation (Rheinwald and Beckett 1980). The conditions that cause terminal differentiation in culture of untransformed keratinocytes were less effective for inducing differentiation of the related tumour cells. The latter

**Table 1**

Origin of tumourigenicity: A multistage genetic process

| | |
|---|---|
| Initial DNA damage | Induced by radiation, chemicals or viruses<br>Leads to:<br>Faulty growth control<br>Loss of chromosome stability |
| Chromosome breakage and rearrangement | Aberrant transpositions occur<br>Chromosome breakages cascades as more and more aberrations arise |
| Selection of successfully growing mutant cells | Chromosome rearrangements produce new phenotypes<br>Selection favours proliferating cells<br>Different mutations and rearrangements succeed in different tissues |

tend in various degrees to continue cycling depending on the cancer cell line, and growth is not completely arrested. *In vivo* the number of cells proliferating could thus be greater at any moment than the number of cells terminally differentiating, the result being a neoplasm which in time could progress to higher states of malignancy.

We see that mechanisms effecting the reversible growth control of fibroblastic cells have their parallel in the irreversible terminal differentiation of certain other cells, and the transformation to tumorigenicity of the two cell types also seem to have elements in common.

*The primordial cell of a tumour is according to my theory a cell which contains, as a result of an abnormal process, a definite and wrongly combined chromosome-complex. This is above all the cause of the tendency to rapid cell proliferation, which is passed on to all of the descendants of the primordial cell, as far as they arise by regular mitotic cell division. But also all other abnormal qualities, which the tumour shows, are involved in the abnormal chromosome combination of the primordial cell and are inherited by all of its descendants. (Boveri 1914; transl. 1929).*

## On the Genetic Basis of Tumour Forming Ability

It has been known since the early 1900s that chromosomes are grossly rearranged in tumour cells. In fact, the available knowledge was summarised in a brilliant piece of deductive reasoning by Theodor Boveri, who proposed that aberrant chromosome arrangements lie at the heart of malignancy. Subsequently, when the transformation of cells by tumour viruses was described, many investigators reported that there too, multiple changes were initiated in the host karyotypes by viral integration (reviewed by Nichols 1981). However, until recently, most investigators have viewed chromosome changes as secondary consequences of malignant transformation rather than as causally related to it. Why should we now change our views and consider the chromosomal aberrations associated with cancer as causally involved in the origin of the disease?

The lines of evidence to be summarised here come from the current work of other investigators as well as from certain of our own experiments. We view the origin of tumour ability as a multistage genetic process, as shown in Table 1.

The first step of carcinogenesis is proposed to be a chromosomal defect in DNA, such as can be caused by radiation, chemicals, or viruses. This step would correspond to the initiation of the initiation-promotion sequence (Berenblum 1975). Initiation itself is not adequate to cause cancer, but must be followed by subsequent events. The need for subsequent events is also indicated from the calculation that mutation rates in rodent and human cells are quite similar, but the appearance of tumours after treatment with carcinogens is far more frequent by orders of magnitude in rodent cells than in human cells (Peto 1977). Thus tests such as those devised by Ames *et al* (1973) are tests for a necessary but not for a sufficient part of the total tumourigenic process. The second step in carcinogenesis involves cell proliferation and continuing chromosome rearrangement, and may correspond to the effects of promoters in the initiation-promotion sequence. We propose that this self-proliferation is necessary to allow chromosome rearrangements to arise and their phenotype effects to be expressed. Most of these re-arrangements will be lethal, but a rare combination will produce a phenotype conducive to survival. A very interesting example of a two stage process has been proposed by Klein *et.al.*(1979) in the origin of Burkitt's lymphoma: infection with Epstein Barr virus must be followed by hyperplasia and non-random chromosome rearrangements in order for the tumours to appear.

The third step is selection of rare cells with phenotypes which permit survival and excessive growth. In an adult human, containing about 10 14 cells, appearance of a productive cancer cell is relatively infrequent during a life-time. Continued chromosome rearrangements account for several properties of tumour cells:

1) Progression and metastasis;
2) The appearance of heterogeneity of appearance and drug resistance in tumours as they grow (Heppner *et.al.* 1978);
3) The gradual loss of tissue specific properties as tumours develop. Initially tumours can be distinguished on the basis of their tissues of origin, and indeed successful survival of the tumour would seem to depend upon a tissue specific combination of normal and modified traits. But as tumours progress these histotypic properties gradually disappear.

It is of course possible that a tumour can arise apparently in a single dramatic step, as following trans formation by certain viruses. Such viruses introduce changes in DNA, first of all by integrating their own genetic material into the host cell, and also introduce the capacity for further rearrangements of host genetic material as discussed more extensively elsewhere (Sager *et.al.* 1981a).

Evidence that damage to DNA plays an initiating role in malignancy comes from many sources: effects of ultra-violet and of ionizing radiation; carcino-genetic potential of known mutagens, and mutagenic potential of known carcinogens; chromosome breakage induced by viral integration, and the genetic predisposition to cancer that occurs in certain hereditary diseases (German 1981).

For example, *Xeroderma pigmentosum* is a disease in which the lack of suitable DNA repair enzymes leads to skin cancer resulting from unrepaired breaks in DNA induced by the UV-radiation in sunlight. It is evident that damage to DNA is causative rather than a secondary consequence of other metabolic events set in motion by the radiation. Similarly, sensitivity of DNA to penetrating X-irradiation, as in *Ataxia telangiectasia* leads to tumours at a wide range of internal sites. In these diseases the DNA damage appears to be randomly located, and is effective in tumour induction because it satisfies two requirements:

1) It leads to loss of chromosome stability, so that continuing genomic changes are generated; and
2) Some of these genomic changes result in faulty growth control, so that some fraction of the damaged cells continue to multiply. Diseases such as retinoblastoma, in which the inherited pre disposition to cancer seems to be a single unique rearrangement, ie. an internal deletion within the long arm of chromosome 13, provide us with especially valuable clues (Knudson *et. al* 1975). New reports of specific rearrangements found in particular genetic diseases are constantly appearing. The importance of these findings is that the chromosome changes are highly non-random. Particular rearrangements are associated with cancer appearing in particular tissues.

The same kind of evidence of non-random chromosome changes associated with particular forms of cancer is also being found in malignant cells arising during the lifetime of the individual, so-called post-zygotic changes in contrast to the pre-zygotic changes in the hereditary diseases (Rowley 1980). As an example, the occurrence of a consistent chromosome change in patients with chronic myelogenous leukemia was first described by Nowell and Hungerford (1960). Subsequently, this chromosomal change was shown to be a translocation between chromosomes 22 and typically 9, the resulting product being referred to as the Philadelphia chromosome. This translocation has been found in 85% of the more than 800 CML patients described by various investigators. When patients with CML enter the terminal acute phase of the disease, further chromosome abnormal ities are observed. Indeed, the new changes in karyotype usually precede the clinical symptoms, and thus they are of diagnostic importance (Rowley 1980).

Taken together, these findings provide strong new evidence of the importance of chromosome rearrangements in the origin of malignancy.

Recent experiments in our laboratory have provided further evidence in support of this hypothesis. CHEF/18 cells are a line of immortal, Chinese hamster embryo fibroblasts that are normal diploids with no detectable rearrangements. They are non-tumourigenic in syngeneic animals and in the nude mouse assay (Sager and Kovac 1978). In a series of mutagenesis studies, these cells were treated with the mutagens EMS and MNNG and the carcinogen 4-NQO and the surviving populations grown and injected into nude mice to test for induced tumour forming ability. No tumours arose at any of the 34 sites each injected with 10 7 CHEF/18. Only three tumours arose in

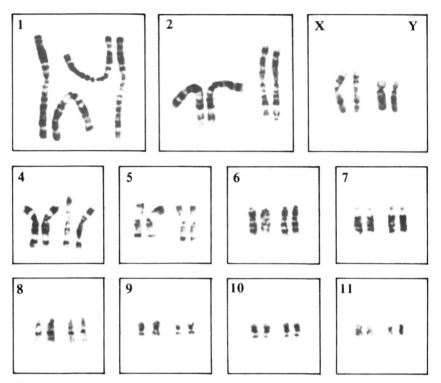

**Figure 3**
Giemsa banding patterns of CHEF/18 and CHEF/16 cells.

30 test sites, and these were so delayed in appearance, (ie. 5-6 months instead of 3-6 weeks seen with tumour-derived cells in this assay) that we can conclude that they resulted from multistep selection in the animals. Thus, no tumours arose in a single step (Smith and Sager 1981).

From the same mutagenized cultures clones were selected that lost the anchorage requirement or the high serum requirement for growth, to test the assumption of other investigators (Shin *et.al.*1975; Barrett and Ts'o 1978) that the loss of these requirements is part of a step-wise progression toward tumourigenicity. In our studies, neither class of mutants showed increased tumourigenicity, relative to the mutagenized unselected population.

The single change that correlated with acquisition of tumour forming ability, was the appearance of chromosome aberrations. Furthermore, tumour-derived cells carried additional aberrations not seen in the injected population. These findings raised the question of whether the further karyotypic changes in the tumour-derived cells arose during tumour growth or by selection of rare pre-existing cells carrying these rearrangements.

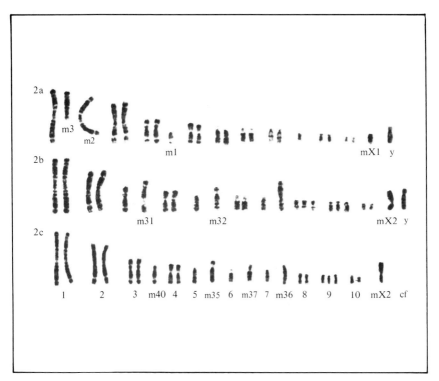

**Figure 4**
Representative Giemsa-banded karyotypes of cells from uncloned tumour-derived populations of CHEF/16 cell origin.

To answer the question, a particular cell line, CHEF/16, consisting of diploid premalignant cells (Sager and Kovac 1978), was studied to compare karyotypes before injection into nude mice and in the derived tumours. The normal karyotype of the premalignant cells is shown in Figure 3, and the rearranged genomes of the stem-lines from three tumours are shown in Figure 4. Although the pre-malignant cells were diploid (Kitchin and Sager 1980a), no diploid cells were recovered from any of the 10 tumours examined (Kitchin and Sager 1980b). Each tumour had a single stem-line (a few had two or three) easily identified by characteristic rearrangements, indicating the clonal origin of each tumour. No universal characteristic change was found, although chromosome 3 was implicated in most of the rearrangements.

These experimental results support our hypothesis that rare modifications in DNA permit later chromosomal rearrangements under conditions of cell growth, and it is these continuing changes which occasionally achieve a conformation allowing the deregulated growth characteristic of tumour cells. We stress the two-step nature of the initial cellular changes - both decreased chromosome stability and decreased growth control being required.

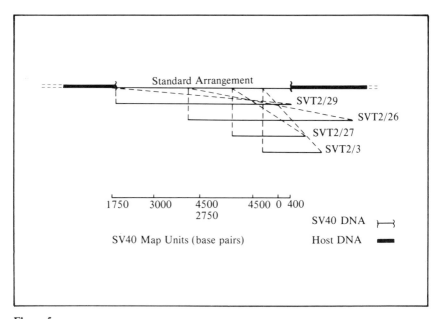

**Figure 5**

Four rearrangements found in SVT2 subclones. The SV40-transformed mouse cell line SVT2 was mapped by restriction site analysis in the region of SV40 integration referred to as Standard Arrangement. Of 20 subclones selected at random, 4 contained tandem duplications as shown in the figure. More than 30 different rearrangements have been mapped in other subclones derived from SVT2 (from Sager *et al* 1981a).

*Should a genome-disturbing event appear, such as by a cancer-inducing agent, the result could be induction of transposition of elements that can serve to control gene action. The insertion of such elements at given loci could initiate those genomic changes that lead to a cancerous state of the cell.*
*(McClintock 1978).*

## Challenges to our Understanding

The central hypothesis being proposed in this paper is that cancer arises as a multistage process in cells that are undergoing genomic rearrangements. External agents that damage DNA are carcinogenic not by virtue of specific point mutations but rather by upsetting chromosome integrity and initiating a successive cascade of further changes. These changes in turn generate pheno typic heterogeneity and thus provide the material basis for natural selection. Tumours arise as clones of cells selected for loss of growth control, and for other properties that facilitate their multiplication.

The process of transposition, discovered by McClintock in the corn plant *Zea mays*, provides a molecular mechanism for the generation of continuing rearrangements. Within the last few years, transpositional elements and the events that they mediate, have been described in bacteria, in yeast, and in

*Drosophila*. We have found evidence by means of restriction enzyme mapping for the occurrence of continuing rearrangements in an SV40 virally-transformed mouse cell line (Sager *et.al.*1981a). Examples of duplications and rearrangements arising in subclones of this cell line are shown in Figure 5. The extraordinarily high rate of rearrangements occurring in this material strongly suggests that it is under the influence of a transposition system. Several investigators have reported that RNA tumour viruses (retroviruses) contain repeat sequences at their ends that facilitate integration, but whether they also transpose has not yet been determined (CSH. Symp. 1981; see Teich, N, this Symposium).

Is there a similarity in molecular mechanisms of normal differentiation and of the defective differentiation seen in cancer cells? McClintock has proposed that the controlling elements which she studied under aberrant conditions do play a role in normal differentiation, but whether transposition *per se* is involved in normal development of higher organisms or whether the elements are normally transacting is now known.

Some recent lines of evidence suggest that rearrangements at the DNA level are not restricted to pathological situations. A flip-flop mechanism has been described in *Salmonella* in which a segment of DNA alternates between a direct and inverted arrangement, leading to alternate expression of two flagellar antigens (Silverman and Simon 1980). In yeast, mating type is determined by alleles of a single locus MAT that codes for mating type specific regulatory genes. Interconversion between the two mating types occurs by genomic rearrangements in which the mating type locus harbours either one of two DNA sequences, so-called 'cassettes', which is excised from its standard location and integrated into the *MAT* locus (Herskowitz and Oshima 1981). Most strikingly, in lymphocyte differentiation, DNA from different regions of the chromosome must be brought together and spliced to produce a suitable sequence for transcription and subsequent immunoglobulin synthesis (Tonegawa *et.al.* 1976). Since the methodology to detect DNA splicing is so new, it is not yet known whether any other systems of differentiation in mammals operate by similar mechanism, but the possibility exists.

Differentiation viewed as a consequence of changes at the chromosome level differs greatly from the widely held and traditional view that developmental changes are non-genetic. Further, some cancer specialists have suggested that the process of malignant transformation itself resembles this postulated non-genetic developmental process (Pierce *et.al.* 1978). Support for this view comes from studies of the teratoma cells formed by certain inbred strains of mice (Stevens 1958). These cells are pluripotent, and can give rise to differentiated cells of all three primary germ layers, as well as to carcinomas, depending upon the environment in which the cells are grown (reviewed by Martin 1980). Because they will form either tumours or differentiated cells, capable of participating in the formation of a normal mouse as shown elegantly by Mintz (1978), it has been proposed that cancer cells can give rise to normal cells. However, this interpretation is not warranted by the data so far available. The cells in question are not yet cancer cells: they are pluripotential cells, with the unusual property of becoming tumorigenic when grown in a particular environment. This unusual property may represent a genetic predisposition to teratoma formation carried by the inbred mice from which the teratoma cells were originally derived.

A novel mechanism operating at the DNA level has recently been implicated in differentiation: DNA methylation (Razin and Riggs 1980). Even the presence of a single methylated cytosine can change a protein-DNA interaction as seen most clearly with restriction enzymes (Smith 1979). Changes in methylation levels do occur in differentiation. For example, differences in methylation of particular sites have been detected in the $\beta$-globin region of mouse DNA extracted from a number of different tissues, but the correlation with gene expression is not clear in this material (Van der Ploeg and Flavell 1980). In the sexual alga *Chlamydomonas*, extensive methylation of chloroplast DNA occurs within a few hours during the differentiation of gametes (Sager *et.al.*1981b).

A remarkable new finding supports the idea that changes in methylation play a significant role in differentiation. Treatment of fibroblasts in culture with the analogue azacytidine can induce differentiation to myoblasts, adipocytes, and chondrocytes (Jones and Taylor 1980); and the mechanism suggested, though not yet proven, is that incorporation of azacytidine into DNA interferes with methylation.

Azacytidine has been used as an anti-cancer drug, but it is also weakly tumourigenic (Benedict *et.al.* 1977). Thus, changes in methylation may be involved not only in normal differentiation but also in tumourigenesis. Evidence of changes in the level of methylation in tumour cells has been reported (Lapeyre and Becker 1979).

One way in which methylation could influence differentiation or tumourigenicity is the following: One might imagine that when a stem cell divides so as to produce a daughter stem cell and a differentiating cell, for example in the bone marrow, the original stem cell is undermethylated, and since its daughter remains in the same environment that cell too retains a low state of methylation. However the differentiating daughter cell moves into another environment, which could cause a higher level of methylation. This higher methylation in turn could inactivate genes that are required for maintaining the undifferentiated stem cell phenotype, and thus cause the cells to enter into differentiation. For further thoughts relating methylation and differentiation see the articles by Holliday and Pugh (1975) and Razin and Riggs (1980).

Looking into the future, the challenge arising from these observations and hypotheses is to build a bridge between the genomic changes and their phenotypic consequences. One consequence of central importance for tumour formation, among the many phenotypic changes that are randomly created, is the loss of growth control. From our evidence, this loss of growth control results from the accumulation of a specific labile protein, whose exquisite sensitivity to external factors particularly suits it for a regulatory role. Our developing ideas of metabolic regulation, combined with new biochemical techniques and the powerful new methodologies of molecular genetics, should enable us to probe this connection between the genome and the phenotype in cancer and in differentiation.

**Acknowledgements**

This work was supported by grants from the National Institutes of Health, DHEW numbers GM 24571 to AB Pardee and CA 24828 to R Sager.

**References**

Ames, B.N., Durston, W.E., Yamasaki, E. and Lee, F.D. *Carcinogens are mutagens: a simple test system combining liver homogenates for activation and bacteria for detection.* Proc. Natl. Sci. USA. *70*, 2281-2285 (1973).

Barrett, J.C. and Ts'o, P.O.P. *Evidence for the progressive nature of neoplastic transformation in vitro.* Proc. Natl. Sci. USA. *75*, 3761-3765 (1978).

Baserga, R. *Multiplication and Division in Mammalian Cells.* Marcel Dekker Inc., New York (1976).

Benedict, W.F., Banerjee, A., Gardner A. and Jones, P.A. *Induction of Morphological Transformation in Mouse C3H/10T Clone 8 Cells and Chromosomal Damage in Hamster A(T$_1$)Cl-3 Cells by Cancer Chemotherapeutic Agents.* Cancer Res., *37*, 2202-2208 (1977).

Berenblum, I. *Sequential Aspects of Chemical Carcino genesis: Skin.* In: F.F. Becker (ed.), Cancer, Vol. *1*, 323-344. Plenum Publishing Corp., New York (1975).

Boveri, T. *The Origin of Malignant Tumors.* Williams and Wilkins Co., Baltimore, (1929) (Translated from the German volume of 1914).

Cold Spring Harbor Symposium. Vol. *45*. Cold Spring Harbor Laboratory, N.Y. (1981).

Dubrow, R., Riddle, V.G.H. and Pardee, A.B. *Different Responses to Drugs and Serum of Cells Transformed by Various Means.* Cancer Res., *39*, 2718-2726 (1979).

Foulds, L. *Neoplastic Development.* Vol. *1 and 2*. Academic Press, London (1969; 1975).

German, J.L. III, (ed) *Chromosome Breakage and Neoplasia,* in press (1981).

Gunn, J.M., Clark, M.G., Knowles, S.E., Hopgood, M.F. and Ballard, F.J. *Reduced rates of proteolysis in transformed cells.* Nature, *266*, 58-60 (1977).

Heppner, G.H., Dexter, D.L., DeNucci, T., Miller, F.R. and Calabresi, P. *Heterogeneity in drug sensitivity among tumour cell subpopulations of a single mammary tumour.* Cancer Res., *38*, 3758-3763 (1978).

Herskowitz, I. and Oshima, Y. *Control of cell type in Saccharomyces cerevisiae: mating type and mating type interconversion. In: The Yeast Saccharomyces cerevisiae* J.N. Strathern, E.W. Jones, and J. Broach (eds), Cold Spring Harbor Laboratory, Cold Spring Harbor, N.Y., in press (1981).

Holliday, R. and Pugh, J.E. *DNA Modification Mechanisms and Gene Activity during Development.* Science, *187*, 226-232 (1975).

Jones, P.A. and Taylor, S.M. *Cellular Differentiation, Cytidine Analogs and DNA Methylation.* Cell, *20*, 85-93 (1980).

Kitchin, R. and Sager, R. *Genetic Analysis of Tumorigenesis: V. Chromosomal analysis of tumorigenic and non-tumorigenic diploid Chinese hamster cell lines.* Somatic Cell Genetics, *6*, 75-87 (1980a).

Kitchin, R. and Sager, R. *Genetic Analysis of Tumorigenesis: VI. Chromosome rearrangements in tumours derived from diploid premalignant Chinese hamster cells in nude mice.* Somatic Cell Genetics, *6*, 615-629 (1980b).

Klein, G. *Lymphoma development in mice and humans: diversity of initiation is followed by convergent cytogenetic evolution.* Proc. Natl. Acad. Sci. USA. *76*, 2442-2446 (1979).

Knudson, A.G. Jr., Hethcote, H.W., Brown, B.W. *Mutation and childhood cancer: A probabilistic model for the incidence of retinoblastoma.* Proc. Natl. Acad. Sci. USA. *72*, 5116-5120 (1975).

Lapeyre, J.N. and Becker, F. *5-Methylcytosine content of nuclear DNA during chemical hepatocarcinogenesis and in carcinomas which result.* Biochem. Biophys. Res. Comm., *87*, 698-705 (1979).

Linkhart, T.A., Clegg, C.H., Hauschka, S.D. *Control of mouse myoblast commitment to terminal differentiation by mitogens.* J. Supramolec. Struc. in press (1981).

Martin, G.R. *Teratocarcinomas and Mammalian Embryogenesis.* Science, *209*, 768-776 (1980).

McClintock, B. *Mechanisms that rapidly reorganize the genome.* Stadler Symp., *10*, 25-48 (1978).

Medrano, E.E. and Pardee, A.B. *A prevalent deficiency in tumour cells of cycle arrest by cycloheximide.* Proc. Natl. Acad. Sci. USA. *77*, 4123-4126 (1980).

Mintz, B. *Gene expression in neoplasia and differentiation.* Harvey Lecture Series, *71*, 193-246 Academic Press, Inc. New York (1978).

Neff, N.T., Ross, P.A., Bartholomew, J.C. and Bissell, M.J. *Leucine in cultured cells.* Exp. Cell Res., *106*, 175-183 (1977).

Nichols, W. *In: Chromosome Breakage and Neoplasia,* J.L. German III ed. in press (1981).

Nowell, P.C., Hungerford, D.A. *A minute chromosome in human chronic granulocytic leukemia.* Science, *132*, 1197 (1960).

Pardee, A.B. *A Restriction Point for Control of Normal Animal Cell Proliferation.* Proc. Natl. Acad. Sci. USA. *71*, 1286-1290 (1974).

Pardee, A.B. and James, L.J. *Selective killing of transformed baby hamster kidney (BHK) cells.* Proc. Natl. Acad. Sci. USA. *72*, 4994-4998 (1975).

Peto, R. *Epidemiology, multistage models and short-term mutagenicity tests.* Origins of Human Cancer, Hiatt, Watson and Weinstein (eds) Cold Spring Harbor Lab., N.Y. 1403-1428 (1977).

Pierce, G.B., Shikes, R. and Fink, L.M. *Cancer: a problem of developmental biology,* Prentice Hall, N.J., (1978).

Prescott, D.M. *The cell cycle and the control of cellular reproduction.* Adv. Genetics, *18*, 99-177 (1976).

Razin, A. and Riggs, A.D. *DNA Methylation and Gene Function.* Science, *210*, 604-610 (1980).

Reddy, G.P.V. and Pardee, A.B. *Multienzyme complex for metabolic channelling in mammalian DNA replication.* Proc. Natl. Acad. Sci. USA. *77*, 3312-3316 (1980).

Rheinwald, J.G. and Beckett, M.A. *Defective Terminal Differentiation in Culture as a Consistent and Selectable Character of Malignant Human Keratinocytes.* Cell, *22*, 629-632 (1980).

Rheinwald, J.G. and Green, H. *Serial Cultivation of Strains of Human Epidermal Keratinocytes: the Formation of Keratinizing Colonies from Single Cells.* Cell, *6*, 331-344 (1975).

Rossow, P.W., Riddle, V.G.H. and Pardee, A.B. *Synthesis of labile, serum-dependent protein in early $G_1$ controls animal cell growth.* Proc. Natl. Acad. Sci. USA. *76*, 4446-4450 (1979).

Rowley, J.D. *Chromosome Abnormalities in Cancer.* Cancer Genetics and Cytogenetics, *2*, 175-198 (1980).

Sager, R. and Kovac, P.E. *Genetic Analysis of Tumorigenesis: I. Expression of Tumor-Forming Ability in Hamster Hybrid Cell Lines.* Somatic Cell Genetics, *4*, 375-392 (1978).

Sager, R., Anisowicz, A. and Howell, N. *Genomic rearrangements and tumour-forming potential in an SV40-transformed mouse cell line and its hybrid and cybrid progeny.* Cold Spring Harbor Symp. Quant. Biol. *45*, (in press). (1981a).

## Questions

*Hahlbrock*

In chloroplasts, it looks as if there is a regular pattern of methylation. Is this methylation here also regular or is it random?

*Sager*

The chloroplast situation is a very special one. That is a stage in the life cycle at which there is probably very little gene expression going on and the methylation that is occurring at that point is methylation which has to do with protecting that DNA against restriction. So it is rather a special case but there is very heavy methylation - yes. What you were seeing there was evidence that there is extensive methylation within each one of the $R_1$ restriction fragments which have been mapped and represent the whole chloroplast DNA map and also that the extent of methylation is extremely variable depending upon which fragment one is looking at.

*Shields*

Since Chinese hamster has such a stable karyotype does it get any less cancer than a Japanese hamster?

*Sager*

I have not the slightest idea. I have never seen a Chinese hamster, healthy or ill, but it is a good point. We know very little about the frequency of mouse cancer in the wild. All we know of are these in-bred lines and so one would really have to compare wild mice and wild hamsters.

*Pardee*

The average wild mouse lives about one day, I am told. So they do not get cancer very often.

*Brooks*

While I tend to share with you the feeling that cancer is associated with chromosomal instability, I could not help recalling that 3T3 has a very unstable karyotype but has a very poor tumour-forming incidence. Would you care to comment on that?'

*Pardee*

Well, they do progress rather rapidly if you are not careful and you have to keep 3T3 at low density, if you let them go to high density they very rapidly lose their control and new cells come up with incredible rapidity. In fact, cultures are not good fore more than a week or so, so they are evolving but we are always throwing away anything that evolves.

*Brooks*

Nevertheless, if you inject them.

*Another*

It depends how you do it. If you inject them on glass beads.

*Brooks*

Yes, but you will get lots more proliferation as well.

*Pardee*

I think it is a very good point and there is something certainly, that we do not understand - something different about *in vitro* and *in vivo*. When you think about it immune systems are needed to keep foreign cells from proliferating so there is also something in there that keeps foreign cells from proliferating too much. You can talk about chalones if you wish (I know they are not very fashionable) but on the other hand I think the cell has to escape from some sort of unknown internal regulatory mechanism in order to become a tumour cell. But something beyond the kinds of growth control we study in culture - you know, the serum-dependence. The second property that is very different in the animal from in culture is this chromosomal instability. Ruth has been culturing these 16 cells in all sorts of culture media and the karyotype remains stable. It is only when they are put in the animal that the karyotype starts explosively changing, so, an animal is not a Petri dish.

*Coffino*

In the slide you showed the hypothetical protein and its hypothetical method of accumulation. You had an experiment with a concentration of zero at zero time and you must therefore have some way of getting rid of it. Do you imagine that this occurs by virtue of its synthesis being restricted at some stage of the cycle or some other event that eliminates it?

*Pardee*

I wish I knew. There are, of course hypotheses (one from Dr Brooks in the audience) that this event may start much earlier. We have not done much about this. We have assumed that the protein is made earlier (let us say in S or $G_2$) and then you might predict that if you stop protein synthesis for a limited time, the protein would decay in $G_2$ as well as $G_1$ but with very different consequences of stopping protein synthesis and allowing decay in $G_2$. There is not much extra delay. You can do it in $G_2$ as compared to in $G_1$ where it was shown many years ago by Schneiderman *et al*, that there is a considerable extra delay. So we do not see any evidence for this protein building up in $G_2$. That does not rule out the possibility that protein synthesis itself is part of a series of events which may start earlier. Again, there were these very nice experiments of Schneiderman of totally stopping protein synthesis for a while and then starting it up again and seeing if something seemed to have decayed and if you did that right at the beginning of $G_1$ there was no appearance of decay. If it was done in the middle of $G_1$ the kinetic evidence showed a lot of decay, so, his data indicated that this process of labile protein synthesis may start around the beginning of the $G_1$ period. They recall, too, that during mitosis there is very little protein synthesis - it is really inhibited quite strongly so a lot of decay could occur then. So I arbitrarily put my curve starting at zero; I could have moved the whole thing up if I had wished - and we get a more elaborate model (which I will not

go into here) but you can account for a number of other things if you add another constant, as usual.

*Borst*

Can I ask a question of the female part of the duet?

*Pardee*

That is you (I guess)

*Sager*

Yes.

*Borst*

Are those specific alterations that you see for putting a piece of SV40 DNA into the chromosome or can you get similar effects by putting a piece of lambda in?

*Sager*

We are in the middle of experiments like that but at the moment I am a little pessimistic about whether or not we will ever get an answer because the methods for putting DNA into cells now, carry with them so many artifacts that it is hard to interpret what you get. Potentially DNA transfer is a very important method and one will certainly have to worry about any bacterial DNA that goes in with it but at the moment, anything that goes in becomes re- arranged and we are just looking at the question of whether you can distinguish re-arrangements of this sort from the re-arrangements which seem to be the artifacts of the method.

*Hartley*

Could I ask a question of Dr Metcalf which is connected with this talk?' If one were to assume that your CSF factors which are slowing up the growth rate of the cells were acting in some way to block the synthesis of this hypothetical labile factor that Dr Pardee is talking about, then your cells could also be blocked at $G_1$ at low levels of this factor. Have you ever looked at that? In other words, if the similar phenomena were acting in your case, your cells would also be blocked in G₁. Is that not a consequence?

*Metcalf*
I am not sure I have followed the argument but the answer is that we have not looked. It is very hard when you have got one cell in 400, to measure things on a flow cytometer. There is a very high background.

*Hartly*
But the slower growing cells should be blocked - that would become the rate-limiting step in division and therefore all the cells (or the large majority of them, under slow growth) should be arrested.

*Metcalf*
Well I do not believe this crap about tumour cells running more quickly than normal cells because having grown up with haemopoietic tumours, in every case you find that the leukaemic cells proliferate more slowly than normal.

*Pardee*
I did not say they proliferated faster

*Metcalf*
I think you had that on one of your earlier slides the interesting difference is that the length of G₁ is the difference between the leukaemic and the normal cell. The leukaemic cell has, in general, a very long G₁ and the rest of the cell cycle is the same for both cells.

*Pardee*
G₀ I would call it. The cells are not growing fast because they are sitting, not dividing for a long time and they have a G₁ DNA content but once they are in cycle I would say they cycle as fast as any other cells. I do not think we are disagreeing. My slides are all wrong or either you did not read it right. You can look at that slide and find out but I am sure I know my slides pretty well (Laughter).

# 6
# Control of Gene Activity

Some of the most elusive questions in development concern the balance between genes and their environment; how, and how strongly, do environmental or cytoplasmic factors influence the genome. In the belief that differentiation is the selective 'unlocking' of parts of the genome by epigenetic factors, one of the goals of developmental biology has therefore been to identify those cytoplasmic factors responsible for specific gene expression and 'Control of Gene Activity' contains illustrations of this.

One of the best known examples is in the control of the transcription of the genes for avian ovalbumin by steriod hormones. Dr Wasylyk introduces this system which is proving so fruitful in suggesting how regulation of the binding between RNA polymerase and specific DNA signal sites may control transcription. Dr Eisen's work is highly relevant here since it concerns the activity of histones in affecting transcription in cells approaching their final stages of differentiation.

A very large problem faced by developmental biologists is how, if at all, the organisation of genes in the genome relates to the temporal sequence of gene switching during development. Although the relationship between nuclear and mitochondrial DNAs is unclear, there have been great strides made in mapping the latter and Dr Borst discusses this as an example of gene organisation.

# Promoter Sequences of Eukaryotic Protein Coding Genes

*Bohdan Wasylyk   Claude Kedinger   Jeff Corden*
*Paulo Sassone-Corsi and Pierre Chambon*

## Introduction

A basic property of all living cells is the ability to switch the expression of their genes on and off, for example, in response to extracellular signals In prokaryotes this switching is mostly controlled at the level of RNA transcription. In complex eukaryotic organisms, although the expression of many different genes is turned on and off during development from the egg, and although this switching continues in the differentiated cells, the importance of control of gene expression at the transcriptional as opposed to post-transcriptional level is still a matter of controversy. In higher eukaryotes, however, there is unequivocal evidence that the expression of at least some genes is controlled at the level of RNA transcription. For example, in the tubular gland cells of the magnum portion of the chick oviduct, the transcription of the ovalbumin and conalbumin (ovotransferrin) genes is turned on by the steroid hormones estradiol and progesterone. Like the genes coding for the other egg white proteins, these genes are not transcribed in the absence of estradiol or progesterone see McKnight and Palmiter (1979); Perrin *et. al.* (1979) and references therein.

## Definition of Promoter and its Properties in Prokaryotes

During the past 20 years some of the basic mechanisms involved in regulation of transcription in prokaryotes and their viruses have been elucidated in molecular terms. It has been learned that transcription is regulated by modulation of the efficiency with which RNA polymerase can recognise and interact with specific DNA signal sequences (promoters and terminators) that specify starting or stopping sites and are involved in the promotion and termination of RNA transcription see Rosenberg and Court (1979 and references therein. The genetic approach has been invaluable in these studies. For instance, it was primarily on genetic evidence that Jacob *et.al.* (1964) first defined the promoter as an initiating element indispensable for the expression of bacterial structural genes. Further progress was made possible by the availability of cell-free systems, reconstructed from purified components, in which the selective *in vivo* transcription events could be accurately duplicated.

In addition to requiring purified RNA polymerase and well-defined templates, such studies *in vitro* also require a detailed knowledge of the transcription unit *in vivo* to determine whether correct initiation and termination of transcription are occurring. The use of such *in vitro* systems, the possibility of purifying specific wild-type and mutant prokaryotic genes and their RNA products, and the availability of DNA and RNA sequencing methods have enabled investigators to analyse the structure and function of certain genes in great detail and to show that prokaryotic promoters are regions of DNA 5' to the structural genes Rosenberg and Court (1979); Losick and Chamberlin (1976).

The messenger RNA (mRNA) start points (the position on a DNA sequence which codes for the first nucleotide of an RNA) of many prokaryotic transcription units have been precisely located by genetic analysis and transcription *in vitro*, and the DNA sequences of these regions have been determined. Pribnow (1975a,b) and Schaller *et. al.* (1975) first noted a sequence homology, related to 5'-TATAATG-3' (T, thymidine; A, adenine: G, guanine), located about 10 base pairs (bp) upstream from mRNA start points (see footnote). Since then about 60 promoters have been sequenced 46 are compiled in Rosenberg and Court (1979), see also Bujard (1980) and the generality of the Pribnow box confirmed. The most conserved nucleotide in the third T, and is identical in all promoters investigated so far. The first TA is also strongly conserved, whilst there is a larger variation in the rest of the heptamer. It may be significant that in the other positions, instead of a single base predominating certain base pairs tend to be excluded see Rosenberg and Court (1979). A second region of homology has been identified around position -35. Interestingly some promoters, known to require additional factors for their function, show little or no homology to the -35 region. A third region of homology exists around the start site of RNA initiation; since this reaction is highly selective with respect to the starting nucleotide. Hence there is often an A in this position, sometimes a G, and much less frequently a C or a U. It has been shown, by both deoxyribonuclease and chemical modification experiments, that RNA polymerase binds to all three conserved sequences of the promoter Rosenberg and Court (1979); Siebenlist *et.al.* (1980).

Several promoter (*in vivo*) mutations have been sequenced, and many of them have been shown to fall within the -10 to -35 region. The most impressive results were some of the promoter-up mutations which increase the efficiency of the lac promoter. This promoter has the Pribnow box sequences TATGTT. A change from G to A in the fourth position increases promoter efficiency 10 fold. Furthermore, mutating the fifth nucleotide as well, from T to A, increases the promoter efficiency another 2.5 fold. This mutation makes the -10 sequence the same as the most probably Pribnow box. Since polymerase binding unwinds a promoter about one helical turn, the change from GC to AT, which reduces hydrogen binding, would be expected to have a positive effect. However that a TA to AT change, which is not expected to influence helix stability, increases the promoter strength suggests that specific sites are important for nucleotide protein interactions.

## In vitro Systems to Study Specific
## Initiation of Transcription of Eukaryotic Genes

In contrast to prokaryotic cells, the molecular mechanisms that underlie the regulation of transcription in eukaryotic cells are still largely unknown, notably because the classical genetic approach is for the most part not possible in these cells. That the mechanism in eukaryotes may not be identical to those in prokaryotes was first suggested 10 years ago by the discovery of the multiplicity of eukaryotic RNA polymerases by our group and Roeder and Rutter for reviews, see Chambon (1975); Roeder (1976). It was subsequently established that cells of both higher and lower eukaryotes contain three structurally and functionally distinct classes of RNA polymerase which are localised in different subcellular fractions. Class A or 1 catalyses the synthesis of ribosomal RNA, class B or 2 that of mRNA, and class C or 3 that of transfer RNA (tRNA) and 5 S RNA for reviews, see Chambon (1975); Roeder (1976). Although highly purified preparations of these enzymes, particularly RNA polymerase B, were available shortly after their discovery, progress has been extremely slow in analysing their role in the control of transcription. The lack of meaningful cell-free transcription systems *in vitro* mostly accounts for this failure. Indeed, because of the complexity of the eukaryotic genome, there was no means to study the transcription of a given gene *in vitro* by incubating the total cellular DNA with purified RNA polymerase. Even when well-defined viral DNA templates such as the Simian virus 40 (SV40) and adenovirus-2 genomes were available, the primary transcription products were unknown, precluding any valid analysis of the factors involved in the control of transcription. Furthermore, intact viral DNA's proved to be very poor templates *in vitro* for the purified RNA polymerase B, which was known to transcribe SV40 and adenovirus genomes *in vivo* Chambon (1975). Several technical breakthroughs were clearly required.

The discovery of restriction enzymes and reverse transcriptase, followed by the advent of molecular cloning and of methods for separating, visualising, and rapidly sequencing DNA and RNA molecules, have made it possible to study, at the nucleotide level, the anatomy of eukaryotic cellular and viral genes and of their primary RNA transcripts Chambon (1978); Breathnach and Chambon (1981). It has now been shown in several instances for example, see Ziff and Evans (1978) and Wasylyk *et.al.* (1980a) for the adenovirus major late transcription unit and for the ovalbumin transcription unit, respectively that the 5′ ends of the RNA primary transcripts and of the mature mRNA's

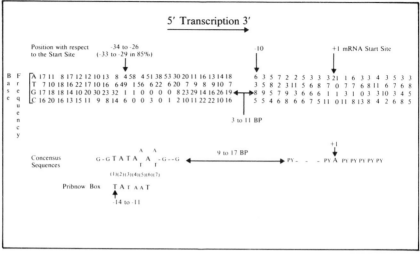

**Figure 1**

Analysis of sequences around and upstream from the mRNA startsite. The sequence of the anti-sense strand of 60 genes has been analysed. The sequences around the mRNA startsite are aligned with respect to the base coding for the first nucleotide of the mRNA (position 1, arrow). The 'upstream' sequences (the numbering is negative upstream from the mRNA start point; numbers in parenthesis below the consensus sequence refer to the position of the individual bases in this sequence) are aligned with respect to the almost invariant A which occurs at position (2) of the upstream consensus sequence. The distance between the T at position (1) in the upstream consensus sequence and the mRNA startsite varies from 26 to 34bp, depending on the gene. More-over 85% of these Ts are located at distances comprised between -29 and -33bp from the startsite. Highly conserved positions are indicated by large upper-case letters; other conserved position (>50%) are indicated by smaller upper-case letters (Py pyrimidine). See Breathnach and Chambon for a list of the references used to compile the concensus sequence.

coincide and therefore that the start point of transcription corresponds to the base coding for the 5' terminal nucleotide of the mRNA's. By analogy to the situation in bacteria, we would expect eukaryotic promotors to be located in the region adjacent to the 5' end of the transcription unit. Indeed, the comparison of several cellular and viral genes has revealed the existence of an AT-rich region of homology centred about 25bp upstream from the mRNA start points Gannon *et.al.* (1979); Cochet *et.al.* (1979); Benoist *et.al.* (1980). This sequence, which is known as the 'TATA' box, was first noticed by Goldberg and Hogness and bears some sequence resemblance to the Pribnow box in prokaryotic promoters Gannon *et.al.* (1979) (see Figure 1).

A second region of homology, 5'-GG CAATCT-3', has been noticed at positions T -70 to -80 of several cellular and viral protein-coding genes Benoist *et.al.* (1980), but its generality remains to be demonstrated. A third region of homology exists around the mRNA startsite (see Figure 1). Rather than having a particular sequence, as suggested previously by comparison of  -

globin and adenovirus major late genes Konkel *et.al.* (1978); Ziff and Evans (1978) the mRNA startsite appears to consist of an A residue (in the anti-sense strand), surrounded by pyrimidines (however, this consensus is certainly biased, since only the 5'-ends of 22 mRNAs all but one of which start with an A have yet been accurately mapped). It is interesting that the 'TATA' box is situated at roughly 3 turns of the DNA helix from the mRNA startsite, whereas the prokaryotic 'Pribnow' box is located at about one helix turn from this site.

These homologous sequences are not found upstream from the start point of genes transcribed by RNA polymerases A Sollner-Web and Reeder (1979) or C Sakonju *et.al.* (1980); Bogenhaden *et.al.* (1980); Pelham and Brown (1980) indicating that the specific transcription of different classes of genes by the distinct classes of eukaryotic RNA polymerases could be due to the specific recognition of sequences characteristic of a class of genes. Although the recognition of sequence homologies is important in suggesting the location of control regions, it is obvious that the actual role of homologous sequences cannot be established without a functional assay, for instance, a cell-free system capable of accurate *in vitro* transcription. technical breakthrough was the establishment in 1978 by Wu (1978) and by Birkenmeier *et.al.* (1978) of accurate cell-free transcription systems for viral and cloned cellular genes transcribed *in vivo* by RNA polymerase C. In these systems the necessary factor, or factors, lacking in the purified RNA polymerase C, are supplied by a cytoplasmic fraction of KB cells Wu (1978) or by a nuclear extract of *Xenopus* oocytes Birkenmeier *et. al.* (1978). Unexpectedly, the groups of Brown Sakonju *et.al.* (1980); Bogenhaden *et.al.* (1980); Pelham and Brown (1980); Birkenmeier *et.al.* (1978), and Birnstiel Kressman *et.al.* (1979) found that the essential information for 5S RNA and tRNA transcription by RNA polymerase C is contained in an intragenic control region, in a position strikingly different from that of promoter regions in prokaryotes.

These observations raised the question whether all eukaryotic promoters are similarly located or whether this location is particular to genes transcribed by RNA polymerase C. Subsequently, Weil *et.al.* (1979) found that a system similar to that of Wu can also be used as a source of factors to promote accurate initiation of transcription by purified RNA polymerase B at the major late adenovirus-2 promoter. Briefly, these workers used a 'truncated template' assay which contains, in addition to a cytoplasmic KB cell extract (S100) and RNA polymerase B, a restriction enzyme-cut DNA fragment containing, at a well- mapped position, the promoter region of the major late adenovirus-2 transcription unit. The RNA's synthesised *in vitro* are labelled with radio-active nucleoside triphosphates and then separated by gel electrophoresis. RNA products of discrete sizes are produced by 'runoff' termination whenever specific initiation occurs. From the length of the 'runoff' transcripts the position of the region coding for the 5' end of the *in vitro* synthesised RNA's can be deduced and compared with the position of the 5' end of the *in vivo* transcription unit. Sequence analysis of the capped *in vitro* synthesised 5' terminus has verified the accuracy of initiation *in vitro* Weil *et al.* (1979). Manley *et al.* (1980) have recently described a second system which will direct specific transcription *in vitro*. This system consists of a whole cell extract that does not require exogenous RNA polymerase B.

We have recently completed a study of the anatomy of the cloned chicken ovalbumin and conalbumin genes and of their transcription units Gannon *et al.* (1979); Cochet *et.al.* (1979); Benoist *et.al.* (1980), and have used the S100 system to demonstrate specific *in vitro* initiation of transcription of these cellular genes at the sites corresponding to the 5' terminal nucleotide of the *in vivo* primary transcripts Wasylyk *et.al.* (1980a). Other studies have demonstrated specific *in vitro* initiation of transcription on a variety of viral and cellular genes Breathnach and Chambon (1981).

## Localisation of Promotor Sequences for In Vitro Transcription by RNA Polmerase B

*Deletion Mutants*

Using deletion mutants of the conalbumin and of the adenovirus-2 major late genes, constructed by *in vitro* genetic techniques, it has been shown that sequences located upstream from the mRNA startpoints are required for the initiation of specific transcription *in vitro* Wasylyk *et.al.* (1980a); Corden *et al.* (1980); Hu and Manley (1980). These sequences are located between positions -12 and -32 the first T of the 'TATA' box of these two genes is located at position -31. A deletion mutant lacking the sequence upstream from position -29 does not promote specific transcription Corden *et.al.* (1980). In addition, it has been found that the -12 to -32 adenovirus-2 major late gene fragment alone, when cloned in the plasmid pBR322, can direct specific *in vitro* initiation of transcription, starting about 25 bp downstream from the 'TATA' box Sassone-Corsi *et. al.* in preparation. *In vitro* transcription of SV40 early gene mutants bearing various deletions located downstream from the 'TATA' box also initiates about 25 bp downstream from the 'TATA' box Mathis and Chambon (1981). The above results indicate that sufficient information for specific initiation of transcription *in vitro* is contained within a 20 bp region including the 'TATA' box, and that transcription initiates about 25 bp down stream from the box. However, in discord with this simple picture, initiation of transcription still occurs on the SV40 early gene region in the absence of the 'TATA' region, but at multiple specific sites Mathis and Chambon (1981), which suggests the existence of function 'TATA' box related substitute elements.

Results obtained with deletion mutants should however be interpreted with caution. Deletion cannot simply be considered as the absence of the deleted sequence, since new DNA sequences are fused at the deletion endpoint,

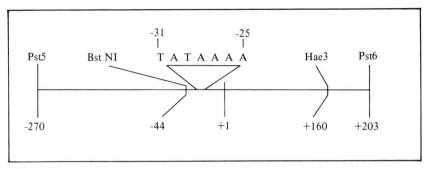

**Figure 2**
Restriction enzyme-map of the conalbumin Pst5-Pst6 fragment. Pst5-Pst6 refer to Pst1 restriction sites previously defined (5). DNA sequences in the direction of transcription (downstream) are numbered with positive integers, whilst sequences 5′ to the startpoint (upstream) are given negative values. +1 represents the position of the base coding for the first nucleotide of conalbumin mRNA. TATAAAA is the sequence of the non-coding DNA strand between nucleotides -31 and -25, and is the conalbumin sequence equivalent to the 'TATA' box consensus sequence found in many eukaryotic genes transcribed by RNA polymerase B taken from Wasylyk *et.al.* (1980b).

making it impossible to rule out that the observed effects are due to an effect of the replacing sequences, rather than to direct alteration of the promoter region. This might lead to a misinterpretation in the identification of the location of the promoter sequences. In order to obtain unequivocal evidence that the 'TATA' box is implicated in the promotion of transcription we have used *in vitro* directed mutagenesis to make single base substitutions in the 'TATA' box.

## Localisation Promotor Sequences for In Vitro Transcription
### *Point Mutations*
#### *Construction and Characterisation of a Mutant Containing a T to G Transversion in the Second T of the Conalbumin 'TATA' Box*
It has been shown Hutchinson *et.al.* (1978); Gillam *et.al.* (1979); Gillam and Smith (1979a,b); Razin *et.al.* (1978) that a specific point mutation can be obtained with a synthetic oligonucleotide differing in one base from a wild-type DNA sequence. This oligonucleotide is first hybridised to the complementary wild-type strand contained in a circular single-stranded DNA vector, extended with DNA polymerase 1, and finally ligated with DNA ligase to complete the other strand. Transfection with these molecules gives rise to clones containing DNA with the desired sequence change. We have used a fd103 phage recombinant containing the conalbumin Pst5-Pst6 fragment (Figure 2) and a synthetic undecanucleotide to construct a mutant containing a single base substitution in the conalbumin 'TATA' box (Figure 3).

The noncoding strand of the conalbumin Pst5-Pst6 fragment (Figure 2) was cloned in fd103 ss-DNA at the position of the unique Pst1 site of the RF DNA. The undecanucleotide, complementary to the 'TATA' box region except for a

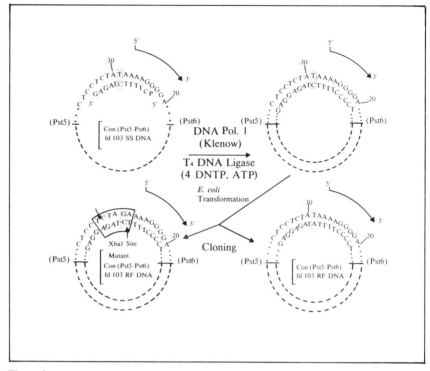

**Figure 3**

Preparation of a mutant containing a single base pair substitution in the conalbumin 'TATA' box. In the figure, conalbumin and fd103 ssDNA are represented by dotted and dashed lines respectively. The individually boxed nucleotides are mismatched (upper circles) and the boxed base pairs (lower circles) are matched. The boxed hexanucleotide sequence (lower left) is the XbaI recognition site. DNA pol. 1 (Klenow) = DNA polymerase I (Klenow fragment); DNTP + deoxyribonucleoside triphosphate; con = conalbumin; Pst5 and Pst6, see Figure 2 and text taken from Wasylyk *et.al.* (1980b).

C (boxed nucleotide in the upper left circle in Figure 3), was synthesised by the triester method, hybridized to the ss-DNA, and used to synthesis the complementary strand (see legend to Figure 3). After cloning, RF DNAs from 50 individual colonies were screened for the presence of an XbaI site, which is conveniently formed by the mutation (see Figure 2). The DNA of two colonies contained an XbaI site. The mutant Pst5-Pst6 fragment was isolated from the fd103 DNA and inserted into the PstI site of pBR322. Recombinants corresponding to the two original clones were selected and on subsequent characterisation were found to give essentially identical results. Figures 4 and 5 demonstrate that the conalbumin mutant differs from the wild-type DNA by the change of the second T of the 'TATA': box to a G. Figure 4 compares the restriction enzyme digestion patterns of mutant and wild-type DNAs. Only the

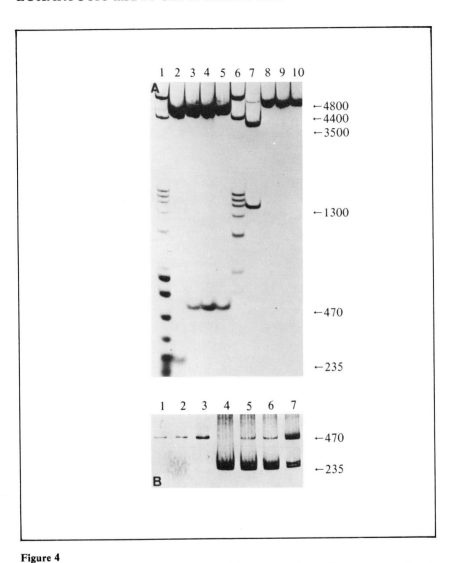

**Figure 4**
Restriction enzyme mapping of mutant and wild-type recombinants. The mutant conalbumin
Pst5-Pst6 fragment was cloned in the Pst1 site of pBR322. (A) The purified recombinant DNA
was digested with the restriction enzymes and analysed on a 1.5% agarose gel. Lanes 1 and 6,
DNA sizes markers; lanes 2, 4, 7, 9 mutant recombinant digested with Pst1 and Xba1, Pst1,
Xba1 and BamH1 and BamH1 respectively; lanes 3, 5, 8, 10 wild-type recombinant digested
with Pst1, Pst1, Xba1 and BamH1 and BamH1 respectively. (B) The mutant conalbumin Pst5-
Pst6 fragment was isolated by sucrose density gradient centrifugation, digested with different
quantities of Xba1 and analysed on a 5% polyacrylamide gel. Lanes 1, 2, 3: .005 μg, .05 μg of
mutant Pst5-Pst6 fragment, respectively, before digestion; lanes 4, 5, 6, 7: 0.5g of mutant
fragment digested with 20, 12.5, 7.5, 2.5, units of Xba1 respectively for 1h at 37°C taken from
Wasylyk et.al. (1980b).

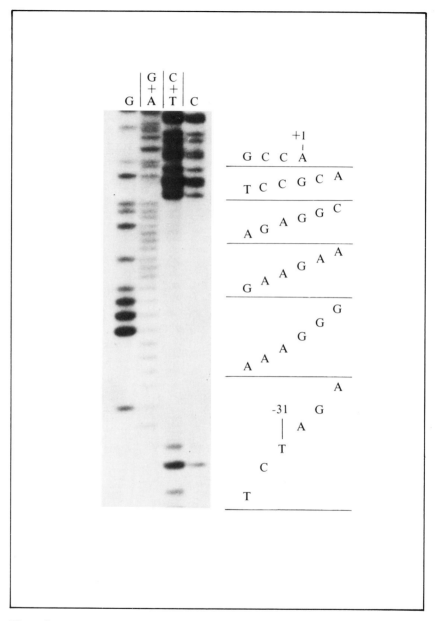

**Figure 5**

Sequences of mutant DNA. The BstN1 (-44)to Hae3 (Cochet *et. al.* 1979) fragment (Figure 1), 5′ end labelled at the BstN1 site, was sequenced by the method of Maxam and Gilbert and the electrophoresed on a 20% acrylamide-urea-gel. -31 and +1 refer to the number of nucleotides from the mRNA startpoint (see Figure 2) taken from Wasylyk *et.al.* (1980b).

mutant, and not wild-type pBR322 recombinant, contained an Xba1 site (Figure 4A, lanes 7-10). As expected, only the Pst5-Pst6 fragment (470 base-pair band) from the mutant DNA contained an Xba1 site (giving the bands at 235 base pairs). To show that the mutant DNA was not contaminated with wild-type fragment we digested 0.5 μg of mutant Pst5-Pst6 fragment with increasing amounts of Xba1 (Figure 4B, lanes 4-7). Comparison of lane 4 (corresponding to the largest amount of Xba1 tested) with lanes 1-3 shows that ≥99% of the mutant Pst5-Pst6 fragment contained the expected Xba1 site. The T -- G transversion was the only modification observed in this region, as shown by the sequence analysis in Figure 5.

*In Vitro Transcription of the Conalbumin 'TAGA' Box Mutant*

By using S1 nuclease mapping and the 'run-off' transcription method it has been shown Wasylyk *et.al.* (1980a) that specific initiation occurs *in vitro* on conalbumin gene DNA. In the 'run-off' assay, RNAs of discrete sizes are produced on restriction enzyme DNA fragments by run-off termination whenever specific initiation occurs. From the length of the run-off transcripts, the position of the 5' end of the RNA can be deduced. As expected (see Figure 2), a major run-off transcript of ≅200 nucleotides (see band labelled with an arrowhead in Figure 6A, lane 3 is obtained with the Pst5-Pst6 fragment as a template. Similarly, for the Hae3-digested Pst5-Pst6 fragment, a specific run-off fragment of about 160 nucleotides was obtained (Figure 6A, lane 4; Figure 6B, lanes 1 and 3).

The RNA run-off transcripts appeared to be slightly shorter than expected, perhaps because of termination of transcription slightly before the end of the fragment or because of slight differences in the electrophoretic properties of the RNA and DNA size markers. Specific run-off transcripts of identical mobility, but weaker intensity, were obtained (Figure 6A) for the mutant Pst5- Pst6 fragment that was intact (lane 1) or was digested (lane 2) with Hae3.

Electrophoresis of the run-off transcript obtained with the mutant Pst5-Pst6 fragment digested with hae3 next to the wild-type transcript on a 5% polyacrylamide/urea sequencing gel (Figure 6B, lanes 1/2 and 3/4) demonstrated that both RNAs had the same mobility. Therefore, it appears that the transcription start site is the same for wild-type and mutant conalbumin genes. By scanning various exposures of the autoradiograms we found that specific transcription on the mutant fragment was about 5% of that of wild-type. Similar results were obtained by using various DNA concentrations (10-50 μg/ml in the assay) and DNA preparations (from both the fd103 and pBR322 recombinants).

The single-base-pair transversion (T to G) at position -29 in the 'TATA' box drastically decreases the efficiency of specific transcription of conalbumin DNA. This down-mutation, together with previous results Wasylyk *et. al.* (1980); Corden *et. al.* (1980) demonstrates that the 'TATA' box is an

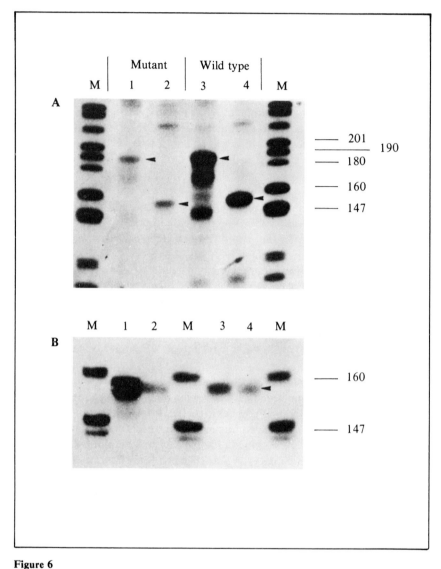

**Figure 6**

*In vitro* transcription of wild-type and mutant conalbumin gene DNA. The wild-type and mutant conalbumin DNA fragments were transcribed *in vitro* as described previously (Wasylyk *et.al.* 1980a). Lanes 1 and 3 transcription with 0.5 μg of mutant and wild-type Pst5-Pst6 fragment, respectively, lanes 2 and 4, 0.5 μg of mutant and wild-type Pst5-Pst6 fragments digested with Hae3, respectively (see Figure 2). (B) The RNA synthesised on Pst5-Pst6 fragment digested with Hae3 was electrophoresed on a 5% polyacrylammide-urea 40cm thin gel (0.3mm). Lane 1, RNA synthesised on the wild-type fragment; lanes 2 and 4, RNA synthesised on the mutant fragment; lane 3, one fifth of the amount of RNA run in lane 1. M, (32p)-labelled DNA size markers. The arrowheads point to the bands discussed in the text taken from Wasylyk *et.al.* 1980b.

important element for initiation of specific *in vitro* transcription. Therefore, it appears that the 'TATA' box fulfills at least one of the criteria used to define prokaryotic promoters. However, we cannot definitely conclude that the 'TATA' box is part of a eukaryotic promoter region because prokaryotic promoters were defined as regions of the DNA that are indispensable for initiation of transcription and to which RNA polymerase binds (see Rosenberg and Court 1979).

The 'TATA' box shares both sequence and functional homologies with the Pribnow box of prokaryotic promoters. Strikingly, all A-T to G-C base substitution in the Pribnow box are promoter-down mutations, and a G-C to A-T base substitution is a promoter-up mutation, suggesting that the Pribnow box mutations are exerting some effect on local DNA melting. However, because A-T to T-A base changes also influence transcription See Rosenberg and Court (1979); Siebenlist (1980) this is probably not the major effect.

These observations raise the question of whether the mutation we have constructed in the 'TATA' box prevents a similar DNA-opening event in eukaryotic transcription or decreases the affinity of RNA polymerase B or factor(s) in the S100 extract for this DNA sequence. Recently we have constructed a point mutation in the conalbumin 'TATA' box with an A instead of the second T (position -29). This is a down mutation which is transcribed even less than the equivalent 'TAGA' mutant. It is interesting that in 56 of 60 known 'TATA' sequences see Breathnach and Chambon (1981) in the third position there is a T, the remaining 4 have an A. These results suggest that this third nucleotide could be a site for some form of specific interaction, for example nucleotide-protein as in the prokaryotic system (B Wasylyk, unpublished results). In preliminary mixing experiments using crude S100 extracts, we have not been able to demonstrate any competition between wild-type and mutant conalbumin DNAs for factor(s) present in the *in vitro* transcription system. However, because we cannot rigorously prove that the DNA is in excess over essential factor(s) in the system, we cannot draw any firm conclusion about the mechanism by which the point mutations affect the efficiency of specific *in vitro* transcription of the conalbumin gene. Studies of the interaction of purified RNA polymerase B and factor(s) present in the S100 extract with the 'TATA' box region will be necessary to answer this question.

### The Role of the 'TATA' Box and other Sequences In Vivo

What is the *in vivo* relevance of the *in vitro* transcription studies? Does the 'TATA' box belong to the promoter region *in vivo* and is there more to the RNA polymerase B promoter than the 'TATA' box and the mRNA startsite? In agreement with the *in vitro* results, studies with sea-urchin histone H2A Grosschedl and Birnstiel (1980) and SV40 early genes Benoist and Chambon (1981); Gluzman *et.al.* (1980), deleted downstream from the 'TATA' box, have shown that the 5'-end of the novel mRNAs synthesised in *Xenopus* oocytes Grosschedl and Birnstiel (1980) or cells in culture Benoist and Chambon (1981); Gluzman *et. al.* (1980) always map about 25 nucleotides downstream from the 'TATA' box.

However, it has been demonstrated in several systems see-urchin histone H2A (Grosschedl and Birnstiel (1980a), SV40 early genes (Benoist and Chambon (1980, 1981), polyoma early genes (Bending *et. al.* (1980) that deletions of regions located around the mRNA startsite, and including the 'TATA' box, do not eliminate transcription *in vivo*. The new RNA species have heterogeneous 5'-ends Grosschedl and Birnstiel (1980); Benoist and Chambon (1981) which in the case of SV40 have been shown to correspond to the 5'-ends of the RNAs synthesised *in vitro* from the same deletion mutants Mathis and Chambon (1981), see above. In addition, there is evidence that sequences situated far upstream from the mRNA startsite are important for *in vivo* transcription of the histone H2A and SV40 early genes. Mutants of SV40 early genes Benoist and Chambon (1981) and the H2A gene Grosschedl and Birnstiel (1980a,b) with intact sequences around the mRNA startsites and 'TATA' boxes, but with deletions mapping more than 150bp upstream, have been constructed *in vitro* and introduced into cells in culture Benoist and Chambon (1981) or *Xenopus* oocytes Grosschedl and Birnstiel (1980a,b). There is very little, if any, *in vivo* transcription of these deletion mutants. Obviously, the interpretation of the results obtained *in vivo* with deletion mutants suffers from the same limitation as the corresponding *in vitro* transcription experiments, since a deletion is more than just the absence of a particular sequence (see above). In vivo experiments with base-substitution mutants constructed *in vitro* by site-directed mutagenesis are required to confirm the interpretation of the results obtained with the deletion mutants. However, if one assumes that none of the new sequences fused at the deletion endpoints of the various mutants affects positively or negatively the functional properties of the remaining wild-type sequence, it appears that the DNA sequences involved *in vivo* in the promotion of specific transcription of eukaryotic protein-coding genes could correspond to larger regions than their prokaryotic counterparts.

Taking together the limited amount of information available at the present time, it appears that at least two elements could be required *in vivo* for specific initiation of transcription at the mRNA start site. One element, which corresponds to the 'TATA' box region, would be involved in the mechanism directing RNA polymerase B to initiate transcription about 25bp downstream at the position corresponding to the 5'-end of the mRNA (the efficiency of initiation being influenced also by the actual DNA sequence around the mRNA startsite), and may correspond to a *sensu strictu* promoter site. In its absence, mRNAs with 5'-terminal sequence heterogeneity would be synthesised (see above). A second element would be located in a region located more than 100bp upstream and its absence would preclude transcription. It could be visualised as a region required to make the downstream sequences accessible to RNA polymerase. It may correspond to binding sites for proteins involved in positive control of transcription. It is also possible that this region is involved in the generation of an 'open', 'active', chromatin structure Mathis *et al.* (1980), since there is evidence that chromatin structure of both viral Wigmore *et.al.* (1980); Saragosti *et.al.* (1980) and refs. therein and cellular WU (1980); Stalder *et.al.* (1980) and refs. therein genes is modified in regions corresponding to their 5'-ends. Such a region would not be required for specific transcription in the *in vitro* cell-free systems, where there is no evidence that a chromatin structure is reconstituted Mathis and Chambon (1981). Alternatively (or in addition) the promoter site could consist of both the 'TATA' box and the indispensable sequence situated further upstream, to both of which the RNA polymerase would bind. In this alternative, a eukaryotic promoter region for RNA polymerase B should be viewed as a folded chromatin structure, since it is unlikely that RNA polymerase B could cover a 150bp linear stretch of DNA. In any case since the 'TATA' box is absent from some genes there should be other sequences which can dictate where transcription should start. In this respect it is worth recalling that in the absence of the 'TATA' box initiation occurs on SV40 early regions both *in vivo* and *in vitro* at multiple sites scattered over a broad area.

## Conclusion

With the development of cell free systems capable of accurate *in vitro* initiation of transcription, it has become possible to study the functional importance of the regions of homology which have been recognised by comparison of the DNA sequences of various genes. Such *in vitro* studies have led to the characterisation of a possible promoter region for RNA polymerase B. However, *in vivo* transcription studies performed by introduction of deletion mutants made *in vitro* into cells in culture or into *Xenopus* oocytes, indicates that the promoter region could be much larger in eukaryotic cells than in prokaryotes. One of the challenging problems for the future is to see to what extent the size of the promoter is related to chromatin structure and whether promoter regions should be viewed in eukaryotes as structures of higher order.

## Acknowledgements

We would like to thank C Wasylyk and C Hauss for excellent technical assistance. The work was supported by grants from the CNRS (ATPs 4160, 3907 and 3558), the INSERM (ATP 72.79.104), la Fondation pour la Recherche Medicale Francaise and la Fondation Simone et Cino del Duca.

208 CELLULAR CONTROLS IN DIFFERENTIATION

# References

Bendig, M.M., Thomas, T. and Folk, W.R. 1980 *Regulatory mutants of polyoma virus defective in DNA replication and the synthesis of early protein.* Cell, *20*, 401-409.

Benoist, C., O'Hare, K., Breathnach, R. and Chambon, P. 1980 *The ovalbumin gene - sequence of putative control regions.* Nucleic Acids Res. *8*, 127-142.

Benoist, C. and Chambon, P. 1980 *Deletions covering the putative promoter region of early mRNAs of simian virus 40 do not abolish T-antigen expression.* Proc. Natl. Acad. Sci. USA. *77*, 3865-3869.

Benoist, C. and Chambon, P. 1981 *The SV40 early promoter region: sequence requirements in vivo.* Nature in press.

Birkenmeier, E.H., Brown, D.D. and Jordan, E. 1978 *A nuclear extract of Xenopus laevis oocytes that accurately transcribes 5S RNA Genes.* Cell, *15*, 1077-1086.

Bogenhagen, D.F., Sakonju, S. and Brown, D.D. 1980 *A control region in the centre of the 5S RNA gene directs specific initiation of transcription: II. The 3' border of the region.* Cell, *19*, 27-35.

Breathnach, R. and Chambon, P. 1981 *Organisation and expression of eukaryotic protein-coding nuclear split genes.* In Ann. Rev. Biochem. *50*, in press.

Bujard, H. 1980 *The Interaction of E. coli RNA polymerase with promoters.* Tibs, 5, 274-278.

Chambon, P. 1975 *Eukaryotic nuclear RNA polymerases in Annual Review of Biochemistry, 44,* (ed. E.E. Snell, Boyer, P.D., Meister, A. and Richardson C.C.), pp 613-638.

Chambon, P. 1978 *The molecular biology of the eukaryotic genome is coming of age.* Cold Spring Harbor Symposia on Quantitative Biology vol. XLIII pp. 1209-1234.

Cochet, M., Gannon, F., Hen, R., Maroteaux, L., Perrin, F. and Chambon, P. 1979 *Organisation and sequence studies of the 17 piece chicken conalbumin gene.* Nature, *282*, 567-574.

Corden, J., Wasylyk, B., Buchwalder, A., Sassone-Corsi, P., Kedinger, C. and Chambon, P. 1980 Science, *209*, 1406-1414. *Promoter sequence of eukaryotic coding gene.*

Engelke, D.R., Ng, S.Y., Shastry, B.S. and Roeder, R.G. 1980 *Specific interaction of a purified transcription factor with an internal control region of 5S RNA genes.* Cell, *19*, 717-728.

Gannon, F, O'Hare, K., Perrin, F., LePennec, J.P., Benoist, C., Cochet, M., Breathnach, R., Royal, A., Garapin, A., Cami, B. and Chambon, P. 1979 Nature, *278*, 428-434.

Gillam, S. and Smith, M. 1979a *Site-specific mutagenesis using synthetic oligodeocyribonucleotide primers: I. Optimum conditions and minimum oligodeoxyribonucleotide length.* Gene, *8*, 81-97.

Gillam, S. and Smith, M. 1979b *Site-specific mutagenesis using synthetic oligodeoxyribonucleotide primers: II. In vitro selection of mutant DNA.* Gene, *8*, 99-106.

Gillam, S., Jahnke, P., Astell, C., Phillips. S., Hutchinson III, C.A., and Smith, M. 1979 *Defined transversion mutations at a specific position in DNA using synthetic oligodeoxyribonucleotides as mutagens.* Nucleic Acids. Res. *6*, 2973-2985.

Gluzman, Y., Sambrook, J.F., Frisque, R.J. 1980 *Expression of early genes of origin-defective mutants of simian virus 40.* Proc. Natl. Acad. Sci. *77*, 3898-3902.

Grosschedl, R. and Birnstiel, M.L. 1980a *Identification of regulatory sequences in the prelude sequences of an H2A histone gene by the study of specific deletion mutants in vivo.* Proc. Natl. Acad. Sci. *77*, 1432-1436.

Grosschedl, R. and Birnstiel, M.L. 1980b *Sopacer DNA sequences upstream of the TATAAATA sequence are essential for the promotion of H2A histone gene transcription in vivo.* Proc. Natl. Acad. Sci., in press.

Hu, S.L. and Manley, J.L. 1980 *Identification of the DNA sequence required for the initiation of transcription in vitro from the major late promoter of adenovirus 2.* Proc. Natl. Acad. Sci., in press.

Hutchinson III, C.A., Phillips, S. and Edgell, M.H. 1978 *Mutagenesis at a specific position in a DNA sequence.* J. Biol. Chem. *253*, 6551-6560.

Jacob, F., Ullman, A. and Monod, J. 1964 *Le promoteur, element genetique necessaire a l'expression d'un operon.* C.R. Acad. Sc. Paris. *258*, 3125-3128.

Konkel, D.A., Tilghman, S.M. and Leder, P. 1978 *The sequence of the chromosomal mouse °-globin major gene : homologies in capping, splicing and poly(A) sites.* Cell, *15*, 1125-1132.

Kressmann, A., Hofstetter, H., Di Capua, E., Grosschedl, R. and Birnstiel, M.L. 1979 *A tRNA gene of Xenopus laevis contains at least two sites promoting transcription.* Nucleic Acids Res. *7*, 1749-1763.

Losick, R. and Chamberlin, M., eds. *RNA polymerase* (1976) Cold Spring Harbor.

Manley, J.L., Fire, A., Cano, A., Sharp, P. and Gefter, M.L. 1980 *DNA-dependent transcription of adenovirus genes in a soluble whole-cell extract.* Proc. Natl. Acad. Sci. USA. *77*, 3855-3859.

Mathis, D., Oudet, P. and Chambon, P. 1980 *Structure of transcribing chromatin.* Prog. Nucleic Acid Res. & Mol. Biol. *24*, 1-55.

Mathis, D. and Chambon, P. 1981 *The TATA box of the SV40 early region, but not the upstream sequences, is required for accurate in vitro initiation of transcription.* Nature, in press.

McKnight, G.S. and Palmiter, R.D. 1979 *Transcriptional regulation of the ovalbumin and conalbumin genes by steroid hormones in chick oviduct.* J. Biol. Chem. *254*: 9050-9058.

Pelham, H.R.B. and Brown, D.D. 1980 *A specific transcription factor that can bind either the 5S RNA gene or 5S RNA.* Proc. Natl. Acad. Sci. USA. *77*, 4170-4174.

Perrin, F., Cochet, M., Gerlinger, P., Cami, B., LePennec, J.P., and Chambon, P. 1979 *The chicken conalbumin gene : studies of the organisation of cloned DNAs.* Nucleic Acids Res. *6*, 2731-1748.

Pribnow, D. 1975. *Nucleotide sequence of an RNA polymerase binding site at an early T7 promoter.* Proc. Natl. Acad. Sci. USA, *72*, 784-788.

Pribnow, D. 1975b *Bacteriophage T7 early promoters : nucleotide sequence of two RNA polymerase binding sites.* J. Mol. Biol. *99*, 419-443.

Razin, A., Hirose, T., Itakura, K. and Riggs, A.D. 1978 *Efficient correction of a mutation by use of chemically synthesised DNA.* Proc. Natl. Acad. Sci. USA. *75*, 4268-4270.

Roeder, R.G. 1976 *Eukaryotic nuclear RNA polymerases, in RNA polymerase* (eds. Losick, R. and Chamberlin, M.1 hp. 285-329 Cold Spring Harbor Laboratory.

Rosenberg, M. and Court, D. 1979 *Regulatory sequences involved in the promotion and termination of RNA transcription.* Ann. Rev. Genet. *13*, 319-353.

Saragosti, S., Moyne, G. and Yaniv, M. 1980. *Absence of nucleosomes in a fraction of SV40 chromatin between the origin of replication and the region coding for the late leader RNA.* Cell, *20*, 65-73.

Schaller, H., Gray, C. and Herrman, K. 1975 *Nucleotide sequence of an RNA polymerase binding site from the DNA of bacteriophage fd.* Proc. Natl. Acad. Sci. USA. *72*, 737-741.

Siebenlist, U., Simpson, R.B. and Gilbert, W. 1980 *E. coli RNA polymerase interacts homologously with two different promoters.* Cell, *20*, 269-281.

Sakonju, S., Bogenhagen, D.F. and Brown, D.D. 1980 *A control region in the centre of the 5S RNA gene directs specific initiation of transcription: I. the 5' border of the region.* Cell, *19*, 13-25.

Sollner-Webb, B. and Reeder, R.H. 1979 *The nucleotide sequence of the initiation and termination sites for ribosomal RNA transcription in X. laevis.* Cell, *18*, 485-499.

Stalder, J., Larsen, A., Engel, J.D., Dolan, M., Groudine, M. and Weintraub, H. 1980 *Tissue-specific DNA cleavages in the globin chromatin domain introduced by DNAaseI.* Cell, *20*, 451-460.

Wasylyk, B., Kedinger, C., Corden, J., Vrison, O. and Chambon, P. 1980a *Specific in vitro initiation of transcription on conalbumin and ovalbumin genes and comparison with adenovirus-2 early and late genes.* Nature, *285*, 388-390.

Wasylyk, B., Derbyshire, R., Guy, A., Molko, D., Roget, A., Teoule, R. and Chambon, P. 1980b *Specific in vitro transcription of conalbumin gene is drastically decreased by single-point mutation in TATA box homology sequence.* Proc. Natl. Acad. Sci. USA, *77*, in press.

Weil, P.A., Luse, D.S., Segall, J. and Roeder, R.G. 1979 *Selective and accurate initiation of transcription at the Ad2 major late promoter in a soluble system dependent on purified RNA polymerase II and DNA.* Cell, *18*, 469-484.

Wigmore, D.J., Eaton, R. and Scott, W.A. 1980 *Endonuclease-sensitive regions in SV40 chromatin from cells infected with duplicated mutants.* Virology, *104*, 462-473.

Wu, C. 1980 *The 5' ends of Drosophila heat shock genes in chromatin are hypersensitive to DNaseI.* Nature, *286*, 854-860.

Wu, G.J. 1978 *Adenovirus DNA-directed trans cription of 5.5 S RNA in vitro.* Proc. Natl. Acad. Sci. USA, *75*, 2175-2179.

Ziff, E.B., Evans, R.M. 1978 *Coincidence of the promoter and capped 5' terminus of RNA from the adenovirus 2 major late transcription unit.* Cell, *15*, 1463-1475.

## Questions

*Sager*

I would like to ask you about your last slide. This has to do with the question of how many bases you can actually delete in the region between the TATA box and the regulatory site. Is there something that is counting the number of nucleotides along there or is it the position of that box upstream or is it its distance that is important?

*Wasylyk*

If you delete sequences downstream from the TATA box there is always a fixed initiation about 30 nucleotides downstream. Now, if you delete the TATA box you always get the same series of initiation sites and they always seem to be at a fixed distance from the point at which you have made the deletion. So it is difficult to interpret because the initiation sites are over a region here of over 200 nucleotides, yet they are always at a fixed distance from the point at which we have made the deletion. It is difficult to know what is directing the sequences *in vivo*. So I will interpret your question that way: what is actually directing initiation when there is no longer the TATA box

*Sager*

What I am really asking you is how many bases can you delete going upstream from the TATA box to this regulatory site which you are inferring is about 100 bases up. Can you delete a lot of material in that region?

*Wasylyk*

You can delete three-quarters of one of the repeats and still get T antigen expression and this deletes everything; the TATA box, the triple repeat and then all you have is one repeat and part of another. So you can delete almost everything.

*Sager*

And you do not replace it with anything. So that the distance has actually been changed.

*Wasylyk*

The distance has actually been changed but you still get this multiple initiation site which to me (it is not my work but it is the way I would interpret it) means that all of this region is actually open and these just happen to be sites which are somehow recognised in a non-specific way but it is always the same sites, it is always the same sequence in this region to code initiation of transcription. In other words, there could be levels of controls. The first level which is the upstream site and then once the region of DNA has been opened then the subset of sites - the TATA box - could be then involved in directing initiation to where exactly it should start.

*Lodish.*

I was wondering if you could comment on the efficiency of various *in vitro* systems. I am concerned about the amount of message or message-like RNA that you make per DNA and how that would reflect on the quantitative effects some of the deletion mutants you have made. How efficient is the system at best?

*Wasylyk*

We have looked at this very carefully and we find that the amount of RNA made is about 1% of that which you would make on single stranded DNA under the same assay conditions. In other words, it is only 1% of the capability of RNA polymerase to make RNA initiating just anywhere. Now, what this means, the extract we use which makes the transcription specific contains many factors and it is very obvious that the moment you can start purifying the system you remove DNA-binding proteins, for example, and other factors. So in this sense, yes we should interpret the results *in vitro* carefully. We should repeat all these experiments once we have the purified factors in the system. Then we probably would not do the same experiments anyway.

*Lodish*

More specifically, is there any reason for believing that what limits the *in vitro* transcription system is the same entity that limits transcription in the cell or looking at it another way, is the reason for believing that indication which reduces *in vitro* transcription by a certain amount would also have that effect in the cell. Any experiments on that?

*Wasylyk*
We are doing that at the moment. It is an obvious possibility that the *in vitro* system just reflects part of the control *in vivo* - this is true of any *in vitro* system.

*Questioner*
Are those initiation sites, the ones you see by your *in vitro* assay, the ones that you designate by arrows there?

*Wasylyk*
Yes, in fact they are - they are exactly the same.

*Questioner*
No, are those obtained by *in vitro* analysis or are they obtained *in vivo?*

*Wasylyk*
These were obtained by *in vivo*, I didn't describe the results obtained *in vitro* using the same deletion mutants, but the answer is that the same (or very close to the same) sites are used by the *in vitro* system. But there is one difference: that is *in vitro* it is the TATA box of the SV40 early region that is important for the initiation of transcription. In other words, if you make mutants from upstream, going down to the TATA box, DNAs which are no longer expressed *in vivo* make correct RNA *in vitro*. So, it seems that the upstream sequences just do not have any role *in vitro* and this could be one of the regulations which are missing *in vitro*.

*Questioner*
One other thing, do you know anything about steroid binding to either of the conalbumin or the ovalbumin genes? Have you done any binding studies with

hormone receptors to these clonal DNAs especially considering the possibility of regulatory sites in SV40?

*Wasylyk*
Yes, one thing we noticed immediately when we started *in vitro* transcription was that ovalbumin was transcribed a lot less than conalbumin and we knew that conalbumin was transcribed constitutively in the liver and that ovalbumin was less transcribed. So we supposed that by adding oestrogen receptor, for example, if we were lucky we could increase the amount of trans cription of ovalbumin compared to conalbumin, and we tried these experiments for a long time and we cannot observe any effect of hormones *in vitro*. So there is no regulation *in vitro* of genes which are normally regulated by hormones *in vivo*.

*Questioner*
How do you select for mutants containing mutations in the TATA box?

*Wasylyk*
Well, if you can generate restriction sites, then if you make the point mutation *in vitro* you can select the mutant, otherwise you just have to sequence and this is a lot of work. This was a convenient source of generating a restriction site by the first mutation we made and then in the next step we could localise the mutation over its nick, to that restriction site.

*Hunt*
What happens if you reconstruct these plasmids into proper mini- chromosomes and then add them into the assay - do they work then?

*Wasylyk*
We have not done those experiments but people have tried. What I can say is that there is no chromatin structure in the *in vitro* system. In other words, the *in vitro* system does not reconstitute chromatin. There are relaxing enzymes; you can

show that all the DNA is relaxed and is in intact, relaxed circles. So in other words, there cannot be any nucleosomes. Then you could say that since it is only 1% of the DNA that has been transcribed - maybe it is that 1% that has chromatin structure. So it is not clear - probably not.

# Distribution and Regulation of Histone H1° in Rodents

*Harvey Eisen R Gjerset and S Hasthorpe*

## Introduction

Although it is generally accepted that the regulation of genetic expression in eukaryotes occurs at the level of the chromatin, little is yet known about the mechanisms involved. This is in part due to fact that chromatin structure is complex and as yet not understood. The core histones (histones 2a, 2b, 3 and 4) have been shown to play a structural role in chromatin, but do not appear to play an obvious role in regulation (Kornberg 1977). The precise role of the H1 histones is not known although they are thought to play a role in determining the higher order structure of the chromatin. The fact that the H1 composition of chromatin varies from tissue to tissue is suggestive of a regulatory role for this family of proteins. Another group of high abundance chromatin proteins, the HMG's (14 and 17) have been shown to be preferentially associated with those regions of the chromatin which are active or potentially active in transcription where their presence confers an increased sensitivity to nuclease digestion (Goodwin *et.al.* 1973; Weisbroud and Weintraub 1979).

*In vitro* systems permitting the accurate and faithful transcription of eukaryotic DNA have been described (Weil *et.al.* 1979; Wasylyk *et.al.* 1980). However the DNA sequences necessary for *in vitro* transcription do not appear to be identical to those required for transcription *in vivo*, and as yet no regulation has been demonstrated *in vitro*. This is not surprising considering the complexity of chromatin. As yet no systems are available for the transcription of chromatin *in vitro*.

Since its discovery (Panyim and Chalkley 1969), the protein H1° has been studied in several laboratories. The distribution and properties of this protein suggest that it may play a role in the regulation of cell proliferation and/or differentiation in mammals.

## The Histone H1°

H1° has been characterised as a very lysine rich histone found mostly in adult mammalian tissues showing little or no cell division (Panyim and Chalkley

1969). The protein purified from ox or mouse liver has been shown to be composed of two polypeptides of identical molecular weight (25000 daltons) but which differ slightly in charge (Smith and Johns 1980a; Gjerset et. al. 1981). The two polypeptides give similar fingerprints after treatment with a variety of proteases and have identical antigenic properties. Although the amino acid composition of H1[0] is similar to that of H1, sequence analysis has shown that the protein is more closely related to histone H5 of avian erythrocytes (Smith et.al. 1980). There is also extensive immunological cross reaction between H1[0] and H5 (unpublished results).

While it is agreed that H1[0] is located on the linked regions of the chromatin there is some disagreement as to whether it is preferentially localised in the active or inactive regions. Smith and Johns (1980b) have demonstrated the presence of a 25K protein on mononucleosomes released from brain nuclei after mild micrococcal nuclease digestion. However similar experiments with rat and mouse liver and with tissue culture cells indicate that the H1[0] is preferentially localised in the fractions which are more resistant to nuclease (Gorka and Lawrence 1979; Keppel et.al. 1979; Gjerset et.al. 1981). It has also been shown to be enriched in DNAase I resistant fractions of mouse liver chromatin.

The presence of H1[0] in mammals appears to be regulated in a rather complex fashion. Most of the solid adult tissues contain relatively large amounts of the protein (7-40% of the very lysine rich histone; Verrichio 1977; Piha and Volkonen 1979). The protein has been shown to appear in the liver after birth and in the pancreas where its appearance followed the arrest of cell proliferation. It has also been shown to decrease in regenerating liver and pancreas (Marsh and Fitzgerald 1973; Benjamin 1971; Gorka, et.al. 1981). In the case of regenerating liver the decrease in H1[0] content followed the onset of DNA synthesis, and is temporally coordinate with the appearance of such foetal specific functions as $\alpha$-foetoprotein and type 3 pyruvate dehydrogenase.

H1[0] has been shown to accumulate in several cell types in culture when they are induced to differentiate. These include mouse Friend virus-transformed erythroleukaemia cells (EL cells), mouse teratocarcinoma, mouse neuroblastoma, mouse melanoma, mouse myeloid leukaemia and rat adrenal cortex (Eisen et.al. 1980). In the case of FL cells variants which do not terminate their differentiation and do not synthesise H1[0] (IP25) have been described, indicating that at least in this case the induction of H1[0] is linked to the differentiation of the cells (Keppel et.al. 1977). It has also been shown that treatment of many cell types in vitro with butyric acid results in the accumulation of H1[0] (Eisen et.al. 1980; d'Anna et.al. 1980). Finally it has been demonstrated that confluent cultures of HeLa cells and mouse neuroblastoma accumulate H1[0] (Pehrson and Cole 1980).

Most work on the distribution and regulation of H1[0] in mammalian tissues has been done by biochemical extraction of lysine rich proteins and analysis by gel electrophoresis. While this procedure gives the overall content of the protein in various tissues, it does not give information on the cellular distribution of the protein or on tissues too small to be analysed. We have thus approached these problems by preparing monospecific antibodies to mouse H1⁰ and examining its distribution in various tissues by indirect immunofluorescence using either frozen sections or cell smears (Gjerset et. al. 1981b). Combining this technique and classical biochemical techniques the following questions have been approached:

1) Is there cellular heterogeneity in the distribution of H1⁰ within a given tissue, and if so does presence of the protein correlate with specific functions expressed by the positive cells?

2) How is H1⁰ regulated during development and in adult animals?

3) What is the distribution of H1⁰ in chromosomes?

**Procedures**

Mouse liver or kidney H1⁰ and H1 were purified as described (Gjerset et.al. 1981a). Antisera were made in rabbits and indirect immunofluorescent staining was performed as described previously (Eisen et.al. 1980). Frozen sections of various mouse and rat organs were cut with a Slee cryostat. Sections were rapidly air dried, fixed for 20 minutes with 4% formaldehyde in PBS, rinsed with PBS, incubated in 0.25% Triton X100 (in PBS) and stored in PBS until stained.

Tissue culture cells were grown in Dubelcco's modified minimal essential medium unless otherwise indicated. For immunofluorescent staining the cells were grown on coverslip or cytocentrifuged and fixed as described above.

Metaphase chromosomes were prepared from colcemid treated cells of clone F4N+2 (Keppel et.al. 1977) grown in the presence of 1.5% dimethyl sulphoxide. The cells were swollen in 0.056 N KCl and then fixed by washing three times in methanol at −20C. They were then resuspended at a cell density of $10^6$/ml in cold methanol and acetic acid was added to a final concentration of 1.5%. The fixed cells were immediately spread on cold dry slides and rapidly dried. They were then formaldehyde fixed and stored in PBS until they were stained.

*Localisation of H1⁰ on Chromatin*

In order to determine whether or not H1⁰ is evenly distributed on chromosomes as in H1 we have stained metaphase chromosomes from cells of strain F4N+2, a defective FL cell variant which grows continually in the presence of inducers of erythroid differentiation. The cells continue to produce H1⁰ under these conditions. The stained chromosomes can be seen in Figure 1. The H1⁰ appears to be distributed in bands and is present on all the chromosomes but not in the centromeres. The pattern of banding is different from that obtained

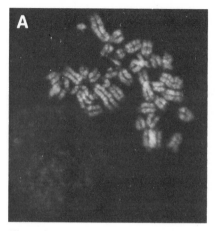
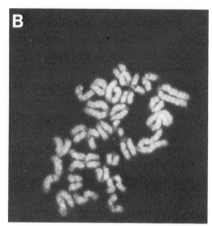

**Figure 1**
Metaphase chromosomes of F4N2 stained with anti H1⁰ serum.

with other techniques such as giemsa or quinocrine staining. We do not know whether this banding pattern represents the accessibility of the antigen or the actual distribution of the $H1^0$ . However since $H1^0$ and H1 have similar localisation on the chromatin and since staining with anti H1 serum gives a uniform pattern it seems likely that the banding seen with anti-$H1^0$ reflects its distribution on the chromatin.

## Tissue and Cellular Distribution of $H1^0$ in Mouse

In order to determine the cellular distribution of $H1^0$ in various mouse tissues, frozen sections were made and analysed by immunofluorescent staining. Sections were also stained with normal rabbit serum to control for auto-fluorescence and with rabbit anti-H1 antiserum to control for false negativity due to failure of antibodies to penetrate the tissues. Table 1 shows a summary of the results. All tissues contain $H1^0$ positive cells. However the proportion of positive cells varies from less than 0.1% in thymus to 80-100% in liver and kidney. With the exception of liver and kidney most tissues examined show cellular heterogeneity for $H1^0$. We have thus far not identified all of the cell types which are positive for $H1^0$, but some indication of the specificity of the protein can be seen from the following examples. Figure 2 shows sections of the cerebellum and hippocampus of adult mouse brain. In the cerebellum it can be seen that the granular cells and stellate cells are positive for $H1^0$ while the purkinje cells appear to contain little or none of the protein. In the hippocampus, $H1^0$ appears to be localised in the pyramidal cells but as can be seen in Figure 1b, not all of the cells are positive. Figure 3a shows a section of adult mouse retina where it can be seen that gangliar cells and the bipolar layer of nuclei contain $H1^0$ while the sensory cell nuclei do not have detectable

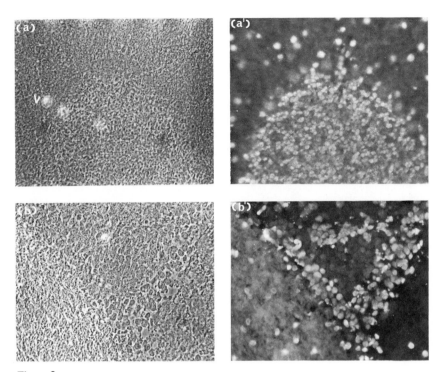

**Figure 2**

Areas of mouse brain stained with anti H1⁰ serum.

a) Cerebellum of adult (9 weeks);

b) Cross-section of hippocampus of adult. Photographs on left are phase contrast. Photograph on right are corresponding fluorescence.

amounts. In testis (Figure 3b) only the interstitial cells (Leydig) contain H1⁰. It seems clear from the remarkable cellular distribution of H1⁰ that its role must be complex.

In tissues showing high cellular turnover the distribution of H1⁰ is different from that seen in solid tissues. Bone marrow contains very few H1⁰ positive cells (0.1-0.3%) none of which has been identified (Wisen *et.al.* 1980). Adult spleen contains 1-3% H1⁰ positive cells amongst which we have tentatively identified the majority which appear to share all known surface antigens with natural killer cells. That these are natural killer cells or their precursors is supported by the finding that spleens from nude mice contain 10-30% H1⁰ positive cells. In thymus H1⁰ was only detected in epithelial cells (Roberts, Waksal and Eisen, unpublished).

In skin and lens, H1⁰ is not present in the undifferentiated stem cells but appears in the post-mitotic cells which are beginning to undergo their terminal differentiation. As shown in Figure 4, H1⁰ is present in a proportion of cells in the peribasal layer while H1 is present in these cells and those of the basal layer. The finding that not all of cells of the differentiating layers of skin have $H1^0$ is puzzling. It is possible that the protein appears only once the cells have begun their differentiation or that it is induced transiently. In lens all of the nucleated fibre cells are positive, as are their post-mitotic precursors.

In the erythropoietic lineage the distribution of $H1^0$ is different depending on the developmental stage of the animal. Embryonic erythrocytes which remain nucleated are strongly positive for $H1^0$. However in the adult, mature erythroid precursors (which can be identified from the pre-globin stage to the normoblast by using antibodies directed to spectrin) do not contain detectable quantities of the protein. This is rather surprising since differentiating FL cells which

**Table 1**
Cellular distribution of H1 and $H1^0$ in various mouse tissues

| Tissue | Cell type | Adult H1 | Adult $H1^0$ | 15 day embryo H1 | 15 day embryo $H1^0$ | 9 day embryo H1 | 9 day embryo $H1^0$ |
|---|---|---|---|---|---|---|---|
| Brain | Neuronal | + | 80% + | + | 5-10% + | | |
| | Glial | + | only cells in optic tract + | | | | |
| | Ganglion | + | + | + | — | | |
| Retin+ | Bipolar | + | + | | | | |
| | Sensory | + | | | | | |
| Lens | Epithelial | + | + | + | — | | |
| | Fiber | + | + | + | + | | |
| Liver | Hepatocytes | + | + | + | 10-15% + | | |
| Kidney | Tubule | + | + | | | | |
| | Glomerulus | + | ±(weakly +) | | | | |
| Muscle | Striated | + | + | + | — | | |
| | Total cells | + | 1-3% + | | | | |
| | T-lymphocytes | + | — | | | | |
| Spleen | B-lymphocytes | + | — | | | | |
| | Erythroblasts | + | — | | | | |
| Bone marrow | | + | 0.1-0.3% | | | | |
| | | 80% | | | | | |
| | Thymocytes | + | — | | | | |
| Thymus | Epithelium | + | + | | | | |
| | germ line | + | — | | | | |
| Testis | Sertoli | + | — | | | | |
| | Leydig | + | + | | | | |
| Foetal erythrocytes | | | | | | | |

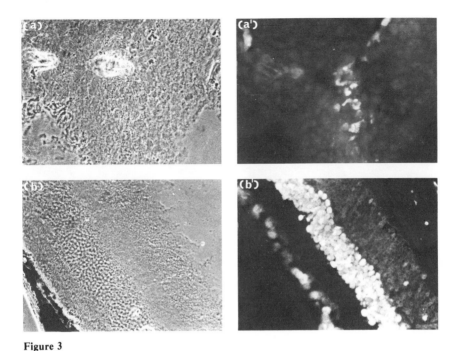

**Figure 3**
a) Adult mouse retina and
b) mouse testis stained with anti H1° serum. Left, phase contrast; right fluorescence.

undergo what appears to be a normal erythroid differentiation accumulate it. We do find the protein in colonies formed *in vitro* by early erythroid precursor cells and its appearance is dependent on the addition of both erythropoietin and burst promoting activity (BPA). These colonies are identified by the fact that they contain haemoglobinised cells. However the H1° containing cells in the colonies are haemoglobin negative. These results suggest that the H1° is appearing in erythroid precursor cells in response to erythropoietin and that it disappears in the more mature cells. This disappearance could be due either to the active removal of the protein or to its dilution through subsequent cell division. The difference between adult and embryonic erythroid cells could be explained by postulating that in the case of the embryo there are fewer cell divisions between the cells in which the H1° is synthesised and the mature erythrocyte.

*Developmental Regulation*
In those cases thus far examined the presence of H1° in cells of solid tissues is linked to their state of maturation. It has been shown that H1° appears in both developing liver and pancreas after birth and after proliferation has ceased. In the case of liver the appearance of H1° is coordinate with the shut-off of foetal

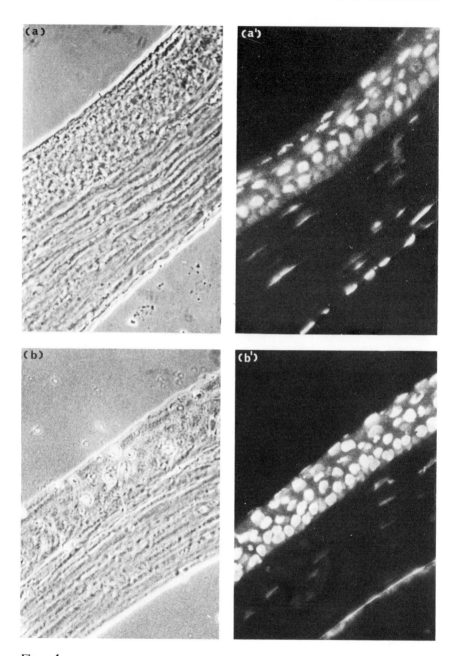

**Figure 4**
Adult mouse cornea stained with
a) anti Hl;
b) anti $H1^0$ ; left, phase contrast; right fluorescence.

functions such as foetoprotein and type 3 pyruvate kinase, and the full expression of albumin. In brain, while most of the neurons of the cortex are arrested at the post-mitotic stage of the cell cycle at birth, they do not contain detectable amounts of $H1^0$. The protein does not appear to be fully present until 3-5 weeks after birth, suggesting that its appearance may be correlated with the maturation of the cells. The same behaviour is seen in the retina where $H1^0$ appears in the ganglion and bipolar cells only after eyes have been opened, even though these cell types are post-mitotic several days earlier. In the retina the signal for $H1^0$ appearance seems to be light since it does not appear in animals maintained in the dark from the time of birth.

$H1^0$ appearance is also linked to cell maturation in skeletal muscle. We are unable to detect it in myotubes of 15 days embryos which are not yet innervated. It accumulates in muscle between birth and three weeks, during which time stable neuro-muscular junctions are formed. It is also interesting that $H1^0$ does not appear in myotubes formed in primary cultures of newborn mouse myoblasts. It is possible that in this case the signal for $H1^0$ accumulation is the formation of stable synapses.

*Hormonal Regulation*
We have examined the expression of $H1^0$ in adult glands, which depend on hormones for their maintenance and function. In all cases the glands were examined before and after surgical removal of the source of the maintenance hormone. It can be seen that for thyroid, adrenal cortex and testis (Leydig cells) hypophysectomy resulted in loss of $H1^0$ within three days. Castration resulted in the loss of $H1^0$ from prostate (Figure 5). Furthermore reinjection of the maintenance hormone for a given four days after its removal resulted in the reappearance of $H1^0$ in that gland within four days. This is shown for prostate in Figure 5. These experiments were done before tissue atrophy could be detected in the glands, and no changes could be detected in the levels of H1. However if castrated mice were left for two weeks before reinjection of testoterone, $H1^0$ could not be detected until the prostate had reached its normal size.

*The Possible Role of $H1^0$*
The findings reported here and by others raise several interesting questions about the possible role of $H1^0$ in mammals. When present in cells it is a major constituent of the chromatin where it has been suggested that it partially replaces H1 (Smith and Johns 1980). It is not present in all cells of a given tissue but rather in specific cell types. It appears in cells of tissues with little cell turnover when the cells are fully mature. In tissues or lineages with high cell turnover it appears in precursors which are beginning their terminal differentiation. Finally, in glands which depend on hormones for their maintenance and activity, the presence of $H1^0$ is strictly dependent on the action of the

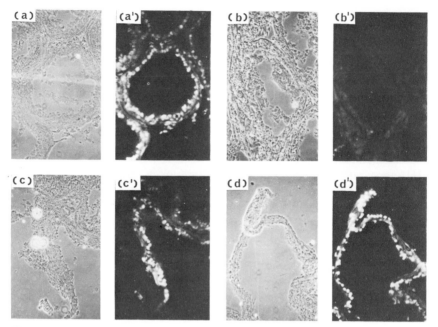

**Figure 5**
Adult mouse prostate stained with anti H1 and anti H1⁰ serum.
a a') normal prostate, anti H1⁰
b b') prostate 4 days after castration, anti H1⁰
c c') prostate 4 days after castration anti H1
d d') prostate 4 days after castration followed by testerone injection for 3 days anti H1⁰

hormone. These results suggest that H1⁰ may play a role in the final stages of the differentiation process. It might, for example, act as a 'lock' in fully differentiated cells, maintaining some inactive regions of the chromatin in a quiescent or condensed state. In tissues where H1⁰ appears before the cells are mature this appearance coincides with the transition from dividing, determined (but not differentiated) cells to terminally differentiated cells. In these cases the H1⁰ could be performing the same role as in fully mature cells of solid tissues. In other words it could again be acting as a lock on inactive chromatin when the developmental program for the terminal differentiation is switched on. It could also be playing a role in the switch.

It has also been suggested that the role of H1⁰ is to block cell proliferation (Panyim and Chalkley 1969; Marsh and Fitzgerald 1978; Marks *et.al.* 1976). Our results and those of others indicate that if this is the case the effect must be indirect rather than direct. Thus far in all cases where the appearance of H1⁰ has been examined in relation to cell proliferation or DNA synthesis, it has been found to occur after the arrest of proliferation. In regenerating rat liver the cells begin to synthesis DNA before any decrease in the level of H1⁰ can be detected. Also some FL cell variants which contain large amounts of the protein grow quite well. These results suggest that the presence of H1⁰ does not prevent proliferation. They do not rule out the possibility that H1⁰ plays a role in preventing the expression of genes whose products are necessary for proliferation.

The regulation of H1⁰ also appears to be perturbed in tumours of tissues whose cells normally contain the protein (Lea *et.al.* 1974; Marks *et.al.* 1975). For example it has reported that the relative contents of H1⁰ in rat hepatomas is inversely proportional to their growth rates and similar results have been reported for human hyperplastic thyroid. These findings have been used to support the hypothesis that H1⁰ plays a role in the regulation of proliferation. However, in general, hyperplastic tissue and tumours also tend to de-differentiate. For this reason it is difficult to distinguish between a correlation of H1⁰ and proliferation or differentiation.

In the case of the FL cells the perturbation of H1⁰ expression appears to be qualitative rather than quantitative. In differentiating FL cells H1⁰ appears coordinately with the erythrocyte specific membrane protein spectrin (Keppel *et.al.* 1977, Eisen *et.al.* 1978). However, *in vivo*, H1⁰ cannot be detected in spectrin containing cells. Our indirect evidence suggests that H1⁰ is present in a more primitive cell of the erythroid lineage, indicating that its synthesis is out of phase in the leukaemic cells. If in fact the protein is playing a role in switching on the genetic programm for the terminal differentiation as we have suggested, it is possible that its synthesis is a target in the transformation of the normal cells.

Thus far all attempts to ascribe a biological role to H1⁰ have been based on correlations. It is clear that more work is required in order to establish causal relationship between the appearance of the protein and *in vivo* phenomena.

## References

Benjamin, W.B. (1971) Nature, *234*, 18-21.

D'Anna, J.A., Gurley, L.R., Becker, R.R., Barham, S.S. and Tobey, R.A., (1980). Biochem, *19*, 4331-4341.

Eisen, H., Keppel, F., Georgopoulos, C.P., Sassa, S.,Granick, J., Pragnell, I. and Ostertag, W. (1978). *In Differentiation of Normal and Neoplastic Haemopoietic Cells.* Ed. Till, J., Clarkson, B. and Marks, P. Cold Spring Harbor Press. pp 277-293.

Eisen, H., Hasthorpe, S., Gjerset, R., Nasi, S. and Keppel, F. (1980). In *In vivo and in vitro Erythropoiesis : The Friend System.* G.B. Rossi Ed. Elsevier Press pp 289-296.

Gjerset, R., Ibarrondo, F., Saragosti, S. and Eisen, H. (1981) Biochem Biophys. Res. Commun. in press.

Gjerset, R., Gorka, C., Hasthorpe, S., Ibbarando, F., Lawrence, J.J. and Eisen, H. (1981b). Proc. Natl. Acad. Sci. U.S.A. submitted.

Goodwin, G.H., Sanders, C. and Johns, E.W. (1973). Eur. J. Biochem., *38*, 14-19.

Gorka, C. and Lawrence, J.J. (1979). Nuc. Acids Res. *7*, 347-359.

Keppel, F., Allet, B. and Eisen, H., (1977). Proc. Natl. Acad. Sci. U.S.A. *74*, 653-656.

Keppel, F., Allet, B. and Eisen, H. (1979). Fed. Proc. *32*, 2119-2135.

Kornberg, R.D. (1977). Ann. Rev. Biochem. *46*, 931-954.

Lea, M.A., Youngsworth, L.A. and Morris, H.P. (1974). Biochem. Biophys. Res. Commun. *58*, 862-867.

Marks, D.B., Kanefsky, J., Keller, B.J. and Marks, A.O. (1975). Cancer Res. *35*, 886-889.

Marsh, W.H. and Fitzgerald, P. (1973). Fed. Proc. *32*, 2119-2135.

Panyim, S. and Chalkey, R. (1969). Biochem. Biophys. Res. Commun. *37*, 1042-1049.

Pehron, J. and Cole, R.D. (1980). Nature, *285*, 43-44.

Piha, R.S. and Walkonen, K.H. (1979). FEBS Letters, *108*, 326-329.

Smith, B.J. and Johns, E.W. (1980). FEBS Letters, *110*, 25-29.

Smith, B.J. and Johns, E.W. (1980). Nuc. Acids Res. *8*, 6069-6079.

Smith, B.J., Walker, J.M. and Johns, E.W. (1980) FEBS Letters, *112*, 42-44.

Varrichio, F. (1977). Arch. Biochem. Biophys. *179*, 715-717.

Waslyk, R., Derbyshire, A.G., Mollo, A., Roget, R., Reoule, R. and Chambon, P. (1980). PNAS, *77*, 7024-7028.

Weil, P.A., Luse, D.S., Segall, J. and Roeder, R.G. (1979). Cell, *18*, 469-484.

Weisbroud, S. and Weintraub, H. (1979). Proc. Natl. Acad. Sci. U.S.A. *76*, 630-634.

## Questions

*Higgins*

Can I ask you more about the prostate's response to removal of steroid and then adding of steroid? I think you implied that $H_1^0$ would re-appear after you gave testosterone during the proliferative phase.

*Eisen*

No.

*Higgins*

In other words, what I am saying, does it come back at the time when you see the response of major tissue-specific antigen dependent proteins or is it after that?

*Eisen*

It comes back after. If you wait two weeks before you re- inject testosterone, $H_1^0$ does not appear until the organ has attained its size. So it is not simply coming back as a response to testosterone but it seems to require the organ to attain its normal size before it comes back. If you inject after short periods when there is no proliferation then it comes back immediately.

*Higgins*

So it is not correlated with the turn-on and turn-off of the antigen-dependence?

*Eisen*

No.

*Bradbury*

If I can just make a comment on the molecule itself. The class of very lysine rich histones $H_1$ consists of three structural domains;

1) a variable, basic N-terminal region (1-39)
2) a conserved globular central region (39-116) and
3) a variable, basic C-terminal region (116-216).

In avian, fish, reptile and amphibian erythrocytes, histone $H_1$ is largely, but not completely, replaced by another class of very lysine rich histones called $H_5$, which is thought to be responsible for the overall suppression of genetic activity of these cells. Although there are substantial sequence differences between $H_1$ and $H_5$, the shape of $H_5$ is very similar to that of $H_1$ except that the N-terminal domain is only 20 residues long. It is significant that the size of the central globular region of $H_5$ is similar to that of $H_1$, although there is only 49% sequence homology. In view of the functional differences between $H_1$ and $H_5$ considerable interest attaches to a recent finding that an earlier observed type of mammalian $H_1$, called $H_1$, has an apolar region which shows considerable sequence homology (70%) with the central globular region of $H_5$. Conformational studies of $H_1$ show that it also has a central globular region of 80 residues with an internal structure similar to that of $H_5$.

$H_1$ and $H_5$ bind to the nucleosome at the entry and exit points of the DNA through their globular regions, and 'seal off' two turns of DNA. It is almost certain that histone $H_1$ has the same mode of binding. This is shown in the figure where the globular structures of $H_1$, $H_1$ and $H_5$ are shown to have the same shape, although the internal structures of $H_1$ and $H_5$ differ from that of $H_1$. A question of major interest relates to the binding strengths of these apolar globular regions to the nucleosome.

*Eisen*

I do not think you can define this one well as you can define $H_1$, because if you put it on trimmed nucleosomes and not the non-trimmed nucleosome and now ask about the sensitivity of these nucleosomes to micrococcal nuclease then with $H_1$ you get the outer regions which are very sensitive. When you look at the $H_1^0$ in the same experiment we do not seem to get that - we get (--) change in the initial rate and then it becomes resistant. And we do not know what to make of this yet. It might be that this is covering more than just the adjacent region; it might be - we just do not know this.

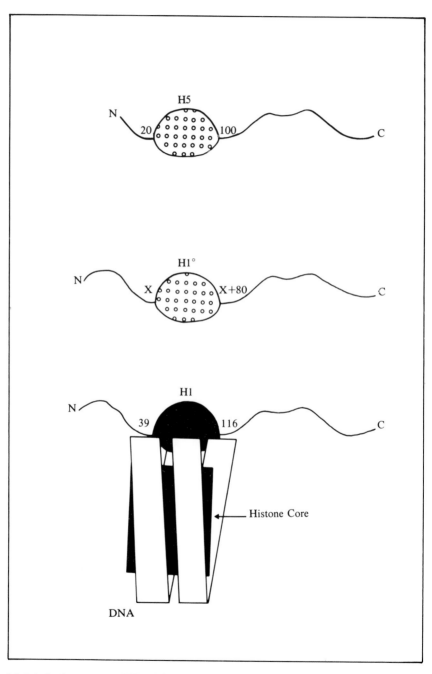

Models for the structure of H1, H1° and H5 and their probable binding site on the nucleosome (taken from Cary *et.al*).

*Bennett*

Do you have any information as to whether there is any difference in the binding pattern given by $H_1^0$ in the same cells and in different cell types which contain it?

*Eisen*

The problem for us, in culture, is that firstly, *in vivo* we cannot do the experiment because we do not see any cells that are dividing. In culture, we have looked at several cell lines where we induce the protein and we do see similarities. The problem is that we see many more differences, but we do not know whether those differences are due to rearrangements within the chromosome or due to something specific. From cell to cell (within the Friend cell) then that pattern seems to be constant but we have looked at neuroblastoma, we have looked at 3T3 fibroblasts, we have looked at mastocytoma cells and the problem is knowing what corresponds to what and we are not good enough yet to do that.

*Questioner*

Is there much species difference in this protein, antigenically or structurally?

*Eisen*

Structurally no; antigenically, yes. The immunology is not quite as straight forward as may be I have presented. The protein only seems to have to or three antigenic sites on it. Even though you can get very high titre antibody, with high affinity, it does not precipitate and so we get little cross-reactivity between antibody we have made to mouse and beef, for example, or in human. There is some cross-reactivity but it is not enough to work with. So we are just in the process of making antibodies to them all. We have made monoclonal antibodies and the only ones that cross-react well turn out to be specific for poly-L-lysine.

*Wolpert*

It would be very interesting to know just how the appearance or disappearance of your protein on the system that was spoken about yesterday - where you could have a virally-infected chondroblast, for example, to go backwards and forwards.

*Eisen*

We have done that on several cell lines which can be induced to differentiate *in vitro*; it includes: teratoma; neuroblastoma; mastocytoma; myoblasts and a couple of others. In vitro are these tumours, if they correspond to a cell which normally has the protein, they do not seem to have it *in vitro* or have very little. In almost every case, one or other of the inducers of the Friend cell will induce it to make it - to induce them to differentiate. There is one of the inducers of the Friend cell which is universal and will induce it in essentially all cells and that is butyric acid. But in almost every case where we have taken a tissue that has it *in vivo*, it doesn't have it *in vitro* but where it can be induced to differentiate you see the appearance of this protein.

*Wolpert*

That is not quite the point. The question is: it should be present in mature chondroblasts.

*Eisen*

Yes, it is.

*Wolpert*

Now if you take chondroblasts and infect them with a virus and then - or, for example with pigment cells they will lose their pigment granules and they will proliferate and may be you will reduce your protein under that situation and it would be very interesting.

*Eisen*

No we have not done that specific experiment. I would like to do it but the antibody to the mouse protein will recognise $H_5$ of chicken but it does not seem to recognise anything in non-avian cells. What I have told you is more or less along those lines; it seems to disappear when these cells are transformed (and most of

them *are* virally transformed) and it seems to come back when the cells are
induced to differentiate.'

# Control of Mitochondrial Biosynthesis

*Piet Borst*

## Introduction

Most of the controls in cellular differentiation are genetically programmed and operate by affecting gene expression. In eukaryotic cells a small fraction of the genes is present in mitochondria and it is therefore appropriate in this Symposium to consider what these genes contribute to differentiation and how the expression of these genes is influenced by differentiation. The relative contribution of mitochondrial genes to the total genetic complexity of mammalian cells is low as Table 1 shows; even in a primitive eukaryote like yeast the mtDNA constitute less than 1% of the cellular genes. Some cells have many mitochondria, however, and the mitochondrial fraction may therefore contain a substantial part of cellular DNA. In toad eggs this is even 99% of all DNA (Table 1).

It is not difficult to find examples of profound alterations in mitochondria associated with differentiation (see Pollak and Sutton 1980), but usually it is not known whether these alterations involve changes in mitochondrial gene expression. Of course, most developmental biologists are well aware of the large contribution that mitochondria make to nucleic acid synthesis in eggs and early embryos, but this is usually considered as a nuisance because mito-

**Table 1**

Contribution of mtDNA to cell DNA

| Source of DNA | Mitochondria per cell | mtDNA (% of total DNA) | | Reference |
| --- | --- | --- | --- | --- |
| | | Amount | Complexity | |
| Mouse L-cell line | $10^2$ | <1 | 0.0005 | Nass (1976) |
| Toad egg | $10^7$ | 99 | 0.0005 | Dawid (1965) |
| Yeast diploid | 2-50 | 15 | 0.6 | Borst and Grivell (1978) |

chondrial poly (A)-RNA interferes with the isolation of the nuclear mRNA of interest. The result is that the section on mitochondria and differentiation will be small in this paper. The main emphasis will be on some of the general questions raised by the very existence of a mitochondrial genetic system and the peculiar properties that this system turns out to have.

## Genes in Yeast mtDNA

Our present knowledge of mitochondrial biogenesis in yeast is outlined in Figure 1 and an inventory of genes in the 70kb, kilobases or kilobasepairs, yeast mtDNA is presented in Table 2. More than 90% of all mitochondrial proteins (both on a weight and a number basis) are encoded in nuclear genes, made on free cell-sap ribosomes and imported by a process that requires intra-mitochondrial ATP (Schatz 1979; Neher *et.al.*1980). The remaining proteins are made by the mitochondrial genetic system and these can be sub-divided in two classes, major and minor proteins. The (quantitatively) major proteins include sub-units of three enzyme complexes and one ribosome-associated protein (Tzagoloff *et.al.* 1979). Only one of the minor proteins has been identified, the *cob* 42kd, kilodaltons, fusion protein; all the others still have the pariah-status of Unassigned Reading Frame (URF) ie. an open reading frame identified by sequencing but without known corresponding protein product of

**Table 2**
A comparison of gene products of yeast and human mtDNA

| Mitochondrial component | Mitochondrial gene product in | |
|---|---|---|
| | Yeast* | Man** |
| Large ribosomal subunit | 21S RNA | 16S RNA |
| Small ribosomal subunit | 15S RNA rib. assoc. protein | 12S RNA ? |
| tRNAs | about 30 | 22-23 |
| Cytochrome c oxidase | Subunits 1 Subunits 2 Subunits 3 | Subunits 1 Subunits 2 Subunits 3 |
| bc₁ | apo-*b* | apo-*b* |
| ATPase complex | Subunits 6 Subunits 9 | Subunit 6 (?) - |
| RNA processing enzymes | *cob* maturase | - |
| URFs | 9 | 8 |

* Borst (1981a)
** Barrell *et.al.*(1981a)

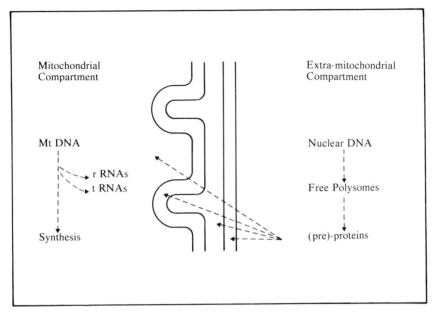

**Figure 1**
Biosynthesis of mitochondrial proteins

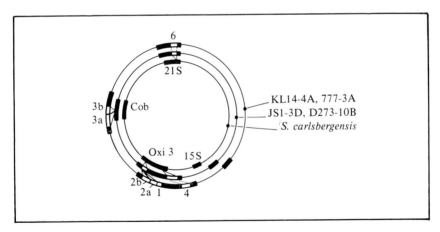

**Figure 2**
The major insertions/deletions in yeast mtDNA that give rise to the strain differences. The circles represent the mitochondrial genomes of *Saccharomyces cerevisiae* KL 14-4A, 777-3A, JS 1-3D and D 273-10B and *S carlsbergensis* NCYC 74. The mitochondrial loci *cob* and *oxi-s* and the genes for the 21S and 15S rRNAs are shown as closed bars. The open bars represent the various large insertions responsible for size differences of mitochondrial loci in different yeast strains. The nomenclature of these is according to Borst and Grivell (1978) apart from insertions 2 and 3 which have since been found to consist of closely adjacent smaller insertions (see Figures 3 and 5). From van Ommen *et.al.*(1980).

clearly defined genetic function. I shall return to the URFs below.

The structural RNAs required for mitochondrial protein synthesis are all gene products of mtDNA. The proteins required for the function of the mitochondrial genetic system, however, appear to be imported, with the exception of at least one of the enzymes involved in RNA processing.

## The Optional Introns in Yeast mtDNA

The first indication for the presence of introns in mtDNA came from a comparison of physical maps of the mtDNAs from a series of *Saccharomyces* strains by Sanders and Heyting in our laboratory (see Borst and Grivell 1978). Although similar in overall restriction maps and gene order, these DNAs differed up to 10% in length due to the presence of large insertions varying in size between about 1 and 3kb. What made these insertions especially intriguing was their apparent location in the neighbourhood of known genes (Figure 2), at that time only coarsely mapped. We first studied the precise location of insert 6 near the single gene for the large rRNA. For nearly a year Heyting wrestled with hybridisation results that seemed to indicate that the insert was within the gene, without being able to come to a definitive conclusion. Then Jeffreys and Flavell (1977) in our laboratory discovered the intron in the $\beta$ globin gene of rabbits and inserts within genes suddenly became respectable.

Like introns in nuclear genes, the mitochondrial intron is transcribed and the intronic sequence is removed by splicing of the precursor-RNA. From the sequence, the exact splice point could be in any of three positions but none of these resembles the consensus sequence for splicing of eukaryotic nuclear transcripts (Table 3). There is no second intron in this gene and there is no detectable difference in function between strains that contain the introns and those that do not. Thus, the intron is optional.

**Table 3**

Sequences at the edges of the ribosomal intron (from refs 11 and 12)

*Saccharomyces* with intron

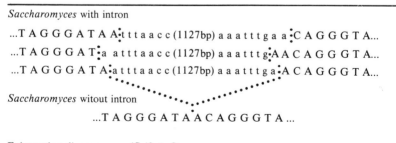

...T A G G G A T A A t t t a a c c (1127bp) a a a t t t g a a C A G G G T A...
...T A G G G A T a a t t t a a c c (1127bp) a a a t t t g A A C A G G G T A...
...T A G G G A T A a t t t a a c c (1127bp) a a a t t t g a A C A G G G T A...

*Saccharomyces* witout intron
                    ...T A G G G A T A A C A G G G T A ...

Eukaryotic splice sequence (Seif *et al*)
                    ...A G g t a a g t ......p y p y x p y a g ...

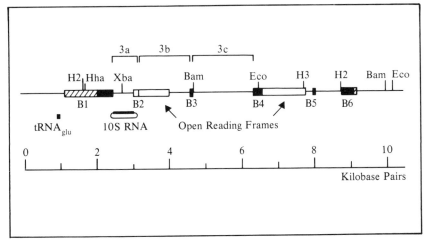

**Figure 3**
The *cob* region in mtDNA from *S cerevisiae* strain KL 14-4A. Cleavage sites for restriction enzymes BamHI (Bam), EcoRI (Eco), HhaI (Hha), HindII (H2), HindIII (H3) and XbaI (Xba) are shown and transcription runs from left to right. Coding sequences for 18S *cob* mRNA, as localised by electron microscopy and DNA sequence analysis, are shown as thickened bars. They are designated B1-B6. The hatched bars are the non-translated regions of the mRNA, the open bars correspond to long open reading frames in introns found by DNA sequence analysis. Modified from Grivell *et.al.*(1980).

The optional intron in the rRNA gene has none of the characteristics of transposable elements in bacterial DNA (*cf* Calos and Miller 1980). It has only been found at a single location in mtDNA, it lacks terminal repeats and there are no repeats of acceptor DNA around the insertion site (see Table 3). This apparent lack of mobility also holds for the other optional introns discussed below. It is possible, however, that these introns had once entered mtDNA as mobile genetic elements, but became immobilised by sequence evolution (Borst and Grivell 1981).

**The Introns in the Gene for Apocytochrome b**
If insert 6 is an optional intron, it seemed not unreasonable to expect that the other inserts might be introns as well. This was first shown for insert 3 in the *cob* region, where the gene for apocytochrome *b* is located. From the work of van Ommen *et al* (1979, 1980) we learnt that this region yields an overlapping series of transcripts. The smallest and most prominent of these, an 18 S RNA (about 2200 nucleotides) was shown to give rise to antigenic determinants of cytochrome *b*, when used to program *in vitro* protein synthesis (Grivell *et.al* 1979). This putative *b* mRNA was mapped on the mtDNA by electron microscopy of DNA.RNA hybrids (Grivell *et.al.*1979) and, more recently, by S1 nuclease protection experiments (JBA Crusius, PH Boer and LA Grivell,

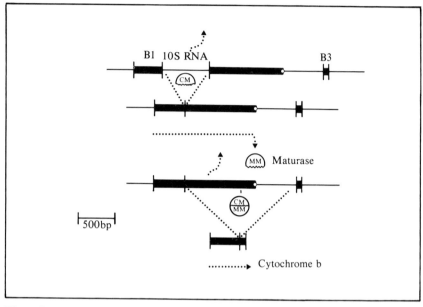

**Figure 4**

Involvement of maturase in splicing of intron B2-B3 of the *cob* gene (adapted from Lazowska *et al* 1980). The figure shows a simplified version of the left half of Figure 3, with only exons B1 and B3. CM is a nuclear-coded, imported RNA processing enzyme ('cytoplasmic maturase') which removes the 10 S RNA from the precursor transcript. MM is the mitochondrial maturase required to splice our the sequences corresponding to the B2-B3 intron. See text for further explanation.

unpublished). This led to the conclusion that the *b* gene in 'long' mtDNAs contains 4 introns, two of which are missing in the 'short' mtDNAs that lack insert 3 (see Figure 2). Further complexities, however, are revealed by the more detailed map in Figure 3 which incorporates sequencing data and the results of the extensive genetic analysis of this gene, mainly carried out by Slonimski and his collaborators. Sequence analysis (Lazowska *et al.*1980) has uncovered the small extra exon B2 (14bp, basepairs) not detectable by electron microscopy. The gene is transcribed into a precursor RNA of about 8kb, which contains all the 6 exons and 5 introns (van Ommen *et al.*1980). An early step in the splicing of this precursor takes out a 10 S RNA (Grivell *et al* 1979) and this fuses onto exon B2 and the long open reading frame in the B2-B3 intron which is continuous with B2. Mutations in this reading frame (the *box* 10 mutations) can lead to the accumulation of a 42kD fusion protein which shares antigenic determinants with cytochrome *b* (Kreike *et.al.*1979). It is now clear that this is an altered version of a protein essential for the processing of transcripts from the *b* gene in 'long' mtDNAs, ie. an 'RNA maturase' (Labowska *et.al.*1980). This hypothesis is schematically illustrated in Figure 4. The removal of the 10 S RNA is presumably catalysed by an imported enzyme (CM in Figure 4) because it also takes place in petite mutants in which mitochondrial protein synthesis has been lost (Church *et.al.* 1979; Halbreich *et al* 1980). The removal of 10 S RNA creates a continuous reading for the synthesis of the maturase. The enzyme (MM) then contributes to further splicing steps which lead to formation of *b* mRNA and which destroy the mRNA on which maturase is made. Mutations in the 3' part of the open reading frame lead to the synthesis of a non-functional maturase. Since the maturase mRNA can not be processed in these mutants, the non-functional maturase is grossly overproduced.

Whether the maturase is a splicing enzyme or only a protein that modifies the specificity of pre-existing splicing enzymes (as indicated in Figure 4) is not yet known. In wild-type cells the protein is present in such low concentrations that it cannot be detected by pulse-labelling (J Kreike, pers. comm.). Presumably, low amounts of this enzyme are sufficient for proper RNA processing. This is also supported by the finding of Dujardin *et.al.* (1980) that some maturase mutations can be suppressed with paromomycin. Suppression by these drugs is always inefficient.

Figure 3 shows also a second long open reading frame in the B4-B5 intron, directly fused in phase to the B4 exon (Nobrega and Tzagoloff 1980). Mutations in this open reading frame (the box 7 mutants) also prevent formation of apocytochrome *b*. It is probable that this reading frame codes for a second maturase, but this remains to be proven.

Finally, it should be noted that the putative mRNA for apocytochrome *b* has a very long leader sequence of about 800 nucleotides. Analogous long leaders have also been found in a number of other putative mRNAs in yeast mitochondria (see Grivell and Borst 1978). The reason for this is unclear.

### The Multiple Introns in the Gene for Sub-unit 1 of Cytochrome C Oxidase

Early attempts to map the transcripts of the *oxi3* gene (which codes for sub-unit 1 of cytochrome *c* oxidase) already resulted in a bewildering array of overlapping transcripts (van Ommen *et.al.* 1979, 1980). Electron microscopy of these transcripts showed some of the prominent ones to be circular (Arnberg *et al.* 1980). Our present knowledge of this complex region is summarised in Figure 5. In a strain with DNA of intermediate length, containing inserts 1 and 4 of Sanders, the coding region of the gene is split in at least 7 exons (Tzagoloff *et al.* 1980). These coding regions are assembled into an 18 S mRNA which also contains about 500 nucleotides untranslated regions (Grivell *et.al.* 1980), but these have not yet been mapped. Long reading frames, fused in phase to exons, fill up most of the first four introns. Insert 2, which is only present in strains with 'long' DNA, splits exon A5 in at least 4 new exons (Grivell *et.al.* 1980). Whether the extra introns 2a-c also contain reading frames is not yet known.

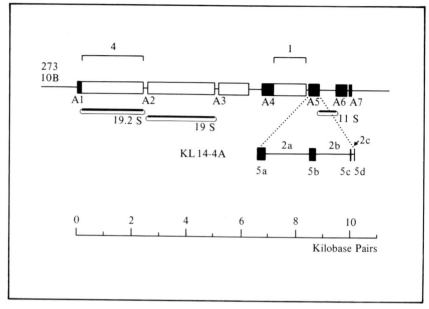

**Figure 5**
The *oxi* 3 region of yeast mtDNA and the circular transcripts derived from it (adapted from Grivell *et.al.*1980; Tzagoloff *et.al.*1980). The upper line shows the gene in *S cerevisiae*, strain 273-10B; the black boxes are the exons (amino acid sequence) A1-A7, the white boxes are long open reading frames in introns. Inserts 4 and 1 are missing in *S carlsbergensis* (see Figure 2) In *S cerevisiae*, strain KL 14-4A, exon A5 is split into 4 separate exons by three additional inserts (2a, 2b, 2c). Transcription is from left to right and the major circular transcripts identified by Grivell *et al.*(1980) are indicated.

In the strains with 'long' DNA 1530bp of exon sequences is spread over nearly 14kb of DNA. Six of these 14kb are contributed by the 5 optional introns. Like in the *b* gene, introns contain open reading frames but in this case no protein or genetic complementation group has yet been detected that could correspond to these extra reading frames.

**Why Circular RNAs?**
Four types of RNA circles have been found thus far by electron microscopy of mitochondrial RNA: the 10 S RNA transcribed from the *b* gene (Halbreich *et al.*1980) and the 3 RNAs shown in Figure 5. All attempts to open these circles by denaturation have been unsuccessful (Arnberg *et.al.*1980) and we think that they are covalently closed, although this remains to be proven by sequencing over the putative joint. Each of the 4 circles is derived from an intron sequence and they could easily arise as a wide-product of splicing. Not all introns give rise to circular splice-products, however, and the concentration of these circles

is high. They may therefore have some function. The possibility that they represent circular mRNAs remains an intriguing one.

## Why URFs?

One of the most unexpected findings of the last two years is that a substantial fraction of the mitochondrial genome is occupied by long open unassigned reading frames (URFs). Many of these URFs are present in introns and fused in phase to sequences which code for part of a known mitochondrial protein (Figures 3 and 5). Not all URFs are located in introns of protein-coding genes, because the intron in the rRNA gene also contains a 705bp URF (Dujon, 1980) and two URFs have been found between genes (Tzagoloff *et.al.*1980). Several of the URFs are in optional introns and therefore code for a protein that is not essential in all yeast mitochondria. URFs are not a peculiarity of yeast, because 6 URFs have been found in human mtDNA (Table 2) and the tight packing of genetic information in this DNA (Barrell *et.al.*1980a) suggests that all 6 must encode an essential function.

No protein product of any of these URFs has been identified yet in wild-type cells and with the exception of the putative *b* mRNA maturase encoded by the B4-B5 intron (Figure 3), none of the URFs has been detected in genetic analyses. The question has therefore been raised whether URFs are genes at all. Further arguments raised against a genetic function are that URFs differ markedly from other protein-specifying genes in their much lower $G + C$ content, their codon usage and their high content of asparagine, tyrosine and lysine residues (Nobrega and Tzagoloff 1980; Tzagoloff *et.al.*1980).

Most of these very properties have also been found by Lazowska *et.al.*(1980), however, for the open reading frame in the B2-B3 intron of the *b* gene (Figure 3). In this case there is no doubt that the reading frame codes for an essential RNA processing enzyme. The unusual properties of URFs must therefore have other reasons. An explanation that I find attractive is that URF products catalyse functions that do not require a very precise amino acid sequence. In a genome that tries to maximise its $A + T$ content this will lead to proteins with a high content of amino acids that are specified by pure AU codons. In fact, the reading frame that specifies the C-terminal part of the *cob* maturase, has only 18 mole % $G + C$ and 180 of the 280 amino acid residues are specified by pure AU codons, ie. phe, leu, ile, tyr, asn, lys. That a strong selection pressure operates to maximise $A + T$ content in yeast mtDNA was already obvious from other data: in protein-coding genes there is a strong preference for A or U in the third position (Nobrega and Tzagoloff 1980); the rRNAs are among the most AU-rich known (see below) and intergenic regions and leader sequences of mRNAs are often >90% $A + T$ (see Borst and Grivell 1978). The nature of the selective force driving yeast mtDNA towards high $A + T$ is unknown, but van Ommen (1980) has speculated that it is due to the absence of an uracil:

DNA-glycosidase, which removes the uracil that results from (chemical) deamination of C. This idea remains to be tested.

What could be the functions of URF gene products that do not require a very precise amino acid function? In addition to RNA processing, these proteins might affect recombination (polarity) or fulfill other regulatory functions not readily detected under laboratory conditions. I consider it unlikely that they contribute to mitochondrial metabolic functions or protein synthesis, because such major enzymatic functions should have been detectable in genetic analysis.

## Why Optional Introns in mtDNA?

Thus far only three genes have been found to contain introns; all the others are continuous (Table 4). In all genes that do have introns, some of these introns are optional. Since we have only looked at a limited number of strains, our present definition of an optional intron is rather arbitrary. All of them might turn out to be dispensable if we look at enough yeast strains. Clearly, many of the explanations proposed for the presence of introns in nuclear genes do not apply here (see Borst 1981b). Two hypotheses seem less far-fetched than the others:

1) Introns allow more efficient intra-genic recombination; this could be useful for the rapid creation of resistant alleles of genes that code for gene products that are targets for inhibitors found in nature (eg. apocytochrome *b* and the large rRNA).

2) Introns allow more precise control of gene expression at the level of RNA processing. This hypothesis is compatible with the observation that some

**Table 4**

Introns in Mitochondrial Genes in Yeast (from Borst 1981a)

| Gene | Number of introns | |
|------|-------|----------|
| | Total | Optional |
| Large rRNA | 1 | 1 |
| Apocytochrome *b* | 5* | 3 |
| Cytochrome *c* oxidase, subunit 1 | 9* | 5* |
| Small rRNA | 0 | 0 |
| tRNAs (10 genes analysed) | 0 | 0 |
| ATPase complex, subunits 6 and 9 | 0 | 0 |
| Cytochrome *c* oxidase, subunits 1 and 2 | 0 | 0 |

*Minimal estimate

mutants in the B1 exon of the *b* gene (see Figure 3) are hypersensitive to glucose repression (see Alexander *et.al.*1979).

## The Diversity of the Mitochondrial Genetic System

Most mtDNAs studied thus far contain genes for tRNAs, rRNAs, the 3 major sub-units of cyt. *c* oxidase, apocytochrome *b* and at least one sub-unit of the ATPase complex (*cf* Table 2). The way these genes are organised, replicated and expressed shows considerable variation, however, in different kingdoms and I shall illustrate this with a few examples:

1) Table 5 shows that the size and structure of mtDNA varies considerably. The smallest mtDNA known is that from sea urchins with only about 14000bp (Piko *et. al.* 1968). The largest mtDNA is the kinetoplast DNA from trypanosomes and related protozoa (see Borst and Hoeijmakers 1979). Figure 6 shows that this DNA consists of large networks containing two types of circles: maxi and mini-circles. The maxi-circles are the equivalent of mtDNA from other organisms; the mini-circles are heterogenous in sequence, not transcribed and their sequence changes very rapidly in evolution. The function

**Table 5**
Size and Structure of mtDNAs (modified from Borst 1977)

| Species | Structure | Mol wt ($\times 10^{-4}$) |
|---|---|---|
| Animals (from flatworm to man) | Circular | 9-12 |
| Higher plants | Circular | 70* |
| Fungi | | |
| Baker's yeast (*Saccharomyces*) | Circular | 49 |
| *Kluyveromyces* | Circular | 22 |
| Protozoa | | |
| *Acanthamoeba* | Circular | 27 |
| Malarial parasite (*Plasmodium*) | Circular | 18 |
| *Paramecium* | Linear | 27 |
| *Tetrahymena* | Linear | 30-36** |
| Kinetoplastidae | Circle network | 2.000-20.000 |
| *Trypanosoma brucei* | Mini-circle | 0.6 |
| | Maxi-circle | 13 |
| *Crithidia luciliae* | Mini-circle | 1.5 |
| | Maxi-circle | 22 |
| Algae | | |
| *Chlamydomonas* | Circular | 10 |

*In several plants the mtDNA consists of several size classes of circles with a combined genetic information content that may exceed $70 \times 10^6$ (Levings *et.al.*1979).
**Size range in different species.

of this major network component is not yet known. Rather complex is also the mtDNA from higher plants, which consists of heterogenous collections of circles up to 35 μm with a complexity equivalent to more than 100 kb (see Levings *et.al.* 1979).

Diversity is not a necessary attribute of organelle genetic systems. The chloroplast DNAs of plants and uni-cellular algae are all circular and differ by less than a factor 2 in contour length with the possible exception of *Acetabularia*.

2) Although the total genetic information in yeast and human mtDNA does not differ much (*cf* Table 2), the gene organisation is very different. Whereas genes in yeast mtDNA are spread over 70kb and often interlaced with long AT-rich non-coding stretches (Figure 7), animal mtDNA looks like a university biochemistry department anno 1980. All genes have been cut to minimum size, there are no introns and the inter-gene distance has been reduced to the barest minimum (Figure 8). One gets the impression that the cell would really like to get rid of the whole DNA molecule but has not found a way yet to do this in a decent fashion. The point is illustrated by the comparison in Figure 9 of the genes and putative mRNAs for apocytochrome *b* in yeast and man. The yeast gene contains 5 introns and the corresponding mRNA contains a long leader sequence of about 800 nucleotides, a trailing sequence of about 100-200 nucleotides and no poly(A) tail. The human gene is 'butt-jointed' to tRNA genes and the corresponding mRNA starts exactly at the initiating AUG codon; the gene ends at a T one nucleotide after the last amino acid and this T is used to make a UAA stop codon by polyadenylation of the mRNA (Barrell *et.al.* 1980a).

3) In human (HeLa cells) mitochondria all transcripts probably start at a single promoter, transcription is completely symmetric and punctuation of the primary transcript with tRNAs (or anti-tRNAs) may play a key role in processing of this transcript (see Figure 8). In contrast, transcription of yeast mtDNA probably starts from at least 5 different promoters (Levens *et.al* 1980) and no defined symmetric transcripts have been detected (see Borst 1981a). Surprisingly, the genes for the two rRNAs in yeast mitochondria are far apart (Figure 7) and probably transcribed independently (contrast Figure 8). With multiple starts for RNA synthesis mitochondrial gene expression in yeast could in theory be differentially controlled at the level of transcription initiation. Whether this occurs in practice is not known.

4) Table 6 shows that there is more diversity in the ribosomes in mitochondria than in the rest of nature. Plant mitochondria still contain ribosomes that look somewhat like bacterial ribosomes, but all other mitochondrial ribosomes lack a 5S RNA and may contain rRNAs much smaller than the ones found elsewhere in nature. The most extreme example of this economy in rRNAs was recently found in trypanosomes where the size of the combined rRNAs has been reduced below 2000 nucleotides and the G + C content to about 20%.

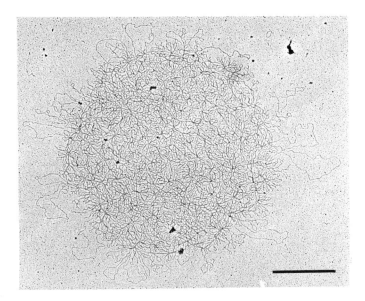

**Figure 6**
Electron micrograph of a kinetoplast DNA network from *Trypanosoma brucei* spread in a protein monolayer. The bar is 1 μm. From Borst and Hoeijmakers (1979).

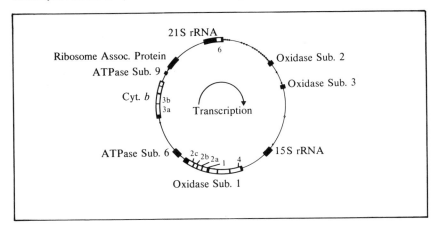

**Figure 7**
A simplified physical map of mt DNA from *Saccharomyces cerevisiae*, strain KL 14-4A. The roman numerals within the circle refer to the large insertions/deletions responsible for the size differences of mitochondrial genes in different yeast strains (see Borst and Grivell 1978). Each of these insertions is now known to be an optional intron (see text). Black bars represent exon sequences of genes, white bars introns. The shaded area drawn for the gene of the ribosome-associated protein (*VAR* 1 locus) reflects the uncertainty in the position of this gene (Butow *et al* 1980). The black dots are tRNA genes, the white dots methionine-tRNA genes. Adapted from Borst (1981a).

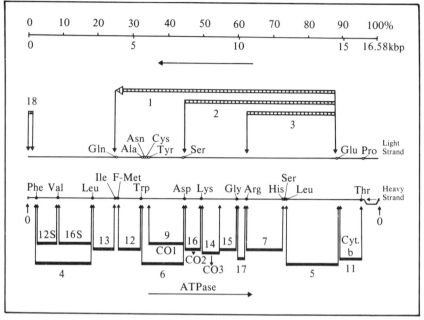

**Figure 8**

Human mtDNA with its genes and transcripts (adapted from Attardi *et.al.*1980; and Barrell *et.al* 1980a). tRNA genes are indicated by the three-letter code of their cognate amino acid; other major transcripts are bracketed by arrows and numbered. The upper and lower horizontal arrows indicate the direction of transcription. 12 S and 16 S are the rRNA genes; CO 2-3 are the genes for sub-units 1-3 of cytochrome *c* oxidase. URFs are unidentified reading frames (see text). Two additional URFs transcribed from the Light strand are not shown.

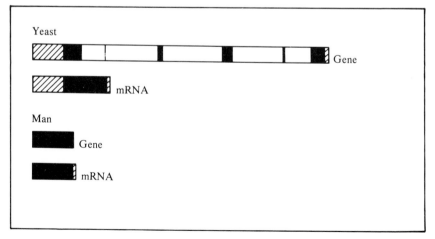

**Figure 9**

Gene and mRNA for apocytochrome *b* in yeast and man. (Adapted from Figures 3 and 8).

5) Mitochondrial tRNAs break all rules previously established for tRNAa outside mitochondria and vary from the rather normal leucyl-tRNA of yeast mitochondria which still has 64% homology with the leucyl-tRNA of *E coli* (Berlani *et.al.*1980) to the bizarre seryl-tRNA in human mitochondria, which is only 62 nucleotides long and lacks the entire 'D-loop and arm' (Barrell *et al* 1980a).

6) Finally the genetic code in mitochondria differs from that elsewhere in nature (Barrell *et al* 1980b; Bonitz *et.al.*1980) and even differs in different organisms (Table 7), a point not usually stressed.

## Why is the Mitochondrial Genetic System so Diverse?

It now looks as if the main gene products of mtDNA are similar throughout nature. Why then are such diverse genetic systems used to produce these gene

**Table 6**
The diversity of mitochondrail ribosomes

| Organism | S-value ribosome | Mole % G+C | Size of rRNAs (b) Large | Small | 5S RNA present | Ref |
|---|---|---|---|---|---|---|
| Higher plants | 78 | 44 | 3600 | 2100 | + | a |
| Yeast (*Saccharomyces*) | 73 | 23 | 3200 | 1600 | — | a |
| Man | 60 | 45 | 1559 | 954 | — | a,b |
| Trypanosomes | ? | $\sim$20 | 1230 | 630 | ? | C |

a Buetow and Wood (1978)
b Eperon *et.al.*(1980)
c Borst *et.al.*(1980)

**Table 7**
The mitochondrial genetic code

| Codon | Usual assignment | Human mitochondria (*) | Yeast mitochondria (**) |
|---|---|---|---|
| UGA | Stop | Trp | Trp |
| (UGG | Trp | Trp | Trp) |
| CUA | Leu | Leu | Thr |
| (ACX | Thr | Thr | Thr) |
| AUA | Ile | Met | Ile |
| (AUG | Met | Met | Met) |

* From Barrell *et.al.*(2980b)
** From Bonitz *et.al.*(1980)

products? This could either reflect the diversity in the primitive endosymbionts from which mitochondria probably arose in the course of evolution or a rapid evolution of mitochondrial sequence. The latter possibility is consistent with the high rate of sequence evolution of mtDNAs. This was already known from studies of total mtDNAs, but it has been confirmed in a striking fashion by the recent sequence analysis of segments of animal mtDNAs. For instance, the large rRNA from mouse mitochondria (van Etten *et.al.* 1980) has only 68% homology with the corresponding RNA from rats (Saccone, pers. comm.). This is even less than the 74% homology found between the 16S rRNAs of *Zea mays* chloroplasts and *E coli* (Schwartz and Kossel). Similarly, the phenylalanine-tRNAs of mouse and human mitochondria have only 70% sequence homology (van Etten *et.al.* 1980).

In my opinion this high rate of evolution of rRNA and tRNA genes is most easily explained by the low demands put on the mitochondrial translation system. This system only produces a very limited number of proteins and usually at a constant relative rate. Such a system may evolve more rapidly than a system which has to produce a large number of proteins at maximal efficiency and subject to various translational controls. A translational system which makes only a few proteins may also survive catastrophic events like an alteration of the genetic code which would be lethal to a protein synthesising system making many proteins.

**Mitochondria and Differentiation**
If we disregard the URFs, all known mitochondrial gene products can be considered indispensable for making functional mitochondria. The proteins that make a liver mitochondrion different from a heart mitochondrion (ie. the presence of urea cycle enzymes), are encoded in nuclear DNA and imported from the cell sap. *A priori*, one would therefore expect that in animal cells RNA synthesis in mitochondria will be more or less the same, whatever the differentiation state of the tissue. This is borne out by the few studies in which this prediction was actually verified. For instance, Battey *et. al.* (1979) analysed the relative amounts of 7 major mitochondrial transcripts in developing *Drosophila* embryos in the period from fertilised egg to larva and found no differences. Likewise, no consistent alterations in mitochondria have been found during the dedifferentiation or defective differentiation observed in cancer cells. In my opinion the sweeping generalisation that cancer cells have normal mitochondria (Borst 1972), still holds.

In some micro-organisms the synthesis of mitochondria can be modulated more subtly than the all or none effects observed in metazoa. For instance, in the presence of high glucose or in the absence of $O_2$, yeast can adjust the synthesis of the components of the mitochondrial respiratory chain to a much lower level and this adjustment is selective, whereas functional cytochrome *c* oxidase is absent in anaerobically-grown cells; the mitochondrion maintains a supply of mitochondrial ribosomes and continues to make the sub-units of the ATPase complex required to render this enzyme oligomycin sensitive (Criddle and Schatz 1969).

One factor that certainly contributes to this selective repression of oxidase formation is assembly control. Woodrow and Schatz (1979) have shown that anaerobic yeast contains the sub-units to make oxidase but these sub-units do not assemble into active holo-enzyme. The block may involve synthesis of haem *a* or the oxidation-reduction state of haem *a* or Cu. In principle, such assembly control could provide a satisfactory, albeit wasteful, mechanism to manipulate the level of individual mitochondrial enzyme complexes: the mitochondrial genetic system produces protein sub-units at a constant rate; whether these can be inserted into the membrane is controlled by an imported protein or other nuclear-controlled factor; sub-units that can not be integrated into the holo-enzyme are degraded.

The system is more complex, however, because after long-term anaerobiosis incorporation of labelled amino acids into oxidase sub-units decreases much more than into another mitochondrial gene product, the ribosome-associated protein *var1* (Woodrow and Schatz 1979). This could be due to a feed-back repression of translation or to other controls on translation, RNA synthesis or RNA processing. As I pointed out before, the genes for apocytochrome *b* and sub-unit 1 are riddled with introns, which requires extensive splicing of precursor-RNA, which is carried out in part by imported enzymes. The cell could therefore modulate the synthesis of these gene products by varying the level of the imported splicing enzymes. Moreover, both genes contain long open reading frames in their introns and presumably all of these must be translated to produce the final gene product. This would make these genes more sensitive than others to an over-all inhibition of translation, eg. by a decreased level of an aminoacyl-tRNA. It should be possible to distinguish between these alternatives by simple experiments, but these have not been completed yet.

African trypanosomes represent a second class of organisms able to completely repress the biosynthesis of a functional respiratory chain. This occurs in the blood-stream of the vertebrate host; in the tse-tse fly a normal mitochondrion is present. It is probable that this repression is selective, like in yeast, and only affects the respiratory chain and not the mitochondrial contribution to the biosynthesis of ribosomes and the ATPase complex (see Borst *et. al.* 1980). We have compared mitochondrial transcripts in blood-stream trypanosomes and cultured trypanosomes (which have a fully developed mitochondrion). We find that the level of all detectable transcripts is about 10-fold decreased in blood-stream trypanosomes but all transcripts are affected to the same extent. The overall decrease might be due to a decrease in mitochondrial RNA polymerase; the complete disappearance of functional respiratory chain components must be due to additional controls at the level of translation or assembly.

In summary, I think that there is good evidence that the contribution of mitochondrial genes to mitochondrial biogenesis can be controlled at the level of assembly of protein complexes. This is a wasteful process, because proteins that cannot be inserted into the complex are destroyed. It is likely that the total level of mitochondrial gene expression can also be controlled at transcription initiation, because the nucleus can decrease the level of the (imported) mitochondrial RNA polymerase (Levens et.al.1980). In yeast there are also indications that the output of mitochondrial transcripts may be decreased by decreasing the number of mitochondrial DNA molecules per cell (see Borst and Grivell 1980). It is, furthermore, an attractive, but speculative possibility that gene expression could be affected at RNA processing. Finally, there is no firm evidence as yet that synthesis of individual mitochondrial transcripts can be *differentially* controlled at the level of transcription initiation.

**Why mtDNA?**
This is one of the most vexing questions in the field and it is embarrassing that no convincing answers have been forthcoming. It is now clear that the mitochondrial genetic system is not used to any extent to translate imported mRNAs. It is also clear that the mitochondrial genetic system is not required because hydrophobic proteins can not reach the inner membrane via import and therefore have to be made inside. The death blow to this idea came when Sebald and coworkers established that the gene for the very hydrophobic sub-unit 9 of the mitochondrial ATPase complex is located on mtDNA in yeast whereas in another fungus, *Neurospora*, the gene is in the nucleus and the (homologous) protein is made on cell-sap ribosomes and imported into the mitochondria (see Tzagoloff et.al.1979). The ATPase complex of chloroplasts resembles that of mitochondria but in this case even more sub-units are contributed by the organelle genome (see Borst and Grivell 1978). If there is any logic in the division of labour between organelle and nuclear genome it certainly does not show up in the synthesis of the ATPase complex.

Since 1970, my favourite explanation has been that the organelle genetic system is an accident of evolution (Borst 1972). According to this hypothesis genetic exchange between organelle DNA and nuclear was extensive in the primitive early eukaryote, leading to a redistribution of genes. Transfer from organelle to nucleus could have been driven by several forces: transfer of the genes for proteins involved in the replication of organelle DNA would potentially increase cellular control over organelle replication; development of a mechanism to import proteins into the organelle would be of great advantage, because it would allow the cell to modify the metabolic pathways in the organelle. Finally, transfer of genes from organelle to nucleus would provide the organelle with the advantages of diploidy and sexuality. Although organelles can recombine their DNA, mitotic segregation leads to elimination of heterogeneity in the organelle DNA population.

The main problem with this hypothesis is that it does not explain why any genes have been retained in the organelle at all and why this should always be more or less the same set of genes. This suggests that at some time in evolution it was advantageous to retain these few genes in the mtDNA and it is not obvious what this selection pressure could have been.

If we cannot provide good reasons why the genes listed in Table 2 and only those should be in mtDNA it may still be possible to find organisms that have a more complex mitochondrial genome which contains genes that reside in the nucleus in yeast or man. The mtDNA of higher plants, which is substantially more complex than the other mtDNAs known (see Table 5), might be a good candidate. On the other hand, one might also hope to find one day a cell in which all genes required to make mitochondria are in the nucleus. Margulis (1975) has actually suggested that the cilia and flagella of eukaryotic cells are derived from such withered endosymbionts. I am intrigued by the possibility that microbodies represent another example of this situation. For a long time it was thought that microbodies bud off from the endoplasmic reticulum, but this has not been confirmed in recent experiments. It now appears that microbody proteins are synthesised on free ribosomes and imported, after completion, into the organelle (see Lazarow *et.al.*1980). In this respect microbodies have more resemblance to mitochondria and chloroplasts than to the other membrane-bound compartments in the cell, which are derived from the endoplasmic reticulum. It seems possible, therefore, that microbodies represent the remnant of an endosymbiont retained by the eukaryotic cell as a handy packaging system for metabolic pathways that require segregation into a separate compartment. The discovery of a microbody in trypanosomes which contains the enzymes of glycolysis (Opperdoes and Borst 1977), provides a simple system to test whether microbody enzymes have prokaryotic characteristics.

### Acknowledgements

I am indebted to students and colleagues in the Amsterdam Laboratory for sharing unpublished experiments with me and for stimulating discussions. I also thank Mr I Eperon (Med Res Council Lab, Cambridge, UK.) and Prof C Saccone (Inst for Biol Chem, University of Bari, Italy) for providing me with unpublished sequences of mtDNAs. The experimental work in our laboratory was supported in part by a grant to PB/LA Grivell from The Netherlands Foundation for Chemical Research (SON) with financial aid from the Netherlands Organisation for the Advancement of Pure Research (ZWO).

## References

Alexander, N.J., Vincent, R.D., Perlman, P.S., Miller, D.H., Hanson, D.K. and Mahler, H.R. *Regulatory interactions between mitochondrial genes.* (1980) J. Biol. Chem. *254*, 2471-2479.

Arnberg, A.C., van Ommen, G.J.B., Grivell, L.A., van Bruggen, E.F.J. and Borst, P. (1980) *Some yeast mitochondrial RNAs are circular.* Cell *19*, 313-319.

Attardi, G., Cantatore, P., Ching, E., Crews, S., Gelfand, R., Merkel, C., Montoya, J. and Ojala, D. (1980) *The remarkable features of gene organisation and expression of human mitochondrial DNA. In: The Organisation and Expression of the Mitochondrial Genome* (Kroon, A.M. and Saccone, C., Eds), North-Holland, Amsterdam, pp. 103-119.

Barrell, B.G., Anderson, S., Bankier, A.T., De Bruijn, M.H.L., Chen, E., Coulson, A.R., Drouin, J., Eperon, I.C., Nierlich, D.P., Roe, B., Sanger, F., Schreier, P.H., Smith, A.J.H., Staden, R. and Young, I.G. (1981) *Sequence of mammalian mitochondria DNA. In: Proceedings of Mosbach Colloquia* (Bucher, Th., Sebald, W. and Weiss, H., Eds), Springer Verlag, Berlin, in press.

Barrell, B.G., Anderson, S., Bankier, A.T., De Bruijn, M.H.L., Chen, E., Coulson, A.R., Drouin, J., Eperon, I.C., Nierlich, D.P., Roe, B.A., Sanger, F., Schreier, P.H., Smith, A.J.H., Staden, R. and Young, I.G. (1980) *Different patterns of codon recognition by mammalian mitochondrial tRNAs.* Proc. Natl. Acad. Sci. US. *77*, 3164-3166.

Battey, J., Rubenstein, J.L.R. and Clayton, D.A. (1979) *Transcription pattern of Drosophila melanogaster mitochondrial DNA. In: Extrachromosomal DNA: ICN-UCLA Symposia on Molecular and Cellular Biology* (Cummings, D.J., Borst, P., Dawid, I.B., Weissman, S.M. and Fox, C.F., Eds), Vol. *15*, Academic Press, New York, pp. 427-442.

Berlani, R.E., Bonitz, S.G., Coruzzi, G., Nobrega, M. and Tzagoloff, A. (1980) *Transfer RNA genes in the cap-oxil region of yeast mitochondrial DNA.* Nucleic Acids Res. *8*, 5017-5030.

Bonitz, S.G., Berlani, R., Coruzzi, G., Li, M., Macino, G., Nobrega, F.G., Nobrega, M.P., Thalenfeld, B.A. and Tzagoloff, A. (1980) *Codon recognition rules in yeast mitochondria.* Proc. Natl. Acad. Sci. US. *77*, 3167-3170.

Borst, P. (1972) *Mitochondrial nucleic acids.* Ann. Rev. Biochem. *41*, 333-376.

Borst, P. (1977) *Structure and function of mitochondrial DNA. In: International Cell Biology.* 1976-1977 (Brinkley, B.R. and Porter, K.R., Eds), The Rockefeller University Press, New York, pp. 237-244.

Borst, P. (1981a) *The biogenesis of mitochondria in yeast and other primitive eukaryotes. In: International Cell Biology* 1980-1981, (Schweiger, H.G., Ed), in press.

Borst, P. (1981b) *The optional introns in yeast mitochondrial DNA. In: idem Barrell et al.* 1981, in press.

Borst, P. and Grivell, L.A. (1978) *The mitochondrial genome of yeast.* Cell *15*, 705-723.

Borst, P. and Grivell, L.A. (1981) *One gene's intron is another gene's exon - a mitochondrial RNA processing protein encoded by an intron.* Nature, in press.

Borst, P. and Hoeijmakers, J.H.J. (1979) *Kinetoplast DNA.* Plasmid *2* : 20-40.

Borst, P., Hoeijmakers, J.H.J., Frasch, A.C.C., Snijders, A., Janssen, J.W.G., and Fase-Fowler, F. (1980) *The kinetoplast DNA of Trypanosoma brucei: Structure, evolution, transcription, mutants. In: idem Attardi et al.* 1980, pp. 7-20.

Bos, J.L., Osinga, K.A., van der Horst, G., Hecht, N.B., Tabak, H.F., van Ommen, G.J.B. and Borst, P. (1980) *Splice point sequence and transcripts of the intervening sequence in the mitochondrial 21S ribosomal RNA gene of yeast.* Cell, *20*, 207-214.

Buetow, D.E. and Wood, W.M. (1978) *The mitochondrial translation system. In: Subcellular Biochemistry* (Roodyn, D.B., Ed.), Vol. 5, Plenum Publ. Com., pp. 1-85.

Butow, R.A., Lopez, I.C., Chang, H.-P. and Farrelly, F. (1980) *The specification of var1 polypeptide by the VAR1 determinant. In: idem Attardi et al.* 1980, pp. 195-205.

Calos, M.P. and Miller, J.H. (1980) *Transposable elements.* Cell, *20*, 579-595.

Criddle, R.A. and Schatz, G. (1969) *Promitochondria of anaerobically grown yeast. I. Isolation and biochemical properties.* Biochemistry, *8*, 322-334.

Church, G.M., Slonimski, P.P. and Gilbert, W. (1979) *Pleiotropic mutations within two yeast mitochondrial cytochrome genes block mRNA processing.* Cell, *18*, 1209-1215.

David, I.B. (1965) *Deoxyribonucleic acid in Amphibian eggs.* J. Mol. Biol. *12*, 581.

Dujardin, G., Groundinsky, O., Kruszewska, A., Pajot, P. and Slonimski, P.P. (1980) *Cytochrome b messenger RNA maturase encoded in an intron regulates the expression of the split gene. III. Genetic and phenotypic suppression of intron mutations.* In: idem Attardi et al. 1980, pp. 157-160.

Dujon, B. (1980) *Sequence of the intron and flanking exons of the mitochondrial 21S rRNA gene of yeast strains having different alleles at the ° and rib1 loci.* Cell, *20*, 185-197.

Eperon, I.C., Anderson, S. and Nierlich, D.P. (1980) *Distinctive sequence of human mitochondrial ribosomal RNA genes.* Nature, *286*, 460-467.

Grivell, L.A., Arnberg, A.C., Boer, P.H., Borst, P., Bos, J.L., van Bruggen, E.F.J., Groot, G.S.P., Hecht, N.B., Hensgens, L.A.M., van Ommen, G.J.B. and Tabak, H.F. (1979) *In: idem* Battey et al. 1979, pp. 305-324.

Grivell, L.A., Arnberg, A.C., Hensgens, L.A.M., Roosendaal, E., van Ommen, G.J.B. and van Bruggen, E.F.J. (1980) *Split genes on yeast mitochondrial DNA: Organisation and expression. In: idem* Attardi et al. 1980, pp. 37-50.

Halbreich, A., Pajot, P., Foucher, M., Grandchamp, C. and Slonimski, P.P. (1980) *A pathway of cytochrome b mRNA processing in yeast mitochondria: specific splicing steps and an intron-derived circular RNA.* Cell, *19*, 321-329.

Hensgens, L.A.M., Grivell, L.A., Borst, P. and Bos, J.L. (1979) *Nucleotide sequence of the mitochondrial structural gene for subunit 9 of yeast ATPase complex.* Proc. Natl. Acad. Sci. US. *76*, 1663-1667.

Jeffreys, A.J. and Flavell, R.A. (1977) *The rabbit beta-globin gene contains a large insert in the coding sequence.* Cell, *12*, 1097-1108.

Lazarow, P.B., Shio, H. and Robbi, M. (1981) *Biogenesis of peroxisomes and the peroxisome reticulum hypothesis. In: idem* Barrell et al. 1981, in press.

Lazowska, J., Jacq, C. and Slonimski, P.P. (1980) *Sequence of introns and flanking exons in the wild type and box3 mutants of the mitochondrial cytochrome b gene reveals an interlaced splicing protein coded by an intron.* Cell, *22*, 333-348.

Levens, D., Lustig, A., Ticho, B., Synenki, R., Merten, S., Christianson, T., Locker, J. and Rabinowitz, M. (1980) *Transcription and processing of yeast mitochondrial RNA. In: idem* Attardi et al. 1980, pp. 265-276.

Levings III, C.S., Shaw, D.M., Hu, W.W.L., Pring, D.R. and Timothy, D.H. (1979) *Molecular heterogeneity among mtDNAs from different maize cytoplasms. In: idem* Battey et al. 1979, pp. 63-74.

Kreike, J., Bechmann, H., van Hemert, F.J., Schweyen, R.J., Boer, P.H., Kaudewitz, F. and Groot, G.S.P. (1979) *The identification of apocytochrome b as a mitochondrial gene product and immunological evidence for altered apocytochrome b in yeast strains having mutations in the cob region of mitochondrial DNA.* Europ. J. Biochem. *101*, 607-617.

Macino, G. and Tzagoloff, A. (1980) *Assembly of the mitochondrial membrane system: Sequence analysis of a yeast mitochondrial ATPase gene containing the oli2 and oli4 loci.* Cell, *20*, 507-517.

Margulis, L. (1975) *Symbiotic theory of the origin of eukaryotic organelles:criteria for proof. In: Symp. of the Soc. Exp. Biol.*: Symbiosis, nr. 29, Cambridge Univ. Press, Cambridge, 1975, pp. 21-38 (Jennings, D.H. and Lee, D.L., Eds).

Nass, M.M.K. (1976) *Mitochondrial DNA. In: Handbook of Genetics,* (King, R.C., Ed.), Vol.5, Plenum Press, New York, pp. 477-533.

Neher, E.M., Harmey, M.A., Hennig, B., Zimmerman, R. and Neupert, W. (1980) *Post-translational transport of proteins in the assembly of mitochondrial membranes. In: idem* Attardi *et al.* 1980, pp. 413-422.

Nobrega, F. and Tzagoloff, A. (1980) *Assembly of the mitochondrial membrane system DNA sequence and organisation of the cytochrome b gene in S. cerevisiae D273-10B.* J. Biol. Chem. *255*, 9821-9837.

Opperdoes, F.R. and Borst, P. (1977) *Localisation of nine glycolytic enzymes in a microbody-like organelle in T. brucei: The glycosome.* FEBS Letters, *80*, 360-364.

Piko, L., Blair, D.G., Tyler, A. and Vinograd, J. (1968) *Cytoplasmic DNA in the unfertilised sea urchin egg: Physical properties of circular mitochondrial DNA and the occurrence of catenated forms.* Proc. Natl. Acad. Sci. US. *59*, 838.

Pollak, J.K. and Sutton, R. (1980) *The differentiation of animal mitochondria during development.* TIBS, *5*, 23-27.

Schatz, G. (1979) How mitochondria import proteins from the cytoplasm. FEBS Letters, *103*, 203-211.

Schwarz, Zs. and Kossel, H. (1980) *The primary structure of 16S rDNA from ZEA mays chloroplast is homologous to E. coli 16S rRNA.* Nature, *283*, 739-742.

Tzagoloff, A., Macino, G. and Sebald, W. (1979) *Mitochondrial genes and translation products.* Ann. Rev. Biochem. *48*, 419-441.

Tzagoloff, A., Bonitz, S., Coruzzi, G., Thalenfeld, B. and Macino, G. (1980) *Yeast mitochondrial cytochrome oxidase genes. In: idem* Attardi *et al.* 1980, pp. 181-190.

van Etten, R.A., Walberg, M.W. and Clayton, D.A. (1980) *Precise localisation and nucleotide sequence of the two mouse mitochondrial rRNA genes and three immediately adjacent novel tRNA genes.* Cell, *22*, 157-170.

van Ommen, G.J.B. (1980) *RNA synthesis in yeast mitochondria.* Academic Thesis, Krips Repro, Meppel.

van Ommen, G.J.B., Groot, G.S.P. and Grivell, L.A. (1979) *Transcription maps of mtDNAs of two strains of Saccharomyces: Transcription of strain-specific insertions; complex RNA maturation and splicing.* Cell, *18*, 511-523.

van Ommen, G.J.B., Boer, P.H., Groot, G.S.P., de Haan, M., Rosendaal, E., Grivell, L.A., Haid, A. and Schweyen, R.J. (1980) *Mutations affecting RNA splicing on the interaction of gene expression of the yeast mitochondrial loci COB and OXI3.* Cell, *20*, 173-183.

Woodrow, G. and Schatz, G. (1979) *The role of oxygen in the biosynthesis of cytochrome c oxidase of yeast mitochondria.* J. Biol. Chem. *254*, 6088-6093.

## Questions

*Slabas*

I would like to ask a question that perhaps Slater can help me out with at the same time. I gather that brown fat adipose tissue has somewhat abnormal mitochondria in that they are slightly uncoupled. What I was wondering was whether the gene expression in those particular mitochondria is different - whether the ratio of things like F1 is slightly different.

*Borst*

Let me try first. Slater is my teacher and I think the students should get a chance first and then whatever is wrong will be corrected by Slater. I do not think anyone has looked in detail into mitochondrial gene expression in brown adipose tissues but I think one can explain what happens there simply by assuming that you have a normal mitochondrion in which one extra protein has been put in which makes a pore for $H+$ ions so that you get a continuous leakage of protons. The proton gradient is dissipated and in that way all the useful energy created by oxidation is lost without getting phos phorylated. I do not know if there is anything Slater wants to add?

*Slater*

No.

*Borst*

In principle it would be interesting to look into this further but everything could be explained by the addition of one extra protein.

*Sager*

If I had not been so weakened by all the delights of being alive here, I think I would do a better job. I think I would like to make a few points. Of course, we are not in total agreement because you hate mitochondria and I love mitochondria. You want to get rid of them and I want to understand them (Laughter). There are a few reasons why I have a more optimistic

hypothesis. Of course they come from things I have worked on. I am very impressed with this whole business of the way in which mitochondria are inherited and it is unfortunate that this all has a sort of sexist sound but I do not really mean it in that sense. There is very strict maternal inheritance and in the systems that I and others have studied and it is clear that the cell/organism/evolution has gone to great pains to develop a very, very complicated mechanism for making sure that only the mitochondria from one of the parents are transmitted to the progeny. Now, I do not understand that any more than you do - may be you understand it better than I. We do not understand the mechanism but we do know that it is a well built-in mechanism with many genes which have evolved for a long time. A different point I would like to make is something I learned from one of my professors, namely, Dobzhanski, who was a great evolutionist, and who said, 'anything that is not useful gets thrown out'. In the course of evolution things are not retained that have a very good function but I think the real challenge is the fact that we still know so little about mitochondria. I will just say one more thing. The most impressive thing about Sanger and his group's total sequencing of mitochondrial DNA is that it only revealed our ignorance. What the sequences which were expected were found and in addition to that half of the genome is not accounted for. Nobody knows what the URFs do. It seems to me that this is something to be concerned about. I will stop with a proposal about what URFs do. I will probably be wrong but until I am proven wrong, its something to think about. Everyone talks about interactions between the nucleus and organelles but that interaction is always described as a one-way process; that is, there are signals from the nucleus telling the organelles what do do. Now, I would like to propose that since one has organelles and they have DNA, they have signalling potential. Lysosomes do not have signalling potential but mitochondria do. That means that they can talk back to the nucleus. My guess is that what some of the URFs are coding for are sequences which are saying something about the level of oxidation, ATP formation or something which is important for the rest of the cell, but nobody has any evidence.

*Borst*

You suggest that these proteins are exported .....

*Sager*

Yes, that the proteins are exported. Now you will tell me that no proteins are exported.

*Borst*

Well, two comments, briefly, I agree that in chloroplasts, impressive methods have been devised to get unilateral gene transfer from organelles. This is not the case in mitochondria usually. In animals, of course there is maternal inheritance. Big deal. You now have these enormous eggs with all these mitochondria and here comes this poor sperm which contributes hardly any mitochondria at all. So, if that is unilateral inheritance, no - I am not impressed. But take yeasts, there is mitochondrial mixing and they are completely equal and there is no sexism in mitochondria in yeast. That is the first point. Second point, about talking back to the nucleus. Well, I agree that we do not know all about what URFs in human mitochondrial DNA do and we also agree that they must do something very essential but I think from the yeast we can say a little more: first, that one thing which was originally there as an URF has been identified as a protein present in very low concentration - essential for RNA processing. Second, that 5 of the 9 URFs that we know are in optional introns, so they are sometimes there, sometimes not. I

suggest they code for functions which are not absolutely essential

*Sager*

But they are not absent in humans

*Borst*

No, not in humans. I am talking about yeast because in yeast we can make strong arguments; in humans we cannot. It is a bad system to do genetics with (Laughter). So, now comes the real point. I think that in yeast the map has really been filled with mutations and it is really striking that one does not have additional complementation groups beyond the ones I have shown on the map. They are several URFs for which one cannot get a complementation group and I think it is very unlikely that there would be an essential function like talking back to the nucleus in one of these genes that we would not have detected it in any way. It is much more likely that these URFs are coding for RNA processing enzymes; that they have overlapping specificities so that under laboratory conditions you can knock out one without making the cell very sick so that you do not detect it as a mutant. Of course, we know that in the animal cells we need a lot of processing because we make these very long transcripts and all the tRNAs have to be cut out - you get all these separate messages - you have to polyadenylate them so that in principle it would not be unreasonable if you had several of these proteins all involved in this complex processing operation. Finally, you know a lot of effort has been put into trying to find proteins that are exported from mitochondria to regulate nuclear genes and I think it is fair to say that all the attempts (and some people have worked for years on this) are negative. You could say they are present in such low concentrations and I agree, that is a negative experiment. It is certainly not conclusive.

# 7
# Differentiating Systems

The preceding papers all deal, in various ways, with molecules and supra-molecular assemblies. However, in considering organismal development it is salutary to reflect upon the enormity of the problem we face in trying to work an appreciation of molecular behaviour into an understanding of development.

The final chapters deal with the opposite end of this scale: the problems of understanding cells as components of larger assemblies.

Dr Gardner suggests how recent techniques are helping to refine issues recognised by experimental embryologists as long ago as the last century; and suggests that we should re-examine the way in which we conceive of 'differentiation' and 'determination'.

Finally Dr Garcia-Bellido presents a comprehensive account of his work on *Drosophila* where the use of mutants promises to reveal more about the mechanism of pattern formation.

# In vivo and In vitro Studies on Cell Lineage and Determination in the Early Mouse Embryo

*Richard L Gardner*

## Introduction

Two related problems continue to command much attention in current experimental embryological research. The first is to establish the *normal* fate of cells of the early embryo in the larva or adult. The second is to find out which structures such cells *can* give rise to in altered circumstances. It is perhaps sobering to reflect that these same problems preoccupied the founders of the discipline roughly a century ago. What has changed in recent years is that introduction of new techniques has enabled such investigations to be tackled with greater precision and in a wider range of organisms than was possible hitherto. As a consequence the distinction between 'mosaic' and 'regulative' development (Davidson 1976) has come to be recognised as a less rigid one than was formerly supposed.

In principle, the best way of studying the fate of embryonic cells is by direct observation of living embryos. This is only practicable in certain organisms that consist of a modest number of cells, and whose embryos develop fairly rapidly in circumstances in which they are amenable to continuous observation. A strikingly successful example of a species in which the fate of cells has been studied in this way is the free-living nematode worm, *Caenorhabditis elegans*, discussed by Sydney Brenner. All the post-embryonic cell lineages have been characterised in this creature (Sulston and Horvitz 1977; Kimble and Hirsh 1979), and rapid progress is being made with the embryonic ones (Deppe, Shierenberg, Cole, Krieg, Schmitt, Yode and von Ehrenstein 1978). Furthermore, since these lineages seem to be invariant, a precise fate map for the species is a legitimate goal in this instance.

In many organisms, including both the mouse and *Drosophila*, lack of stable reference points in eggs, and variability in cell arrangement combined with high cell number and/or inaccessibility of embryos conspire to make the above approach to cell lineage impracticable. It is therefore necessary to resort to more devious means of following the fate of cells. The continuity necessary for tracing lineages in these species can only be achieved by marking cells indelibly so that all their mitotic descendants can be identified at any stage later in development. Genetic polymorphisms provide the markers of choice because of their heritability from one cell generation to the next. They can be exploited readily in *Drosophila* by using selective chromosome loss or X-ray-induced mitotic recombination to change the genotype of single embryonic cells *in situ* (Gehring 1978; Garcia-Bellido this Symposium). Unfortunately, this is not the case in the mouse in which one must combine cells from different embryos in order to harness genetic markers (Tarkowski 1961; Mintz 1965; Gardner 1968 1978a). The precision with which the fate of cells can be followed by this strategy obviously depends both on the size of the grafts and the spatial resolution of the assay used to distinguishable donor from host cells. Graft size is not a problem in the mouse. Indeed, experience with transplanting single cells has shown that it is a very favourable species in which to undertake strict clonal analysis of development (Gardner and Lyon 1971; Gardner and Rossant 1979; Kelly 1975). It is, at present, the lack of a really satisfactory cell autonomous genetic marker that has prevented exploitation of the full range of possibilities offered by this approach to mammalian development. Electrophoretically distinguish allozymes of glucose-phosphate isomerase provide the only ubiquitous genetic marker currently available in the mouse, and have therefore been used in virtually all transplantation experiments discussed in the following pages. The principal shortcoming of this enzyme as a marker is that tissue architecture has to be disrupted prior to electrophoretic analysis. Hence, one can only determine the proportions of donor and host cells in a sample and not their spatial arrangement. This is a particularly serious limitation in the case of organs like the placenta which cannot be separated into their constituent tissues prior to analysis (Gardner 1978b). A more detailed discussion of existing genetic markers in the mouse is provided by McLaren (1976).

In recent years, the relationship between cell lineage and differentiation has been investigated principally in two ways in the early mouse embryo. The first, as indicated above, is by transplantation or recombination of genetically labelled cells or tissues followed by return of the chimaeric embryos to the uterus for further development. This provides the best approach that is currently available for elucidating the normal fate of cells, particularly if single cells are transplanted orthotopically. It can also be adapted for investigating the developmental potency of cells in altered circumstances (eg. Rossant 1975a). The second approach, which has been addressed largely to the problem of potency, entails culture of early embryos and isolated tissues or cells *in vitro*. Before considering the rather different conclusions emerging from the *in vivo* versus *in vitro* studies, it is perhaps worthwhile drawing attention to one semantic and two technical problems that relate to them.

## Problems

### Determination

The semantic problem concerns use of the word *determination*. Its original definition was a purely operational one, cells or tissues being regarded as determined if they were found experimentally to be restricted in developmental potential. Recently, there has been a tendency to regard determination as representing a specific cellular state that is attained by a quantal step some time before the onset of differentiation (see Johnson 1979; for discussion). These unwarranted attributes appear to have been acquired largely through adoption of the behaviour of insect imaginal disks as a paradigm. There is considerable evidence in the classical embryological literature that restrictions in potency can be gradual rather than abrupt. Indeed, the rather unfortunate term 'labile determination' was introduced in recognition of this fact (eg. Huxley and de Beer 1934). Concerning the question of the temporal relationship between determination and differentiation, one can hardly do better than quote Weiss (1939):

'We can say, therefore, that parts which have started to develop as *equals* become gradually *determined* in various directions, which makes them *intrinsically unequal*, although this inequality, at first remains latent and only in time becomes manifest and discernible. However, the distinction between latent and manifest differentiation cannot be fundamental. For, if two cells which were originally alike become 'determined' to develop in different directions, we must assume that their physical and chemical constitutions have undergone divergent changes, even if there is no external criterion for this. One could almost call *determination 'invisible differentiation'*. It is to be hoped in some future time application of sensitive physico-chemical tests will detect differences among cells which escape mere microscopic observation. Until then, one must keep in mind that visible histological differentiation of a cell follows its 'determination' with a certain lag.'

Johnson and his colleagues (Johnson, Handyside and Braude 1977; Johnson 1979) have advocated use of 'commitment' or 'behaviour' in place of determination. However, strict adherence to a policy of abandoning terms once they have been abused is likely to lead eventually to enhancement of the confusion that it is designed to reduce. Hence, determination will be retained here and used, as originally, to denote restrictions in developmental potential. Such restrictions provide a useful series of experimentally definable points in the history of cell lineages to which other differentiative events can be related.

### Staging of Embryos and Isolation of Defined Cell Populations from them

With extension of the range of investigative techniques, an increasingly complicated pattern of morphological, physiological and biochemical changes is emerging during the course of early development. Obviously, it is necessary to establish both the order in which such changes occur and their cellular distribution before one can begin to search for causal relationships between them. The effectiveness with which this can be achieved depends on the accuracy with which embryonic material can be staged and separated into its constituent cell populations.

*a) Staging of Embryos*

The staging of intact living embryos merits discussion because it presents some problem, even prior to implantation. Up to the early 8-cell stage it is a simple matter to count the total number of blastomeres. Thereafter, however, cells begin to form extensive contacts with their neighbours so that their individual boundaries can no longer be discerned (Ducibella 1977). This *compacted* state persists throughout the remainder of cleavage, precluding cell counts on intact morulae. Onset of cavitation, marking the transition from morula to blastocyst, represents the next clear morphological change, and appears to take place almost exclusively in embryos consisting of between 28 and 33 cells (Smith and McLaren 1977). The staging of growing blastocysts also poses problems, especially prior to loss of the zona pellucida. Blastocysts within their zonae are often classified according to degree of expansion of the blastocoele. However, the latter seems to bear a somewhat tenuous relationship with cell number (see eg. Table 1, Handyside 1978), suggesting that the volume of the blastocoele may be subject to cyclic fluctuation *in vivo* as well as in culture (Cole 1967). Nadijcka and Hillman (1974) have attempted a more rational classification of the blastocyst phase of development into four substages. Unfortunately, their scheme is of limited value in classifying living embryos because it is based primarily on ultrastructural characteristics.

In many studies, morulae and blastocysts are categorized according to age rather than morphology. Untreated or hormonally-primed females are usually placed with males during the latter part of one day and checked for evidence of mating next morning. Development is then timed from the mid-point of the dark period in untreated females and from human chorionic gonadotrophin (HCG) injection in those that have been primed. However, the actual time of ovulation varies by about 3 hours within groups of females that have received HCG and by 8 hours or more in those not primed, though it is usually preceded by mating in both cases (Snell, Fekete, Hummel and Law 1940; Edwards and Gates 1959; Bingel and Schwartz 1969; Bronson, Dagg and Snell 1966). Since ovulation of a complete clutch of eggs takes 1 hours or less (Edwards and Gates 1959; Bronson *et. al.* 1966), one might expect less variation in development between embryos from the same female than from different ones. This has indeed been found to be the case (McLaren and Bowman 1973). One way of reducing the variability between females is to restrict mating to a define interval when all those destined to ovulate are very likely to have done so (eg. McLaren and Bowman 1973; Nicol and McLaren 1974). This strategy may, however, be of limited value in random-bred matings because studies on inbred mice have revealed that the interval between coitus and fertilization can vary significantly as a function of both paternal (Krzanowska 1964; Hoppe 1980) and maternal genotype (Nicol and McLaren 1974).

Fertilisation *in vitro* is probably the best way of initiating development synchronously in batches of embryos (Hoppe 1980). However, homogeneity of embryonic material cannot be achieved even if the time of fertilisation is controlled very precisely because there is asynchrony in cell division within individual embryos from the 2-cell stage (Kelly, Mulnard and Graham 1978). Thus, embryos composed of 3, or between 5 and 7, 9 and 15, or 17 and 31-cells are found routinely *in vivo* (Lewis and Wright 1935), despite the fact that all cells appear to be cycling (Barlow, Owen and Graham 1972; McLaren and Bowman 1973), and cell death is not normally encountered before the blastocyst stage (Copp 1978). Furthermore, overlap in S phase of successive cycles has been detected in embryos composed of more than 8-cells (Barlow *et al* 1972). Nevertheless, synchrony is not lost altogether during cleavage because, when the frequency of embryos is plotted against cell number, distinct peaks are evident at 16 and around 32 cells (Smith and McLaren 1977). Several factors may contribute to the complete absence of a peak corresponding to 64-cells (Smith and McLaren 1977), such as the increasing prominence of $G_1$ and $G_2$ (Barlow *et. al.* 1972; Mukherjee 1976), and withdrawal from cycle of cells that are destined to endo-reduplicate their DNA or die (Barlow *et.al.* 1972; Copp 1978).

A further complication emerging from recent work is that both the pattern and extent of this asynchrony in cell division within embryos varies from one to another (Kelly *et.al.* 1978). Thus, the interval between division of the two blastomeres in intact 2-cell embryos in culture ranges from 1 minute or less to 180 minutes. Similar or greater variation was seen between the first and last blastomere to divide from the 4 and the 8-cell stage (Kelly *et.al.* 1978).

Hence, a certain amount of difficulty will be encountered in attempting to relate developmental events to the cell cycle using single embryos. Such difficulty will be enhanced by pooling embryos prior to analysis, even if they are carefully matched for stage. This problem can only be circumvented by studying single cells that are defined in terms of both stage of cycle and number of cycles they have completed. This is feasible with cleaving embryos because blastomeres can continue to divide and differentiate following isolation (Tarkowski and Wroblewska 1967; Sherman and Atienza-Samols 1979), and because the number of cycles they have completed can be deduced from their size. However, these valuable characteristics are evidently lost shortly after blastulation.

*b) Tissue Isolation*

Single cells from preimplantation embryos can form very large clones following aggregation with blastomeres or injection into blastocysts (Kelly 1975; Gardner and Lyon 1971; Gardner and Rossant 1979). It is therefore vital to avoid contamination when attempting to isolate specific types of cells from early embryos in order to study their normal fate or potency. Unfortunately, this important point has not always received the attention that it deserves.

Initially, microsurgical techniques were devised for isolating trophectoderm and inner cell mass (ICM) tissues from the blastocyst (Gardner 1971; Gardner and Johnson 1972), and for separating primitive endoderm from ectoderm in the mature ICM (Gardner and Rossant 1979). The obvious disadvantages of these techniques are that they require special equipment and are rather time-consuming (Gardner 1978a; Papaioannou 1981). However, their overriding virtue is that tissue separation is monitored visually throughout so that contaminated specimens can be readily identified and discarded. Furthermore, a high rate of normal development is found in blastocysts that have been reconstituted from microsurgically isolated trophectoderm and ICM tissue (Gardner, Papaioannou and Barton 1973). Culture of isolated blastomeres provides an alternative way of obtaining trophectoderm vesicles which, though small, are capable of producing normal trophoblastic giant cells (Tarkowski and Wroblewska 1967; Sherman 1975).

Simpler ways of obtaining various tissues from pre and peri-implantation embryos have been implemented or suggested during the past few years. Those for obtaining trophectoderm depend on the greater sensitivity of the ICM or its precursor cells to lethal damage by drugs (eg. Rowinski, Solter and Koprowski 1975; Sherman and Atienza 1975) or ionizing radiation (Snow 1973; Goldstein, Spindle and Pedersen 1975). Trophectoderm cells obtained thus can form giant trophoblasts that are indistinguishable by various criteria from those produced manipulatively (Sherman and Atienza 1975). The ability of trophectoderm to form terminal polyploid cells may indeed account for its differential survival, and therefore cannot be regarded as proof that it retains the capacity for normal development following isolation by these selective procedures.

The junctions between trophectoderm cells appear to form an effective barrier against entry of macromolecules into the blastocyst (Ducibella, Albertini, Anderson and Biggers 1975; Magnuson, Jacobson and Stackpole 1978). This has been exploited ingeniously by Solter and Knowles (1975) who showed that sequential exposure of blastocysts to anti-mouse serum and complement could be used to achieve selective lysis of trophectoderm cells. The elegance and simplicity of 'immunosurgery' has led to its adoption as the method of choice for isolating ICMs and, as discussed later, for ridding the ectodermal cores of cultured ICMs of their investing endoderm. It has the further virtue of enabling isolation of ICMs or 'inside cells' from earlier stages than can be tacked microsurgically (Handyside 1978). However, it is important to bear in mind that immunosurgery depends on the use of undefined reagents which will obviously differ between batches and laboratories. The antisera employed have been raised by immunizing rabbits variously with spleen cells (Solter and Knowles 1975), spermatozoa (Harlow and Quinn 1979), or foetal homogenates (Handyside 1978) of murine origin. Also, experience seems to differ regarding both the source of complement (Solter and Knowles 1975; Spielman, Jacob-Muller and Beckord 1980) and its treatment prior to use (eg. Solter and Knowles 1975; Handyside 1978; Hogan and Tilly 1978a). In addition, different workers have adopted dissimilar protocols for reasons that are seldom explicitly stated. Finally, the surface antigenic profile of trophectoderm appears to change as the blastocyst matures (Jenkinson and Billington 1977) and it can also differ among cells in individual embryos (Willison and Stern 1978). It is perhaps not surprising, therefore, that the efficacy of the technique has proved to be rather variable (McLaren and Smith 1977; Magnuson *et. al.* 1978; Harlow and Quinn 1979).

Handyside and Barton (1977) undertook a critical and comprehensive evaluation of immunosurgery on blastocysts, using a variety of different ways of assessing the purity of ICMs obtained thereby. Their data provide compelling evidence that immunosurgery *can* yield pure ICMs. Unfortunately, in the majority of published studies in which the technique has been used to investigate the developmental potential of isolated ICM or primitive ectodermal tissue, the possibility of contamination due to incomplete lysis of the outer cell layer has not been rigorously excluded.

Finally, Surani, Tochiana and Barton (1978) have found that the ionophore A23187 can also be used to obtain viable ICM tissue by inducing lysis of trophectoderm cells. However, its efficacy has not been examined closely, and its mode of action if obscure. It is unlikely that it works simply by exclusion because it has a low molecular weight (523 daltons) and is relatively ineffective in lysing cells of isolated ICMs (Surani *et. al.* 1978; Harlow and Quinn 1979).

## Studies on early Development

### *Differentiation of ICM versus Trophectoderm*
Kelly (1975) was able to demonstrate retention of totipotency by both daughters of blastomeres isolated from 4-cell embryos by recombining them individually with groups of blastomeres of a different genotype. Earlier studies indicating that the lability of blastomeres persists into later cleavage (reviewed in Gardner 1978b) have been confirmed by more recent experiments. Thus, morphologically normal blastocysts can be formed both by groups of outside and of inside cells from late morulae, and from the ICMs of early blastocysts

(Rossant and Vijh 1980; Handyside 1978; Hogan and Tilly 1978a; Spindle 1978; Rossant and Lis 1979). Hence, cell determination does not seem to occur prior to blastulation, although a number of differences between inside and outside cells of the embryo have been discerned before this stage (Handyside and Johnson 1978; Johnson, Pratt and Handyside 1981). Earlier microsurgical studies suggested that trophectoderm and ICM represented distinct populations of determined cells in blastocysts composed of approximately 60 cells (Gardner and Johnson 1972; Rossant 1975a, 1975b, 1976). The results of three recent studies on *in vitro* deveopment of immunosurgically isolated ICMs are consistent with this conclusion (Handyside 1978; Spindle 1978; Rossant and Lis 1979). However, those of a fourth study (Hogan and Tilley 1978a, 1978b) indicate that ICM cells may retain the capacity to regenerate trophectoderm or form trophoblasts beyond the 60-cell stage. This discrepancy has yet to be explained. It might be indicative of genotypic differences in the timing of differentiative events. However, for reasons discussed earlier, the possibility that it is due to incomplete immunosurgical destruction of the trophectoderm cannot be dismissed.

Early studies by Mintz (1965) on aggregated embryos suggested that differentiation of trophectoderm versus ICM depends on disparate cellular micro-environments established during cleavage. This view was endorsed by Tarkowski and Wroblewska (1967) who proposed specifically that trophectodermal differentiation was precipitated by an external location and ICM differentiation by an internal location of cells in the morula. Results of various experimental studies on cleaving embryos support this 'inside-outside' hypothesis (see Gardner and Rossant 1976), particularly those involving manipulation of the relative position of labelled blastomeres (Hillman, Sherman and Graham 1972). Recently, Graham and his colleagues have tackled the difficult problem of how cells are normally allocated during cleavage. They first examined division order in intact and dissociated embryos, and found that the first cell to divide from the 2-cell stage tended to produce descendents which divided ahead of those of its partner and which made a larger contribution to the ICM (Kelly, Mulnard and Graham 1978). In further elegant studies, they obtained evidence that the effect of division order on allocation may be mediated by the extent of contact between cells. First, they found that cells dividing earlier during a particular cleavage tended to form contacts with a greater number of cells than those dividing later, and therefore more often form deep or inside cells. Second, deep cells contribute more frequently to the ICM than superficial cells (Graham and Deussen 1978). Finally, the observed patterns of cell contact appear to be established and maintained by continuous interactions between blastomeres (Graham and Lehtonen 1979). The question still remains as to what is responsible for the divergent differentiation of inside and outside cells.

The dramatic change in cell relations occurring at compaction has led to the proposal that it may be instrumental in establishing critical differences in the microenvironments of inside and outside cells (Ducibella 1977). Cleaving embryos can be maintained in a decompacted state without disturbing cell division by culturing them in the presence of rabbit antisera directed against mouse teratocarcinoma cells (Kemler, Babinet, Eisen and Jacob 1977; Johnson, Chakraborty, Handyside, Willison and Stern 1979). Brief inhibition of compaction is compatible with normal subsequent development (Kemler *et al.* 1977; Johnson *et. al.* 1979) while more prolonged culture in antiserum results in the formation of abnormal blastocysts in which the ICM is reduced or disorganised (Johnson *et. al.* 1979). Hence, compaction does seem to be important for normal morpho genesis, though Johnson, Handyside and Pratt (1981) consider that it may play a rather different role from that envisaged by Ducibella (1977).

*Partitioning of ICM Cells into Primitive Endoderm*
*versus Primitive Ectoderm*
According to Orsini and McLaren (1967) blastocysts from matings between mice belonging to a random-bred stock are invariably still encased within their zonae pellucidae at 92 hours after the estimated time of ovulation, the vast majority hatching very shortly thereafter. The ultrastructural studies of Nadijcka and Hillman (1974), also on blastocysts of random-bred origin, suggest that the primitive endoderm has usually formed before loss of the zona pellucida. The distinction at this stage of development between primitive endoderm cells that are organised as a single layer on the blastocoelic surface of the ICM and the remaining ICM cells (primitive ectoderm cells) is a rather subtle one. It depends on the former cells displaying more extensive rough endoplasmic reticulum than the latter, part of which consists of somewhat enlarged cisternae. Discontinuous deposits of amorphous material are evidence between the ectoderm and endoderm (Nadijcka and Hillman 1974), although separation of the tissues by a continuous basement membrane does not seem to occur for at least another 24 to 36 hours (Bartel 1972; Adamson and Ayers 1979; Wartiovaara, Leivo and Vaheri 1979; Leivo, Vaheri, Timpl and Wartiovaara 1980).

Blastocysts are clearly attached to the luminal epithelium of the uterus by 4 days post-coitum (*pc.*) and various changes characteristic of early implantation have taken place (Finn and McLaren 1967). At this stage the primitive endodermal cell monolayer is readily discernible by light microscopy at this stage, both in conventional histological preparations and in living blastocysts. It is no longer confined to the free surface of the ICM, some cells having migrated around the inner surface of the mural trophectoderm to form the distal or parietal endoderm. The remaining primitive endoderm cells continue to invest primitive ectoderm, and also surround the invaginated part of the polar trophectoderm (Copp 1978), as the proximal or visceral layer of the extraembryonic endoderm. Cells of these two endoderm layers differ markedly in their contacts with neighbouring cells and, somewhat later, also in biosynthetic activity (Table 1).

*In vivo* and *in vitro* studies on the early steps in differentiation within the ICM outlined above will be considered separately because they have yielded very different results.

*a)In vivo Studies*

Most if not all cells of dissociated i.e. 4 day *pc.* ICMs can be assigned unequivocally to one of two morphological classes, 'rough'(R) or 'smooth'(S). Equivocal or intermediate (I) cells account for the remainder. Furthermore, by separating ICMs into their constituent tissues prior to dissociation, R cells can be assigned to the primitive endoderm and S cells to the primitive ectoderm. When present, I cells can be found in either or both tissues (Gardner and Rossant 1979). Single R and S cells yield different patterns of colonization of host conceptuses following injection into blastocysts (Table 2). These distinct patterns are maintained even when the donor contribution is raised considerably by injecting several R or S cells into each blastocyst. Individual I cell clones conform to one or the other distribution. No single case of a clone extending across the demarcation line shown in Table 2 has been encountered so far (Gardner and Rossant 1979; Gardner 1981). Two conclusions have been drawn from these experiments and from additional studies on post-natal chimaeras (Gardner 1978c). Firstly, primitive endoderm cells form only the extraembryonic endoderm of the mouse conceptus, the entire soma of the foetus, its germ-line, and all extraembryonic mesoderm originating from the primitive endoderm. Secondly, the two types of cell are differentiated at 4½

**Table 1**
Some differences between cells of the parietal and visceral endoderm

| Characteristic | Parietal Endoderm | Visceral Endoderm | Source of information |
|---|---|---|---|
| Extent of contact between adjacent cells | +/— | +++ | Enders, Given and Schlafke (1978) |
| Prominence of dilated endoplasmic reticular cisternae | +++ | + | Hogan and Tilly (1981) |
| Synthesis of α-foetoprotein (AFP) | — | + | Dziadek and Adamson (1978) |
| Synthesis of fibronectin | + | +++ | Hogan and Tilly (1981) |
| Synthesis of type 4 collagen | +++ | + | Adamson and Ayers (1979) Hogan and Tilly (1981) |
| Synthesis of laminin | +++ | + | Hogan and Tilly (1981) |

days *pc.* with respect to properties that either ensure their precise partitioning in the ICMs of host blastocysts or which permit them to proliferate only if they happen to reach the correct location.

As noted earlier, primitive endoderm cells differentiate on the free surface of the ICM facing the blastocoele. If ICMs are isolated and aggregated in pairs prior to endodermal differentiation, all external cells and only the external cells exhibit the ultrastructural characteristics of primitive endoderm 24 hours later (Rossant 1975b). Furthermore, if ICMs of early blastocysts continue to develop *in vivo* after their cell number is reduced experimentally, they invariably give rise to extraembryonic endoderm. Only if their post implantation development is more extensive do they form primitive ectodermal derivatives as well (Gardner 1975). In addition, early rat ICMs injected into mouse blastocysts typically spread over the surface of the host ICM, and contribute disproportionately to extraembryonic endoderm later in development (Gardner and Johnson 1975). Finally, the ICM seems to undergo 'compaction' prior to endodermal differentiation (Nadijcka and Hillman 1974; Enders, Given and Schlafke 1978). These observations, together with others on differentiation in clumps of embryonal carcinoma cells in culture (Martin and Evans 1975), suggest that the 'inside-outside' hypothesis may be applicable to differentiation within the ICM as well as the morula. Early ICM cells would be expected to exhibit the following properties if this is indeed the case:

1) They should be labile with respect to primitive endodermal versus ectodermal differentiation.

**Table 2**
Maximal tissue distribution of different classes of ICM cell clones following blastocyst injection

| Host Tissue Colonised | | | | | |
|---|---|---|---|---|---|
| Donor cell type | Parietal Endoderm | Visceral Endoderm | Extra-embryonic Mesoderm | Amniotic Ectoderm | Foetal Soma + Germ-line |
| Primitive endoderm (R cells) | ▓▓▓▓ | ▓▓▓▓ | | | |
| Primitive ectoderm (S cells) | | | ▓▓▓▓ | ▓▓▓▓ | ▓▓▓▓ |
| Early ICM | ▓▓▓▓ | ▓▓▓▓ | ▓▓▓▓ | ▓▓▓▓ | ▓▓▓▓ |

Filled blocks denote tissues that are colonised by donor cells, and empty blocks those that are not. Based on data of Gardner and Rossant (1979) and Gardner (1981), and of unpublished data of J Rossant and RL Gardner.

2) It should be possible to make them differentiate as primitive ectodermal cells by surrounding them, and as primitive endodermal cells by placing them on the outside of groups of cells.

Preliminary blastocyst injection experiments failed to reveal the existence of early ICM cells that were able to contribute mitotic descendants to derivatives of both the primitive endoderm and primitive ectoderm (J Rossant and RL Gardner, unpublished results). However, current experiments, using daughter cell pairs obtained during brief culture of early ICM cells, have yielded positive results. Furthermore, both daughters can yield the same pattern of colonization when injected into different blastocysts, thereby excluding the possibility that each early ICM cell is programmed to produce one primitive endodermal and one primitive ectodermal daughter (RL Gardner, unpublished results).

Cleavage stage embryos are currently being used to test the effect of position on differentiation of early ICM cells because they evidently do not possess an inside environment until the 8-16 cell stage (Barlow, Owen and Graham 1972). Hence, by varying the stage of the host embryo and in later cleavage, the site of injection, one can readily control how long, if at all, the donor cells remain in an outside location. Donor cells are labelled genetically, but can also be located shortly after transplantation because of their small size relative to host blastomeres. A method for handling donor embryos has been devised that enables selection of ICM cells for transplantation that are defined in terms of the number of cycles they have completed since fertilization, and the total cells in the embryo from which they were derived. In most recent experiments short-term culture of donor cells prior to injection has been used to obtain daughter cell pairs. The importance of this additional step is that it allows the two products of one cell to be assayed under the same or different conditions, and hence facilitates distinction between positionally-dependent differentiation and cell selection.

The results to date on injection of single cells and daughter cell pairs into 2-cell embryos are consistent with the 'inside-outside' hypothesis. Thus, all except 2 of a total of 22 chimaeric conceptuses have exhibited exclusively extraembryonic endodermal colonisation by donor cells. The two exceptions displayed chimaerism in derivatives of both the primitive endoderm and primitive ectoderm. Use of 8-cell host embryos has yielded rather confusing results so far since, though primitive ectodermal contributions are found, they are less common than primitive endodermal ones (RL Gardner, unpublished data). At present, attempts are being made to determine whether this is due to donor cells not being 'inside' at the critical stage, or to the fact that the internal environment provided by the morulae is inappropriate for primitive ecto-dermal differentiation.

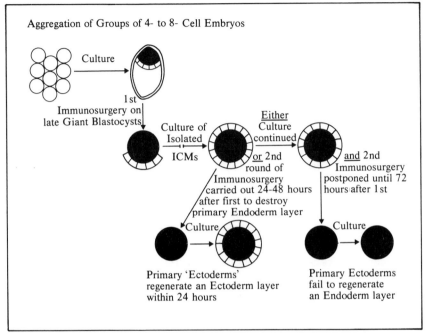

Aggregation of Groups of 4- to 8- Cell Embryos

Culture

1st
Immunosurgery on
late Giant Blastocysts

Culture of
Isolated
ICMs

Either
Culture
continued

or 2nd
round of
Immunosurgery
carried out 24-48 hours
after first to destroy
primary Endoderm layer

and 2nd
Immunosurgery
postponed until 72
hours after 1st

Culture

Culture

Primary 'Ectoderms'
regenerate an Ectoderm layer
within 24 hours

Primary Ectoderms
fail to regenerate
an Endoderm layer

**Figure 1**
Scheme of experimental protocol used by Pedersen, Spindle and Wiley (1977) to demonstrate regeneration of endoderm from primitive ectoderm.

## b) In vitro Studies

Pedersen and his colleagues (Pedersen, Spindle and Wiley 1977) used the protocol outlined in Figure 1 to investigate the developmental potential of primitive ectodermal tissue in culture. ICMs were isolated immunosurgically at the late blastocyst stage and cultured in bacteriological dishes to prevent their attachment and outgrowth. They were subjected to a second round of immunosurgery 24 hours after the first in order to destroy the outer layer of primitive ectoderm. The response of the resulting secondary ICMs (Figure 1) to a further period of 48-72 hours in culture depended on the number of cleavage stage embryos that had been used to make the giant blastocysts from which they were derived. All those obtained from blastocysts composed of 2 embryos degenerated. However, regeneration of a new surface layer of endoderm occurred in 11%, 58% and 74%, respectively, of secondary ICMs from blastocysts composed of 4, 8 and 10 embryos. In further experiments on blastocysts consisting of 10 cleavage stage embryos, regeneration of endoderm was observed consistently if the second round of immunosurgery was deferred until 48 hours, but not if it was carried out at 72 hours after the first

(Figure 1). Pedersen *et al* (1977) concluded from these studies that primitive ectoderm retains the option to differentiate into endoderm for at least 48 hours after primitive endodermal differentiation has taken place in the blastocyst.

Recently, Dziadek (1979) found that by initiating *in vitro* culture at the 8 rather than the 2-cell stage, she could obtain endoderm regeneration routinely from secondary ICMs isolated from blastocysts composed of 3 embryos. Furthermore, she discovered that while few if any endoderm cells of primary ICMs were stained by immunoperoxidase using a specific anti-AFP serum, the majority of those regenerated by secondary ICMs showed strong reactivity (see Table 1). Extrapolating to normal development, Dziadek (1979) proposed that the first layer of endoderm formed by the blastocyst is parietal, and that it induces the primitive ectoderm to produce a second distinct visceral endoderm layer. This model is in conflict with results of the blastocyst injection experiments discussed earlier (Table 2) because it requires the existence of clones which specifically embrace both primitive ectoderm derivatives and visceral endoderm and precludes those spanning both parietal and visceral layers of the extraembryonic endoderm.

Although it is unlikely from the *in vivo* studies that primitive ectoderm cells contribute normally to extraembryonic endoderm, the foregoing experiments nevertheless raise the interesting possibility that their programming can be altered by prolonged exposure to outside conditions *in vitro*. However, other explanations for these findings must be excluded before the idea of repro-gramming can be entertained seriously. Regeneration might, for example, be an artifact attributable simply to delayed differentiation of internal cells in the physiologically aberrant conditions obtaining within giant ICMs in culture. Adverse effects of prolonged *in vitro* culture on both the growth and differentiation of ICM tissue are evident from the literature (eg. Bowman and McLaren 1970; McReynolds and Hadek 1972; Handyside 1978; Spindle 1978). This explanation has been made less likely by a recent report that a minority of secondary ICMs isolated from standard blastocysts can exhibit endoderm regeneration, particularly if the culture dishes are pretreated with medium that has been conditioned by a parietal endoderm-like cell line of teratocarcinoma origin (Atienza-Samols and Sherman 1979).

The further possibility must also be considered that not all endoderm cells are being destroyed by immunosurgery, either because they are resistant to complement-mediated lysis (Harlow and Quinn 1979), or because some are protected from exposure to the reagents. Concerning the latter, it is note worthy that in all studies undertaken so far, embryos have been recovered before the estimated time of primitive endodermal differentiation and the isolated ICMs have been cultured for at least 24 hours thereafter before immunosurgical destruction of this layer is attempted. *In vivo*, the endoderm appears to be growing faster than the ectoderm during its initial phase, a substantial proportion of its cells spreading around the mural trophectoderm.

If a similar differential in growth rate is maintained *in vitro* in conditions in which the cells are denied the option of spreading on the substratum, it is conceivable that the endoderm might soon consist of more than a single layer of cells. Thus, some endodermal cells could thereby be protected from immuno-surgical destruction and, if spread on the surface of the primitive ectoderm, also elude detection by light microscopy, which is the only check for contamination employed so far.

Hence, *in vitro* studies undertaken to date do not provide compelling evidence that ectoderm cells retain the capacity to differentiate as extra-embryonic endoderm. Proof can only be obtained by demonstrating endoderm regeneration from ectoderms that have been isolated under conditions in which they can be shown to be devoid of cells exhibiting the ultrastructural characteristics of primitive endoderm. Furthermore, the ectoderms should be derived from blastocysts that have attained the stage of endodermal differ-entiation *in vivo*.

## The ICM in Delayed Implantation

Gestation may be prolonged in mice that mate during post-partum oestrus because concurrent lactation can postpone implantation and thus lead to slowing or arrest of development at the blastocyst stage (McLaren 1968). This natural interruption of development can be mimicked by ovariectomizing mice early in pregnancy and maintaining them on progesterone (Bergstrom 1978). Delay can be terminated by a single injection of oestrogen Bergstrom 1978), or by removing the suckling young (McLaren 1968). According to Copp (1978), the total number of cells in delayed blastocysts is similar to that of non-delayed blastocysts just before they implant, though the former contain more tro-phectoderm and fewer ICM cells than the latter. The vast majority of cells are arrested in $G_1$, and although DNA synthesis is resumed fairly rapidly following reactivation, mitoses are not seen for more than 24 hours (Sherman and Barlow 1972; Copp 1978). If the delyaed mouse blastocyst lacks primitive endoderm cells, as appears to be the case in the rat (Baevsky 1963; Schlafke and Enders 1963) the above observations suggest that it might provide ideal material for closer examination of the initial stages of differentiation within the ICM.

## Subsequent Differentiation within the Extra Embryonic Endoderm

Visceral endoderm cells from 5.5 day *pc.* postimplantation embryos can colonize the endoderm layer of the visceral yolk sac of host conceptuses following injection into blastocysts (Rossant, Gardner and Alexandre 1978). However, the frequency with which they do so is very low, despite trans-plantation of between 6 and 10 cells *per* blastocyst. Most unexpectedly, further experiments have revealed that this is because transplanted *visceral* cells contribute exclusively to the *parietal* endoderm in most chimaeras

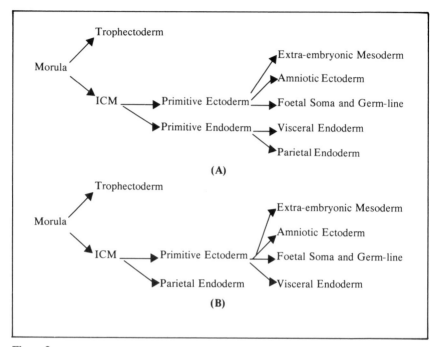

**Figure 2**
Alternative lineages proposed a) by Gardner and Papaioannou (1975) and b) by Dziadek (1979) for the origin of parietal and visceral endoderm cells.

(Gardner 1981), even when they are taken from the region of 6.5 day *pc.* embryos which is actively engaged in AFP synthesis (Dziadek and Adamson 1978). Independently, Hogan and Tilly (1981) have provided both morphological and biochemical evidence that visceral endoderm cells of 7th day embryos can transform into parietal endoderm cells *in vitro.* It is not clear at present whether the ability to undergo such a dramatic change in phenotype is a general property of the visceral endoderm or restricted to relatively immature cells within it. Nevertheless, the above findings raise the interesting possibility that the parietal endoderm may normally grow by recruitment of cells from the visceral layer. They also lend further support to the scheme of cell lineage illustrated in Figure 2a. Attempts to ascertain whether parietal endoderm cells can colonize visceral endoderm derivatives following blastocyst injection have so far yielded negative results. However, both the frequency and level of chimaerism obtained with parietal cells have been much lower than with their visceral counterparts (Gardner 1981).

**Conclusion**
I have tried to outline the various ways in which the lineage and time of

determination of cells in the early mouse embryo are currently being investigated, and have considered some of the principal conclusions to which they have led. While an intelligible pattern is beginning to emerge, it is clear that certain important issues have still to be resolved. Thus, conflicting data have been obtained concerning the time of determination in both the ICM and primitive ectoderm, and the origin of visceral endoderm cells. At present, one cannot neglect the possibility that these discrepancies may be attributable to difficulties in staging embryos and isolating specific tissues from them. I have placed particular emphasis throughout on the need to study cells in the intact embryo, since it is only in this context that their normal fate or full potency is likely to be realised (Gardner 1978c). However, despite the fact that chimaeras have been obtained with both visceral endoderm and extra-embryonic cells (Rossant, Gardner and Alexandre 1978) blastocyst injection has major limitations as a method of studying cells of post implantation embryos. Firstly, the consequences of increasing disparity in age between donor and host cells are difficult to assess. Secondly, attempts to obtain colonisation by later primitive ectoderm cells have been unsuccessful so far (J Rossant, personal communication). Fortunately, alternative strategies are emerging, notably the grafting of small groups of marked cells between postimplantation embryos maintained in short-term culture (Beddington 1981).

## Acknowledgements
I wish to thank Rosa Beddington, Wendy Gardner, Chris Graham and Jo Williamson for help in preparing the manuscript and The Royal Society and Medical Research Council for support.

## References

Adamson, E.D. and Ayers, S.F. *The localisation and synthesis of some collagen types in developing mouse embryos.* Cell, *16*, 953-965 (1979).

Atienza-Samols, S.B. and Sherman, M.I. *In vitro development of core cells of the inner cell mass of the mouse blastocyst: effects of conditioned medium.* J. Exp. Zool. *208*, 67-71 (1979).

Baevsky, U.B. *The effect of embryonic diapause on the nuclei and mitotic activity of mink and rat blastocysts. In Delayed Implantation* (ed. A.C. Enders), pp. 141-153. Chicago: University of Chicago Press (1963).

Barlow, P., Owen, D.A.J. and Graham, C. *DNA synthesis in the preimplantation mouse embryo.* J. Embryol. exp. Morph. *27*, 431-445 (1972).

Bartel, H. *Electron microscopic observations of the inner cell mass of a mouse embryo.* Acta Anat. *83*, 289-301 (1972).

Beddington, R.S.P. *An autoradiographic analysis of the potency of embryonic ectoderm in the 8th day postimplantation mouse embryo.* J. Embryol. exp. Morph. (in press) (1981).

Bergstrom, S. *Experimental delayed implantation. In Methods in Mammalian Reproduction* (ed. J.C. Daniel), pp. 419-435. New York: Academic Press (1978).

Bingel, A.S. and Schwartz, N.B. *Timing of L H release and ovulation in the cyclic mouse.* J. Reprod. Fert. *19*, 223-229 (1969).

Bowman, P. and McLaren, A. *Cleavage rate of mouse embryos in vivo and in vitro.* J. Embryol. exp. Morph. *24*, 203-207 (1970).

Bronson, F.H., Dagg, C.P. and Snell, G.D. *Reproduction. In Biology of the Laboratory Mouse* (ed. E.L. Green), pp. 187-204. New York: McGraw-Hill (1966).

Cole, R.J. *Cinematographic observations on the trophoblast and zona pellucida of the mouse blastocyst.* J. Embryol. exp. Morph. *17*, 481-490 (1967).

Copp, A.J. *Interaction between inner cell mass and trophectoderm of the mouse blastocyst. I. A study of cellular proliferation.* J. Embryol. exp. Morph. *48*, 109-125 (1978).

Davidson, E.H. *Gene Activity in Early Development,* 2nd ed. New York: Academic Press (1976).

Deppe, U., Schierenberg, E., Cole, T., Krieg, C., Schmitt, D., Yoder, B. and Von Ehrenstein, G. *Cell lineages of the embryo of the nematode Caenorhabditis elegans.* Proc. natn. Acad. Sci. USA *75*, 376-380 (1978).

Ducibella, T. *Surface changes of the developing trophoblast cell. In Development in Mammals,* vol *1* (ed. M.H. Johnson), pp 5-29. Amsterdam: North Holland (1977).

Ducibella, T., Albertini, D.F., Anderson, E. & Biggers, J.D. *The preimplantation mammalian embryo: characterisation of intercellular junctions and their appearance during development.* Devl. Biol. 45, 231-250 (1975).

Dziadek, M. *Cell differentiation in isolated inner cell masses of mouse blastocysts in vitro: onset of specific gene expression.* J. Embryol. exp. Morph. *53*, 367-379 (1979).

Dziadek, M. and Adamson, E.D. *Localisation and synthesis of alphafoeto-protein in post-implantation mouse embryos.* J. Embryol. exp. Morph. *43*, 289-313 (1978).

Edwards, R.G. and Gates, A.H. *Timing of the stages of the maturation divisions, ovulation, fertilisation and the first cleavage of eggs of adult mice treated with gonadotrophins.* J. Endocrin. *18*, 292-304 (1959).

Enders, A.C., Given, R.L. and Schlafke, S. *Differentiation and migration of endoderm in the rat and mouse at implantation.* Anat. Rec. *190*, 65-78 (1978).

Finn, C.A. and McLaren, A. *A study of the early stages of implantation in mice.* J. Reprod. Fert. *13*, 259-267 (1967).

Gardner, R.L. *Mouse chimaeras obtained by the injection of cells into the blastocyst.* Nature, Lond. *220*, 596-597 (1968).

Gardner, R.L. *Manipulations on the blastocyst.* Adv. Biosci. *6*, 279-296 (1971).

Gardner, R.L. *Analysis of determination and differentiation in the early mammalian embryo using intra- and inter-specific chimaeras: In The Developmental Biology of Reproduction. 33rd Symposium of the Society for Developmental Biology* (ed. C.L. Markert and J. Papaconstantinou), pp. 207-238. New York: Academic Press (1975).

Gardner, R.L. *Production of chimaeras by injecting cells or tissue into the blastocyst. In Methods in Mammalian Reproduction* (ed. J.C. Daniel), pp. 137-165. New York: Academic Press (1978a).

Gardner, R.L. *The relationship between cell lineage and differentiation in the early mouse embryo. In Genetic Mosaics and Cell Differentiation: Results and Problems in Cell Differentiation,* vol. 9, (ed. W. Gehring), pp. 205-241. Berlin: Springer-Verlag (1978b).

Gardner, R.L. *Potency of normal and neoplastic cells of the early mouse embryo. In Birth Defects: Proceedings of the Fifth International Conference,* (ed. J.W. Littlefield and J. De Grouchy), pp. 154-166. Amsterdam: Excerpta Medica (1978c).

Gardner, R.L. Manuscript in preparation (1981).

Gardner, R.L. and Johnson, M.H. *An investigation of inner cell mass and trophoblast tissues following their isolation from the mouse blastocyst.* J. Embryl. exp. Morph. *28*, 279-312 (1972).

# CELL LINEAGE AND DETERMINATION 275

Gardner, R.L. and Johnson, M.H. *Investigation of cellular interaction and deployment in the early mammalian embryo using inter-specific chimaeras between rat and mouse.* In Cell Patterning. Ciba Foundation Symposium 29 (New Series), pp. 183-200. Amsterdam: Elsevier (1975).

Gardner, R.L. and Lyon, M.F. *X-chromosome inactivation studied by injection of a single cell into the mouse blastocyst.* Nature, Lon. *231*, 385-386 (1971).

Gardner, R.L. and Rossant, J. *Determination during embryogenesis.* In Embryogenesis in Mammals. Ciba Foundation Symposium 40 (New Series), pp. 5-18. Amsterdam: Elsevier (1976).

Gardner, R.L. and Rossant, J. *Investigation of the fate of 4.5 day post coitum mouse inner cell mass cells by blastocyst injection.* J. Embryol. exp. Morph. *52*, 141-152 (1979).

Gardner, R.L., Papaioannou, V.E. and Barton, S.C. *Origin of the extoplacental cone and secondary giant cells in mouse blastocysts reconstituted from isolated trophoblast and inner cell mass.* J. Embryol. exp. Morph. *30*, 561-572 (1973).

Gehring, W. *Genetic Mosaics and Cell Differentiation: Results and Problems in Cell Differentiation* vol.9. Berlin: Springer-Verlag (1978).

Goldstein, L.S., Spindle, A.I. and Pedersen, R.A. *X-ray sensitivity of the pre-implantation mouse embryo in vitro.* Rad. Res. *62*: 276, 287 (1975).

Graham, C.F. and Deussen, Z.A. *Features of cell lineage in preimplantation mouse development.* J. Embryol. exp. Morph. *48*, 53-72 (1978).

Graham, C.F. and Lehtonen, E. *Formation and consequences of cell patterns in preimplantation mouse development.* J. Embryol. exp. Morph. *49*, 277-294 (1979).

Handyside, A.H. *Time of commitment of inside cells isolated from preimplantation mouse embryos.* J. Embryol. exp. Morph. *45*, 37-53 (1978).

Handyside, A.H. and Barton, S.C. *Evaluation of the technique of immuno surgery for the isolation of inner cell masses from mouse blastocysts.* J. Embryol. exp. Morph. *37*, 217-226 (1977).

Handyside, A.H. and Johnson, M.H. *Temporal and spatial patterns of the synthesis of tissue-specific polypeptides in the preimplantation mouse embryo.* J. Embryol. exp. Morph. *44*, 191-199 (1978).

Harlow, G.M. and Quinn, P. *Isolation of inner cell masses from mouse blastocysts by immunosurgery or exposure to the calcium ionophore A23187.* Aust. J. Biol. Sci. *32*, 483-491 (1979).

Hillman, N., Sherman, M.I. and Graham, C.F. *The effect of spatial arrangement on cell determination during mouse development.* J. Embryol. exp. Morph. *28*, 263-278 (1972).

Hogan, B.L.M. *High molecular weight extracellular proteins synthesised by endoderm cells derived from mouse teratocarcinoma cells and normal extra embryonic membranes.* Devl. Biol. *76*, 275-285 (1980).

Hogan, B.L.M. and Tilly, R. *In vitro development of inner cell masses isolated immuno-surgically from mouse blastocysts. II. Inner cell masses from 3.5 to 4.0 day p.c. blastocysts.* J. Embryol. exp. Morph. *45*, 107-121 (1978a).

Hogan, B.L.M. and Tilly, R. *In vitro development of inner cell masses isolated immuno-surgically from mouse blastocysts. I. Inner cell masses from 3.5 day p.c. blastocysts incubated for 24 h before immunosurgery.* J. Embryol. exp. Morph. *45*, 93-105 (1978b).

Hogan, B.L.M. and Tilly, R. *Cell interactions and endoderm differentiation in cultured mouse embryos.* J. Embryos. exp. Morph. (in press) (1981).

Hoppe, P.C. *Genetic influences on mouse sperm capacitation in vivo* aKelly, S.J. *Studies of the potency of early cleavage blastomers of the mouse.* In The Early Development of Mammals. 2nd Symposium of The British Society for Developmental Biology (ed. M. Balls and A.E. Wild), pp. 97-105. Cambridge: Cambridge University Press (1975).

Huxley, J.S. and de Beer, G.R. *The Elements of Experimental Embryology.* Cambridge: Cambridge University Press (1934).

Jenkinson, E.J. and Billington, W.J. *Cell surface properties of early mammalian embryos. In Concepts in Mammalian Embryogenesis* (ed. M.I. Sherman), pp. 235-266. Cambridge: MIT Press (1977).

Johnson, M.H. *Intrinsic and extrinsic factors in preimplantation development.* J. Reprod. Fert. 55: 255-265 (1979).

Johnson, M.H., Handyside, A.H. and Braude, P.R. *Control mechanisms in early mammalian development. In Development in Mammals,* vol.2 (ed. M.H. Johnson) pp. 67-97. Amsterdam: North-Holland (1977).

Johnson, M.H., Pratt, H.P.M. and Handyside, A.H. *The generation and recognition of positional information in the preimplantation mouse embryo. In Cellular and Molecular Aspects of Implantation* (ed. S. Glasser and D. Bullock). Plenum Press (in press) (1981).

Johnson, M.H., Chakraborty, J., Handyside, A.H., Willison, K. and Stern, P. *The effect of prolonged decompaction on the development of the preimplantation mouse embryo.* J. Embryol. exp. Morph. *54,* 241-261 (1979).

Kelly, S.J., Mulnard, J.G. and Graham, C.F. *Cell division and cell allocation in early mouse development.* J. Embryol. exp. Morph. *48,* 37-51 (1978).

Kemler, R., Babinet, C., Eisen, H. and Jacob, F. *Surface antigen in early differentiation.* Proc. natn. Acad. Sci. USA *74,* 4449-4452 (1977).

Kimble, J. and Hirsh, D. *The postembryonic cell lineages of the hermaphrodite and male gonads in Caenorhobditis elegans.* Devl. Biol. *70,* 396-417 (1979).

Krzanowska, H. *Time interval between copulation and fertilization in inbred lines of mice and their crosses.* Folia biol., Krakow *12,* 231-244 (1964).

Leivo, I., Vaheri, A., Timpl, R. and Wartiovaara, J. *Appearance and distribution of collagens and laminin in the early mouse embryo.* Devl. Biol. *76,* 100-114 (1980).

Lewis, W.H. and Wright, W.S. *On the early development of the mouse egg.* Contr. Embryol. Carnegie Instn. Washington *148,* 114-147 (1935).

Magnuson, T., Jacobson, J.B. and Stackpole, C.W. *Relationship between intercellular permeability and junction organisation in the preimplantation mouse embryo.* Devl. Biol. *67,* 214-224 (1978).

Martin, G. and Evans, M.J. *Differentiation of clonal lines of teratocarcinoma cells: formation of embryoid bodies in vitro.* Proc. natn. Acad. Sci. USA *72,* 1441-1445 (1975).

McLaren, A. *A study of blastocysts during delay and subsequent implantation in lactating mice.* J. Endocr. *42,* 453-462 (1968).

McLaren, A. *Mammalian Chimaeras.* Cambridge: Cambridge University Press (1976).

McLaren, A. and Bowman, P. *Genetic effects on the timing of early development in the mouse.* J. Embryol. exp. Morph. *30,* 491-500 (1973).

McLaren, A. and Smith, R. *Functional test of tight junctions in the mouse blastocyst.* Nature, Lond. *267,* 351-352 (1977).

McReynolds, H.D. and Hadek, R. *A comparison of the fine structure of late mouse blastocysts in vivo and in vitro.* J. exp. Zool. *182,* 95-118 (1972).

Mintz, B. *Experimental genetic mosaicism in the mouse. In Preimplantation Stages of Pregnancy: Ciba Foundation Symposium* (ed. G.E.W. Wolstenholme and M. O'Connor) pp. 194-207. London: Churchill (1965).

Mukherjee, A.B. *Cell cycle analysis and X-chromosome inactivation in the developing mouse.* Proc. Natn. Acad. Sci. USA *73,* 1608-1611 (1976).

Nadijcka, M. and Hillman, N. *Ultrastructural studies of the mouse blastocyst substages.* J. Embryol. exp. Morph. *32,* 675-695 (1974).

Nicol, A. and McLaren, A. *An effect of the female genotype on sperm transport in mice.* J. Reprod. Fert. *39,* 421-424 (1974).

Orsini, M.W. and McLaren, A. *Loss of the zona pellucida in mice, and the effect of tubal ligation and ovariectomy.* J. Reprod. Fert. *13*, 485-499 (1967).

Papaioannou, V.E. *Micromanipulation and microsurgery of cells and early embryos. In Techniques in Cellular Physiology* (ed. P.F. Baker). Amsterdam: Elsevier: North Holland (in press) (1981).

Pedersen, R.A., Spindle, A.I. and Wiley, L.M. *Regeneration of endoderm by ectoderm isolated from mouse blastocysts.* Nature, Lond. *270*, 435-437 (1977).

Rossant, J. *Investigation of the determinative state of the mouse inner cell mass. I. Aggregation of isolated inner cell masses with morulae.* J. Embryol. exp. Morph. *33*, 979-990 (1975a).

Rossant, J. *Investigation of the determinative state of the mouse inner cell mass. II. The fate of isolated inner cell masses transferred to the oviduct.* J. Embryol. exp. Morph. *33*, 991-1001 (1975b).

Rossant, J. *Investigation of inner cell mass determination by aggregation of isolated rat inner cell masses with mouse morulae.* J. Embryol. exp. Morph. *36*, 163-174 (1976).

Rossant, J. and Lis, W.T. *Potential of isolated mouse inner cell masses to form trophectoderm derivatives in vivo.* Devl. Biol. *70*, 255-261 (1979).

Rossant, J. and Vijh, K.M. *Ability of outside cells from preimplantation mouse embryos to form inner cell mass derivatives.* Devl. Biol. *76*, 475-482 (1980).

Rossant, J., Gardner, R.L. and Alexandre, H.L. *Investigation of the potency of cells from the postimplantation mouse embryo by blastocyst injection: a preliminary report.* J. Embryol. exp. Morph. *48*, 239-247 (1978).

Rowinski, J., Solter, D. and Koprowski, H. *Mouse embryo development in vitro: effects of inhibitors of RNA and protein synthesis on blastocyst and post-blastocyst embryos.* J. exp. Zool. *192*, 133-142 (1975).

Schlafke, S. and Enders, A.C. *Observations on the fine structure of the rat blastocyst.* J. Anat. *97*, 353-360 (1963).

Sherman, M.I. *The role of cell-cell interaction during early mouse embryogenesis. In The Early Development of Mammals: 2nd Symposium of The British Society for Developmental Biology* (ed. M. Balls and A.E. Wild), pp. 145-165. Cambridge: Cambridge University Press (1975).

Sherman, M.I. and Atienza, S.B. *Effects of bromodeoxyuridine, cytosine arabinoside and colcemid upon in vitro development of mouse blastocysts.* J. Embryol. exp. Morph. *34*, 467-484 (1975).

Sherman, M.I. and Atienza-Samols, S.B. *Differentiation of mouse trophoblast does not require cell-cell interaction.* Exp. Cell Res. *123*, 73-77 (1979).

Sherman, M.I. and Barlow, P.W. *Deoxyribonucleic acid content in delayed mouse blastocysts.* J. Reprod. Fert. *29*, 123-126 (1972).

Smith, R. and McLaren, A. *Factors affecting the time of formation of the mouse blastocoele.* J. Embryol. exp. Morph. *41*, 79-92 (1977).

Snell, G.D., Fekete, E., Hummel, K.P. and Law, L.W. *The relation of mating, ovulation and the estrous smear in the house mouse to time of day.* Anat. Rec. *90*, 243-253 (1940).

Snow, M.H.L. *Abnormal development of preimplantation mouse embryos grown in vitro with 3 H thymidine.* J. Embryol. exp. Morph. *29*, 601-615 (1973).

Solter, D. and Knowles, B.B. *Immunosurgery of mouse blastocysts.* Proc. natn. Acad. Sci. USA *72*, 5099-5102 (1975).

Spielmann, H., Jacob-Muller, U. and Beckord, W. *Immunosurgical studies on inner cell mass development in rat and mouse blastocysts before and during implantation in vitro.* J. Embryol. exp. Morph. *60*, 255-269 (1980).

Spindle, A.I. *Trophoblast regeneration by inner cell masses isolated from cultured mouse embryos.* J. exp. Zool. *203*, 483-490 (1978).

Sulston, J.E. and Horvitz, H.R. *Post embryonic cell lineages of the nematode, Caenorhabditis elegans.* Devl. Biol. *56*, 110-156 (1977).

Surani, M.A.H., Tochiana, D. and Barton, S.C. *Isolation and development of the inner cell mass after exposure of mouse embryos to calcium ionophore A23187.* J. Embryol. exp. Morph. *45*, 237-247 (1978).

Tarkowski, A.K. *Mouse chimaeras developed from fused eggs.* Nature, Lond. *190* : 857-860 (1961).

Tarkowski, A.K. and Wroblewska, J. *Development of blastomeres of mouse eggs isolated at the four- and eight-cell stage.* J. Embryol. exp. Morph. *18* : 155-180 (1967).

Timple, R., Rohde, H., Robey, P.G., Rennard, S.I., Foidart, J. M. and Martin, G.R. *Laminin-a glycoprotein from basement membranes.* J. Biol chem. *254* : 9933-9937 (1979).

Wartiovaara, J., Leivo, I. and Vaheri, A. *Expression of the cell surface-associated glycoprotein, fibronectin, in the early mouse embryo.* Devl. Biol. *69* : 247-257 (1979).

Weiss, P. *Principles of Development.* p. 296. New York: Henry Holt and Company (1939).

Willison, K.R. and Stern, P.L. *Expression of a Forssman antigenic specificity in the preimplantation mouse embryo.* Cell *14* : 785-793 (1978).

## Questions

*Weiss*

Do you get any differences in the frequency of conversation depending upon the strain or origin of the mouse?

*Gardner*

We are doing all these with a random-bred strain which has just been selected to be homozygous for the two GP1 variants. We have at one time tried to fiddle around with combinations because rather than inject several cells if you want to see whether partitioning is real, it would be much nicer if you could generate much larger clones. By analogy with the minute technique of *Drosophila*, you could get cells that had a very high proliferative advantage but we have never found any consistent or predictable effects when we do this and the striking thing, anyhow, using these experiments which, again, would fit in with the clonal work in *Drosophila*, is that the size of the clones you get when you take a series of cells from the same inner cell mass then they are very heterogenous indeed. Some are absolutely huge, in particular if you inject the cells into the cleavage stage embryo you can get the whole of the extraembryonic endoderm derived from the mitotic descendants of one cell; in other cases they may contribute to 10% of the total cell population so it is very heterogenous indeed.

*Weiss*

One other question. Since you can to some extent manipulate the cells you are going to inject before you inject them, can you use colchicine or something to make them tetraploid - can you use that as a marker?

*Gardner*

Well, there has been a lot of work on inducing tetraploidy with cytochalasin B during cleavage, done by Tarkofsky in Warsaw and Michael Snow in London. In the latter case, it was with the specific aim of using it as a marker but there seem to be packing problems with these larger cells and if you aggregate the tetraploids with the diploids the former just end up by being pushed out into the trophectoderm. He did actually get some straight tetra ploids going through to birth but he was concerned with both the efficiency with which he could recognise the cell size differences and the very low viability and poor performance of the tetraploids in that combination. So it does not look like being a very promising marker although it does have interesting effects when you want to try to make tubules and things like that – the cells really have problems in undergoing certain morphogenetic processes.

# From the Gene to the Pattern: Chaeta Differentiation

*Antonio Garcia-Bellido*

## Introduction

The generation of form in biological systems remains a major unresolved problem. In viruses, and possibly in some cell organelles such as membranes, flagella, myosin fibres, etc., the basic building principle is self assembly; i.e. as in organic cystals, the properties of the individual elements determine their interactions and organisation in specific three-dimensional structures. In multicellular systems the degrees of freedom of these interactions seem to be higher and the spatial organisation of these elements seems to require a global building principle, referred to as positional information in modern terminology. However, whereas in simple systems we know in some depth the properties of the elements involved in the structure, in multicellular systems we know very little of the properties of cells in the morphogenetic period. Specifically, we know almost nothing about how genetic instructions within cells determine their behaviour in supracellular communities. In the present paper we will discuss the genetic mechanism at work in the specification of the chaeta pattern in the adult cuticle of *Drosophila*. This is a two-dimensional pattern. But such patterns may be more than simple models for studying morphogenesis. In many instances of animal development, as in the nervous system, multilayered organisations derive from cellular monolayers and possibly result from specification of cells as they are in the monolayers.

The cuticle of insects results from differentiation of monolayers of epidermal cells of ectodermal origin. Cells in this monolayer become specialised in the production of specific cuticular organs, trichomes, chaetae, scales, sensillae, etc., which appear, in the final structure, in fixed and characteristic positions.

Formally, the generation of this two-dimensional pattern can be described by two operations: the cytodifferentiation of the different elements and spatial distribution of these elements in the cuticular surface. A mechanistic explanation of the final pattern requires an understanding of the extent to which cyto-differentiation is a response to the position of the cell in the system or alternatively, whether position is defined by cell to cell inter actions and is a consequence of genetic activity in the individual cells. We will report results of clonal and genetic analysis of the chaeta pattern of *Drosophila*, which support the second interpretation.

**The Cell Lineage of Chaetae**
Chaetae are sensory organs, mechano- and chemoreceptors, which consist of two external, cuticular elements: the base or socket (tormogen) and the shaft (trichogen), and two internal nervous elements: one or several bipolar neurons in the base of the socket, and supporting glia-like cells surrounding the axons (see Lawrence 1966). The different chaetae have specific patterns of central nervous system projections (Ghysen 1979). Externally, the different chaetae can be distinguished by shaft structure, colour, and texture under high power magnification. Under low power magnification they are readily distinguishable into small chaetae (microchaetae, also called 'hairs' in early papers) and large chaetae (macrochaetae, or 'bristles'). Both size and position are regular and constant enough to permit identification of individual chaetae (especially macrochaetae) and the use of their interspecific variations in taxonomy (Figure 1).

Chaetae differentiate from the same population of epidermal cells which will give rise to 'non-innervated' cuticular elements, as trichomes, during the proliferation period of the imaginal discs. Clonal analysis (in gynandromorphs) has shown that even neighbouring chaetae can derive from different lineages separated already in the early zygote (Sturtevant 1929). Mitotic recombination clones initiated in early stages of development embrace chaetae and trichomes (Stern 1936). However, clones initiated about 4 division cycles prior to the end of the proliferation period of the notum contain either chaetae or trichomes (Garcia-Bellido and Merriam 1971a). In clones initiated early, the probability of two chaetae being differentiated within the same clones is roughly proportional to the size of the clone and the final distance between the chaetae. Thus, the final chaeta pattern, within a particular cuticular region, does not result from segregation of chaetae of the same lineage. Chaetae appear, as a rule, within the clone of epidermal cells in which they were originated. There are however, interesting exceptions. The sex-comb area in the male foreleg rotates relative to the same area in female (Tokunga 1962). In the abdominal tergites chaetae appear at regular intervals, but in clones, individual marked chaetae may appear separated from the marked sister epidermal cells and vice versa, non-marked chaetae appear within the clone of marked epidermal cells (Garcia-Bellido and Merriam 1971b). Comparable migrations have been found in the chaeta pattern of legs (Lawrence *et.al.* 1979). Thus, short migrations of already specified chaetae might be involved in their arrangement in a pattern. It is not known how important this mechanism is in chaeta pattern formation.

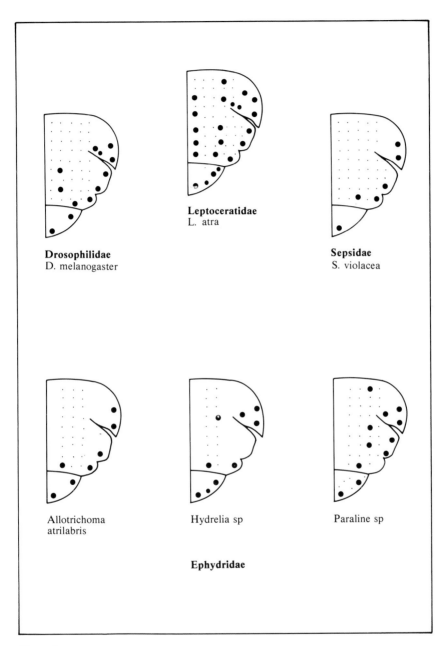

**Figure 1**
Schematic representation of the chaeta pattern in the notum (dorsal mesothorax) of different genera (*Acalyterata*) related to *Drosophila*. Heavy dots: macrochaete; small dots: microchaete.

## Variations of the Chaeta Pattern

The study of the mechanisms involved in the generation of the normal chaeta pattern begins with the analysis of its variations. The regularity of chaeta patterns, such as that of the notum, permits the ready detection of variants. It is an old observation that the chaeta pattern is invariant in flies reared under extreme temperature conditions and in small flies emerging from crowded cultures. Most of the variants known are of genetic origin.

Comparative anatomy of higher Diptera, especially in genera related to *Drosophila* (Sturtevant 1970) also uncovers a constant chaeta pattern in the notum (Figure 1). We do not know how far this constant pattern is maintained by selective pressure or by the very mechanism of its formation. Sturtevant found high correlations in variations of macrochaetae and of microchaetae but no correlation between macrochaeta and microchaeta variations. This suggests the existence of, at least partially, independent genetic control for both types of chaetae (see below). Analysis of the patterns of macrochaetae of a sample of genera (Figure 1) indicates that they have a common underlying pattern. It is impossible however to arrange them in a linear series. It is formally easier to derive each of them from the most complex pattern (*Leptocera*) by suppression of chaetae in certain positions than to explain the seriation by independent addition of chaetae starting from a naked type. The most complex pattern is moreover the most regular, and can be viewed as a grid formed by rows of chaetae. Without experiment, this consideration remains speculation, but it is worth emphasising that comparative anatomy of related species represents a powerful analytical tool for inferring the existence of invariant properties in development susceptible of being proved by genetic analysis in one of them (*Drosophila melanogaster*).

Studies on selection of quantitative characters have used chaeta patterns as model systems. The spontaneous appearance of flies with extra chaetae or with fewer chaetae than normal can be used to start selection lines. As for other quantitative traits, selection is effective in the first generations. The base of this selection is assumed to be the existence in the genome of genetic 'modifiers'. In the subsequent generations of selection a plateau is usually reached, unless new variability is introduced by mutation. Genetic analysis in outcrosses of these selected lines uncovers the existence of 'major' (discrete and mappable genetic factors) and 'minor' (multiple factors which can only be detected in combinations) modifiers (Thoday 1958). It is questionable however, whether all these modifiers are alleles of genes whose primary function is to control chaeta differentiation or positioning. In some cases these major modifiers have been found to correspond to alleles of known mutants (for example *hairy*, see below) but in other cases no genetic analysis of their loci has been undertaken.

In some chaeta patterns, like that of the macrochaeta of the notum, selection for extra chaetae is difficult; this barrier to variation is explained by assuming that the wild type pattern is 'canalised' (Rendel 1968). Selection on mutant strains that affect the chaeta pattern, such as *scute* (see below), which remove some macrochaetae, is more efficient than in wildtype, presumably because the mutation destabilises the canalisation (Rendel 1968). The study of major modifiers found in outcrosses of wildtype and mutant selected lines permits the assignment of these major modifiers to an additive class or to a class of loci which are specific for the mutant or for the canalised phenotype. In this way regulatory genes in the process of pattern have been proposed (Latter 1973, Fraser 1967, Rendel 1976).

The study of the patterns affected by selection shows very localised effects. Thus, for example, selection for extra scutellar chaetae could lead to flies with more chaetae, but these appear only on the scutellum, the characteristic pattern of other regions remaining unaffected (Rendel and Evans 1978). This suggests that the modifiers being selected have local, rather than general effects on pattern or chaeta differentiation. Their effects have been interpreted as due to lowering the threshold of response of presumptive chaeta cells in a region to an invariant underlying prepattern (Sondhi 1962). In some cases the new pattern may be reminiscent of patterns found in other genera of *Drosophilidae* (Sondhi 1962). To my knowledge, experiments have not been performed trying to select for changes in position of extant chaetae.

It is obvious that selection experiments represent sources of variation useful both in uncovering the logic of the construction of patterns and in detecting genetic factors at work in the mechanism of this construction. However, to derive full benefit from these experiments they should be accompanied by developmental and genetic analysis of the loci involved.

The most accessible source of variation in pattern formation is mutation. The regular distribution of chaetae in the cuticle of *Drosophila* permits the ready detection of chaeta pattern mutants, and many such are known. They can formally be classified as those which remove and those which add chaetae to the normal pattern. It is, in principle, conceivable that many of these mutations produce their effect on chaetae as part of a complex pleiotropic syndrome or as secondary consequences of non-specific gene misfunction. It is also conceivable that genes involved in chaeta differentiation and/or positioning might have only, or mostly, lethal alleles. The sorting out among visible mutation and among lethals of those loci pertinent to chaeta pattern formation is a heavy task. The problem is compounded by the fact that the understanding of a gene function relation to other genes. In the following we discuss work, carried out in this laboratory, related to the developmental and genetic analysis of chaeta pattern formation.

### The Achaeta-Scute Gene Complex
Among the mutations which remove chaetae are those of two closely linked loci, *achaeta* (*ac*) and *scute* (*sc*), on the tip of the X chromosome. Many mutants at these loci have been accumulated through the years, and a rich

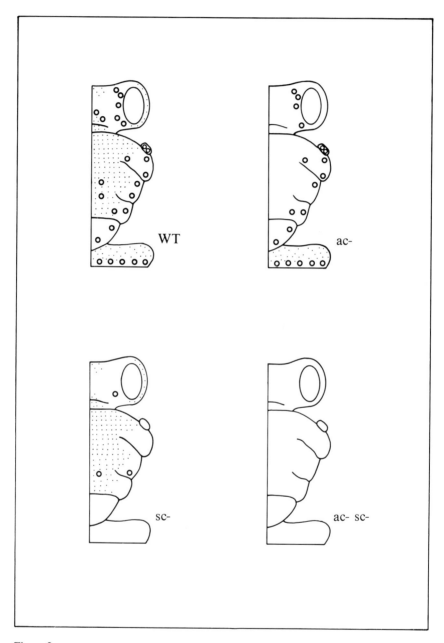

**Figure 2**

Schematic representation of the chaeta pattern in mutants of the *achaeta-scute* complex. WT: wild type; *ac-* deficient for *ac(In(1)y³PLsc⁸R)*; *sc-*: deficient for *scα(In(1)sc⁸Lsc⁴R)*; *ac- sc-*: deficient for both *(In(1)y³PLsc⁴R)*.

literature about the genetics of this genes is available. What makes these mutants especially interesting is that they show allele-specific patterns of effects. Whereas alleles of the *achaeta* locus mainly remove microchaetae, alleles of the *scute* locus remove only macrochaetae (Figure 2). All these mutations are recessive, and there is an almost complete complementation between *achaeta* and *scute* alleles, suggesting partially independent functions. Alleles of the *scute* locus may differ in the pattern of chaetae removed, and scx/scy doubly heterozygous files show non-complementation for chaetae affected by both loci and complementation for the allele-specific ones. This finding led to the suggestion that the scute gene is in turn a complex gene with independent functions related to specific chaeta sites (Dubinin 1933). When more alleles are incorporated into this study the picture of gene-site sp?cificity blurs, and a different interpretation emerges. It is possible to seriate the different chaetae sites (without relation to topological position) in such a way that the different alleles affect contiguous sites in this seriation, in most cases starting from the same origin - the most sensitive site (Garcia-Bellido 1979). Thus chaeta-site specificity in mutants may result from variable amounts of wild type function and positional threshold requirements.

The *scute* and *achaeta* loci are complex. Mutant flies with chromosomal rearrangements with breakpoints in the lBl-lB4/5 polytene-chromosome region may show *achaeta* or *scute* phenotypes of different extent in the chaeta-site seriation (Muller 1965, Garcia-Bellido 1979). Combining the elements of these chromosomal rearrangements in heterozygous condition we can generate flies with genetic duplications and deletions within the region. Whereas the duplications are wild type, except for a *Hairy wing* (*Hw*) phenotype (see below) the deletions have a more or less extreme pattern of chaeta removal depending on the elements used. Based on the phenotype caused by these deletions a linear map of breakpoints can be built. This map is linearly correlated with the order of breakpoints as. visualised in the polytene chromosomes (Garcia-Bellido 1979). The *achaeta-scute* gene complex can thus be subdivided into different regions (Figure 3): an *achaeta* region(s) related to microchaeta differentiation, two *scute* ($\alpha$ and $\beta$) regions (the deletion of either of which has the same pattern of removal of macrochaetae) and a lethal (lethal of *scute*) region located between the two *scute* regions. The functional relations among these regions are remarkable in the sense that

1) *Scute* point mutants will not complement with deficiencies of either of the two *scute* regions and
2) Flies doubly-heterozygous for rearrangements with one breakpoint in the *scute* $\alpha$ and the other in the *scute* $\beta$ region have mutant phenotypes. This genetic behaviour of *achaeta-scute* mutants has led to the suggestion that this region contains different functions, each of which is necessary for chaeta differentiation, and which act in a combinatorial way (possibly by a polymeric

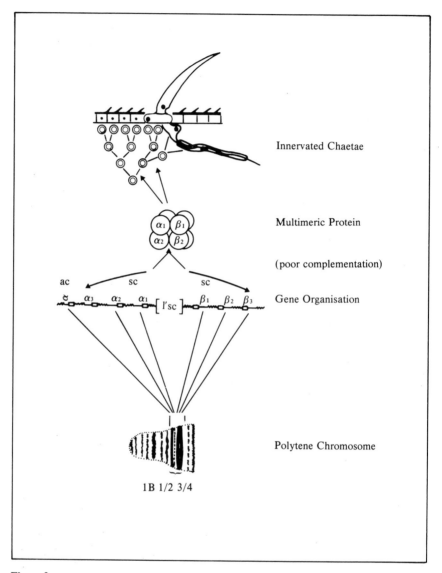

**Figure 3**

Hypothetical gene organisation of the *achaeta-scute* gene complex and its products. in the bottom, the chromosome bands which contain the gene complex and the linear organisation of the different functions based on the phenotype of chromosomal rearrangements with breakpoints in this region. $\gamma_1$, $\alpha_3$, $\alpha_2$, etc., the independent coding regions affected by the breakpoints, separated by non-coding regions. l'sc: *lethal of scute* region. The poor completion found in heterozygous rearrangements suggest that the product of *scute* is a multimer. In the top, the cell divisions giving rise to epidermal cells and innervated chaetae; the two arrows correspond to the possible steps where the *achaeta* and *scute* mutant insufficiently affect chaeta differentiation.

product). Moreover, transcription (and translation) of the entire region, of the order of 250Kb, must occur preferentially *cis*-coupled to explain the poor complementation observed (Garcia-Bellido 1979).

The subdivisions found in the genetic map of the gene complex and the cytological appearance of the chromosome bands (Figure 3) in this region, are compatible with the idea that diversification of function originated with tandem repetition of the same original sequence (Garcia-Bellido 1979). Developmental analysis of the *achaeta-scute* complex indicates that it plays a role in nervous system differentiation. The deletion of the entire gene complex is zygotic lethal but it is viable in clones of epidermal cells. Within these clones cuticular differentiation is otherwise normal but all and only the innervated chaetae and sensillae of the cuticle are absent (Garcia-Bellido and Santamaria 1978). The gynandromorph lethal focus of the deletion embryos maps to the embryonic central nervous system (Garcia-Bellido and Santamaria 1978). Jimenez and Campos-Ortega (1979) and White (1980) have shown that these embryos are normal in all germ layer derivatives but lack cuticular sensory organs and the central nervous system after some neuroblast divisions enters histoloysis and disappears. From these results it can be speculated that the *achaeta-scute* gene complex is involved in the segregation of an epidermal and a nervous pathway, from the ectoderm germ layer, in the formation of both the central and the peripheral nervous systems of larval and imaginal cuticular organs. The same final phenotype can be accounted for if the wild type function of these genes is to implement or to maintain the differentiation of nervous elements, i.e. the final differentiation of chaetae, once the individual cells of the epidermis have been singled out to become chaetae.

### The Production of Extra Chaetae

It is interesting that some mutations in the same *ac-sc* complex lead to the formation of more chaetae, i.e. to the conversion of otherwise non-innervated cuticular elements into innervated extra chaetae. Such mutations carry the genetic name of *Hairy-wing* (*Hw*). The same phenotype can be caused by point mutants (*Hw*[49]c), small rearrangements within the complex (*Hw*[1]), internal duplications of the gene (see above) and by gene variegation due to the proximity of part of the gene to centric heterochromatin. Except for the supposed point mutant - it could be a small rearrangement - the general feature of all of them is the decompensation in doses of different regions of the *achaeta-scute* complex. A complete duplication of the complex has a wild type phenotype. *Hw* mutations are dominant in flies with one or several wild type doses of the entire complex; they behave therefore as overproducers or derepression mutations. The *Hw* extra chaetae are microchaetae and they appear in the notum, wing surface (as those shown in Figure 5) and other

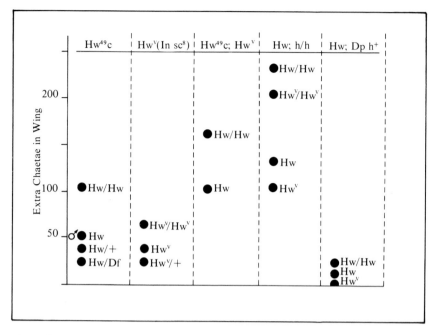

**Figure 4**

Effect of different genetic constitutions on the number of extra chaetae in the wing, in male (*Hw*) or females (*Hw/\**). *Hw⁴⁹c*: a point mutant *Hwv*: *Hw*-variegated in the *X(In(1)sc⁸)* or the *Y(sc⁸Y)*. *Hw; h/h*: combinations with *hairy;* *Hw; Dp* (3)*h:* combination with an extra dose of the wild type allele of *hairy*. (A tandem duplication).

regions of the body. As expected from mutations of the depression type *Hw* is not dosage compensated; the number of extra chaetae is the same in the hemizygous males and heterozygous females, and this number is half that in homozygous females. The number of extra chaetae can increase further in flies which carry *Hw* and either one or two duplications with *Hw*-variegated (In(1)sc⁸) mutations, or are simulataneously homozygous for a mutant (*hairy*) in the third chromosome (Figure 4).

Thus, changes in the *achaeta-scute* complex lead to changes in the chaeta pattern, to removal of chaetae attributable to insufficiency of gene function and to appearance of extra chaetae owing to excess of function. This finding indicates that this gene complex is involved not only in the mechanism of implementation of chaeta differentiation but also in that of the decision to differentiate chaetae. How much the new pattern that emerges by excess of function results from response to an underlying pattern of position or is a consequence of cell to cell interaction? The study of other mutants and of the developmental stages when these decisions are taken sheds light on this question.

## Gene Interactions with the Achaeta-Scute Complex

A recessive mutation in the third chromosome, *hairy* (*h*) in homozygous condition causes the appearance of extra microchaetae, distributed in a pattern indistinguishable from that of *Hw* (Figure 5). The extra chaetae are also innervated (Stern 1938). The locus *hairy* has interesting interactions with the *achaeta-scute* complex. Sturtevant (1970) already showed that *ac* mutants are dominant suppressors of *hairy*. Flies homozygous for *h* and heterozygous for *ac* show a reduction of extra chaetae; if they are also homozygous for *ac* as they lack the extra chaetae as well as all the normal chaetae of the *achaeta* pattern (Garcia-Bellido and Merriam 1971c) (Figure 5). Of all the internal deletions of the *achaeta-scute* complex only the *achaeta* region has this effect. This result is compatible with *achaeta* being the structural gene necessary for the expression of *hairy*. In fact *h/h* flies with one or more extra doses of the wild type *achaeta-scute* gene complex (as duplications in the genome) show increasing numbers of extra chaetae (Figure 6). Especially relevant for subsequent discussion is the finding that, whereas the number of these extra chaetae increases linearly in the wing surface with the number of $ac+$ -$sc+$ doses, it reaches a maximal amount in the notum, above which more $ac+$ doses lead to fewer microchaetae than normal (Figure 5) (Moscoso del Prado and Garcia-Bellido, unpublished).

The interactions between *h* and *Hw*, mentioned above, are especially relevant; *h* and *Hw* double mutants show a superadditive effect in the formation of extra chaetae (Figure 4) (see Neel 1941). Reciprocally, *Hw* flies (no matter if point mutants or of the *Hw*-variegated type) which have three doses of the wild type allele of *hairy* have reduced numbers of extra chaetae (Figure 4). These results are consistent with the formal hypothesis proposed by Falk (1964) that *hairy* is a regulator gene of the *achaeta-scute* complex and *Hw* equivalent to an operator-constitutive mutation in the system. This control would be by repression of the structural gene, the *achaeta-scute* complex, and more specifically of the *achaeta* region of it. Obviously *Hw* mutants do not correspond to total derepression because their expression can be modulated by manipulating the dosage of the *hairy* locus. Gene-dosage analysis of the interaction between the two loci has yielded an interesting result: *hairy* becomes dominant when *h* heterozygous flies contain more than two wild type doses of the *achaeta-scute* complex (Figure 6). Apparently one dose of the wild type allele of *h* is insufficient to repress three or more doses of the *achaeta* structural gene (Moscoso del Prado and Garcia-Bellido, unpublished). The latter finding is of special relevance, because it can be used as an operation to detect mutations anywhere in the genome with similar effects, in heteroygous condition, i.e. in the first generation following mutagenesis. This approach has led to the discovery of several (5) new mutants which produce extra microchaetae. All are alleles of *hairy*, suggesting that this may be the only locus in the genome with dose dependent interactions with achaeta.

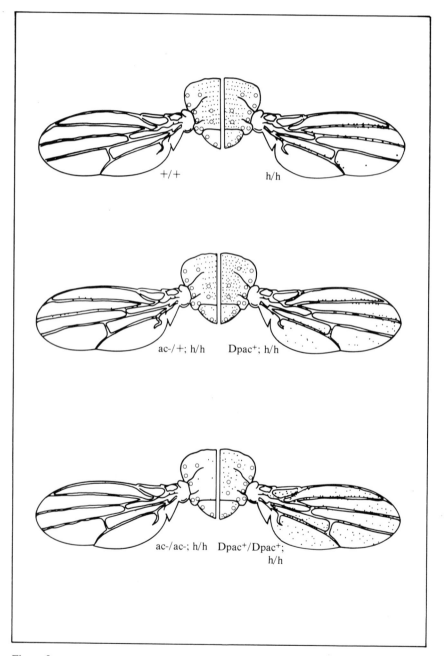

**Figure 5**

Phenotype of different genetic combinations of the *achaeta* and *hairy*, in notum and wing. *Dp ac+* is actually *Dp(1;2)sc19*.

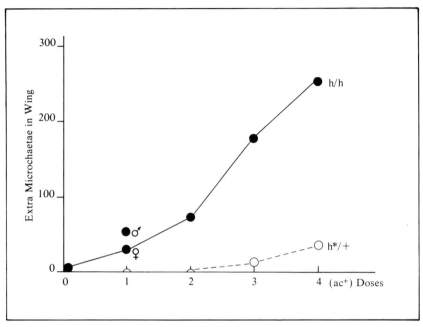

**Figure 6**

Number of extra microchaetae in wings of flies with different doses of the $ac+$ locus ($Dp(1;2)sc^{19}$) in otherwise homozygous or heterozygous mutant flies for *hairy*.

In this search, however, other mutations which lead to the appearance of extra macrochaetae were also found. All are recessive in both males and females but in heterozygous condition in flies with three doses of the *achaeta-scute* complex they show extra macrochaetae in the notum, head and tergites. All the mutants so far found (5) are alleles at a locus designated extra macrochaetae (*emc*) in the tip of the left arm of the third chromosome, far separated from *hairy*. They arose in recessive lethal chromosomes, but in double heterozygotes some combinations are viable. Heterozygous flies (*emc/emc²*) show a pattern of macrochaetae in the notum that resembles the pattern of the genus *Leptocera* (comp. Figures 1 and 7). Flies with the same genotype with respect to *emc* but with three or four wild type doses of the *scute* complex shows more extra macrochaetae arranged in a regular pattern (Figure 7) of longitudinal rows. In these flies however, the microchaeta pattern remains normal. Macrochaeta differentiation requires the function of the *scute* genes. In fact *scute* deletions but not *achaeta* deletions suppress the *emc* phentotype. This genetic behaviour is consistent with the *emc* locus coding for a specific repressor of the *scute* subset of the gene complex (Moscoso del Prado and Garcia-Bellido, unpublished). If this is the correct interpretation, an archetypic pattern of macrochaetae could appear by derepression.

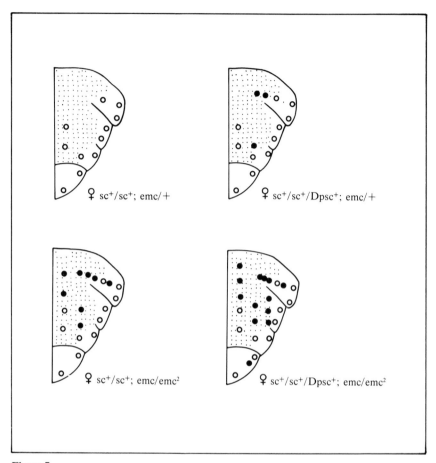

**Figure 7**

Phenotype of flies with different doses of the *scute* gene and homozygous or heterozygous for the mutant extramacrochaetae . (*emc* and *emc²*, two different mutant alleles).

No other mutant loci have been so far found in this search for dose dependent phenotypes. Other mutants so far analysed, known to affect the chaeta pattern, *Tuft*, polychaetoid, (see Lindsley and Grell 1968) are not sensitive in their expression to the number of doses of wild type *achaeta-scute* complexes. The extra chaetae caused by these mutations disappear in mitotic recombination clones homozygous for the *achaeta-scute* deletion (Moscoso del Prado and Garcia-Bellido, unpublished). This result indicates that the formation of innervated chaetae (*Tuft* chaetae are innervated, I. Deak unpublished) has no alternative developmental pathway to that passing through the *achaeta-scute* gene function.

## Developmental Genetics of the Chaeta Pattern

*Cell Autonomy*

A developmental analysis of these mutants is necessary for understanding the conditions in which the functions of their wild type alleles determine cell differentiation and patterning. It is of overall importance to recall that these mutants are cell autonomous in genetic mosaics (Sturtevant 1932, Stern 1954). Mitotic recombination clones of the mutant genotype express the phenotype that corresponds to the same location in the whole mutant fly. This applies to point mutants of the *achaeta-scute* complex (Stern 1954), to the partial or total deletion of it (Garcia-Bellido and Santamaria 1978) to *Hairy wing* (Gottlieb 1964) and to *hairy* (Garcia-Bellido and Merriam 1971c, Garcia-Bellido 1977). As with normal chaetae, extra chaetae caused by the last two mutations are not related by lineage (Garcia-Bellido 1979, and unpublished). This cell autonomy indicates that it is the genetic constitution of the individual cells, with respect to those genes, that determines the response of whether to differentiate or not a chaeta in the normal position or to form extra chaetae.

The classical work of Stern (1954) on *achaeta* mosaics (see also Roberts 1961) showed that when an *ac* clone covers the position of an *achaeta* site no chaeta is formed. However, if the clone borders runs through that region, a non-mutant chaeta from the surrounding heterozygous cells population, or even a mutant chaeta, may differentiate at some distance from the normal site. Slight effects of *Hairy wing* mutant territories upon neighbouring cells in mosaics have also been reported (Gottlieb 1964). This finding of locally restricted non- autonomy led Stern to suggest that any chaeta position is first defined as a region to be later narrowed down to a single cell. It is conceivable that the singling out of a chaeta-forming cell among neighbouring, equally competent, cells result from cell interactions, competing for a diffusible inducer or for the depletion of a diffusible inhibitor (Wigglesworth 1940, Ghysen and Richelle 1979).

*Cell Interactions*

We can now state the question of the role of the cell genotype in chaeta pattern formation. Does the pattern result from the response of cells to a non-homogeneous ('prepatterned') distribution of morphogens?, or alternatively is the cell population homogenous so that it is the genetic constitution of the cells which determines - through cell interactions - the final positioning of the chaeta-forming cells? Put in other words: is there in the anlage a series of positional signals to which the individual cells respond, or is position a consequence of the genetic constitution of the cells? For the purpose of discussion we will distinguish in the notum the microchaeta pattern which is affected by *achaeta* mutations, and the macrochaeta pattern affected by *scute* mutations, and in the tergites the chaeta pattern (mostly microchaetae) affected by *scute* mutations.

The pattern of microchaetae in the notum is basically one of regular spacing of elements. We have seen that mutations in Drosphila melanogaster can reduce the chaeta density (*ac*) or increase it *h* and *Hw*. Comparative analysis of this microchaeta pattern in different genera (Figure 1) shows that the variations are mostly in density, although when reduced to a minimum (in Ephydridae) the chaetae appear in anterior-posterior rows running in the central part of the heminotum. The same *Drosophila melanogaster* mutants lead also to the appearance of chaetae (extra chaetae) in scutellum, pleura and wing, normally void of them. It is, therefore, interesting to mention here that Sturtevant (1970) in his survey of 57 genera found 39 with chaetae in pleura and 20 with chaetae in the *scute*llum. These results suggest that the same chaeta pattern caused by mutation in *Drosophila* can appear in evolutionarily-related species.

We have seen that the density of microchaetae in notum and wing can be modulated by the number of doses of the *achaeta-scute* complex present in otherwise homozygous *h* flies (Figure 5) and *Hw* flies (Ghysen and Richelle 1979). More over, we have seen that whereas the density of extra chaetae in the wing increases linearly with the amount of *achaeta* function, this increase has a limit in the notum above which the density drops to less than in wild type (Figure 5). This finding suggests that neighbouring cells compete for morphogens (either diffusible chaetogen, or inhibitors, or both) and it is in line with the local non-autonomy shown in mosaics. Whatever the formal model we use (see Wigglesworth 1940, Meinhardt and Gierer 1974) to explain it, this microchaeta pattern is monitored by the function of the *achaeta* gene and implemented by cell interactions. The monotonic chaeta pattern of the tergites may follow the same morphogenetic rules (see Wigglesworth 1940, Lawrence 1973, Santamaria and Garcia-Bellido 1972). It is interesting that in *scute* mutants, which do not fully remove tergite chaetae, the remaining chaetae appear at regularly spaced intervals, and that *emc* mutants increase the density of the tergite chaetae. These results indicate that position of microchaetae varies with density and this in turn varies with the amount of *achaeta* wild type function of the cells.

The *Drosophila melanogaster* macrochaeta pattern in the notum is not regular. It is, therefore, important to recall

1) That the *melanogaster* pattern may derive from a more primitive and more regular one (Figure 1) and
2) That the depression of *scute* (caused by *emc*) leads to a regular pattern of a similar configuration to that found in the presumed archetypic one (Figure 7). The irregular, reduced, pattern of *D. melanogaster* may result from insufficient *scute* function. Why this insufficiency is expressed in certain sites

could be defined by local variations in concentration of 'inducer' molecules. However, the fact that the derepression of *scute* leads to the uncovering of new sites rather than the accumulation of extra macrochaetae around extant ones, argues against the existence of prepatterned inducers. Thus, it is still possible that the specific pattern of macrochaetae results from cell interactions, with different spatial solutions depending on the amount (or type) of *scute* function of the cells.

In order to evaluate these cell interactions we have to know which is the distribution of presumptive chaeta-forming cells when they become singled out from the remaining epidermal cell population in the anlage. In the adult notum compartment there are about 10,000 epidermal cells, 100 microchaetae and eleven macrochaetae. Clonal analysis of the normal notum showed that microchaeta-forming cells are separated from other epidermal cells about 40 hours before pupation, i.e. about 4.5 division cycles before cell division ceases in the anlage. Clones contain either chaetae or trichomes but not both (Garcia-Bellido and Merriam 1971 a). Shortly after pupation the cuticular elements of the chaeta are already visible histologically (Lees and Waddington 1942). Since divisions occur every 8. hours during the cell proliferation period and affect all cells (with the possible exception of chaeta-forming cells), micro-chaeta-forming cells become segregated from other epidermal cells when the notum compartment contains about 500 cells. Whatever the genetic basis of this clonal segregation we can estimate when the genetic decision becomes irreversible. Whereas early induced clones of homozygous *achaeta-scute* deletion cells show spots void of chaetae, mutant microchaetae appear in clones initiated later than 24 hours before pupation (Garcia-Bellido and Santamaria 1978). At this time the notum anlage contains about 1000 cells, and therefore the density of microchaetae is 1/10. In clones of the same genetic constitution, macrochaetae start appearing at about 48 hours before pupation, when there are about 250 cells in the anlage, corresponding to a density of one in about 20 cells (Figure 8). Therefore the spacing of the cells when they become genetically determined to differentiate into chaetae, is in radial distances of only two or three cells. Moreover, if the extra microchaetae caused by the derepression of *achaeta* (*Hw* and *h* mutations) or of *scute* (*emc* mutations) are determined at the same time this density must increase considerably. In this anlage a prepatterned distribution of inducers should show discontinuities between neighbouring cells. It is therefore possible that the genes-*scute* first and *achaeta* later - are active in all cells of the anlage and as a consequence of cell to cell interactions some of them become macro- and microchaetae.

Chaeta differentiation can still be perturbed later in development. Child (1935 1936) has shown that the mutant pattern of *scute* alleles, can be modified by changes in temperature during the last day of larval development.

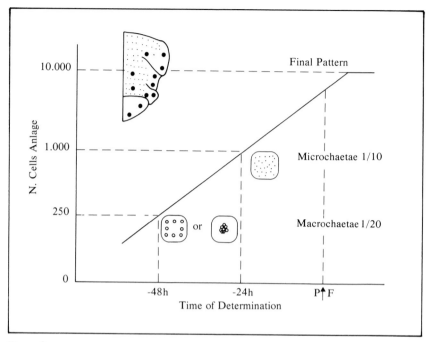

**Figure 8**
Densities and distribution of chaeta forming cells and epidermal cells at the time of chaeta determination in the notum anlage.

X-irradiation applied during the same time causes irreversible loss of individual macrochaeta (Garcia-Bellido and Santamaria 1978). In the mutant shibiri, temperature pulses applied around the time of pupation can also cause suppression of chaetae and even appearance of extra chaetae in the notum. (Poodry *et al.* 1976). The extra chaetae caused by *Hw* and *h* mutations are only irreversibly determined about 8 hours before pupation (Garcia-Bellido and Merriam 1971c). Thus, the process of cell interaction, leading to the final chaeta differentiation, may last several hours. During that time intercalary growth of epidermal cells continues, and this may lead to region specific spacing (see Murphy and Tokunga 1971).

### From the Gene to the Pattern: A Working Hypothesis
From the genetic point of view we envisage the wild type chaeta pattern of Drosophila melanogaster as caused by the precise amount of *achaeta* and *scute* gene function in individual cells, modulated by both the internal amount of repressor products of the genes *hairy* and *extra macrochaetae* and by cell interactions. These cell interactions, (possibly consisting of short range diffusible products) may reinforce or reduce the activity of these genes in

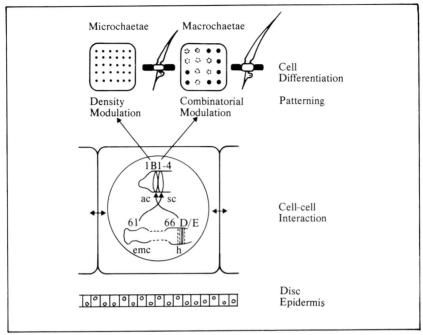

**Figure 9**
Schematic representation of the elements involved in chaeta patterning. See text for discussion.

neighbouring cells and thus lead to the discontinuity which is expressed as a pattern (Figure 9). Mutant or species variations are expressed in the micro-chaeta pattern, mainly, in chaeta density variations and consequently in variations in position. Mutant or species variations in the macrochaeta pattern are expressed in the lack or presence of chaetae in certain positions. However, we have seen that the *scute* gene is a complex gene whose products work in a combinatorial way. This might explain why different *scute* mutants affect to a variable extent, the same seriation of chaeta sites, and why different temperatures change the pattern of sites affected by a particular *scute* mutant. It is possible that site-specificity of species and mutants results from variations of the combinatorial products of *scute* modulated again by cell interactions.

Previous considerations have dealt with the role of the *achaeta-scute* complex in the patterning of chaetae. Its relation to the earlier described role played by this gene complex in the differentiation of innervated elements in the central nervous system and in the peripheral system remains unexplained. It may be relevant to recall that the deletion of the *achaeta-scute* complex causes the disintegration and histolysis of already formed neuroblasts in early embryos (Jimenez and Campos-Ortega 1979). It is possible that these two developmental operations, nervous cell differentiation and patterning or supracellular organisation, are related.

The problem of chaeta differentiation and patterning is obviously more complex than outlined above. For one thing, mutants other than those discussed here affect it. They, however, could represent non-specific perturbations of the growing systems, interference with normal cell interactions or affect the implementation steps of the studied ones. Genetic and developmental analysis hopefully will sort them out into a logical frame of interactions, susceptible to later verification in molecular terms.

## Acknowledgements

I wish to thank J Moscoso del Prado for allowing me to quote unpublished results and for fruitful discussions; LH Throckmorton for showing me his collection of dipteran species related to *Drosophila*, from which the schemes of Figure 1 were made, and DL Lindsley, J Modolell and L Robbins for comments to the manuscript. This work was supported by grants of the Spanish CADC and CAICYT.

## References

Child, G. (1935) *Phenogenetic studies on scute-1 of Drosophila melanogaster II. The temperature effective period.* Genetics, *20*, 127-155.

Child, G. (1936) *Phenogenetic studies on scute-1 of Drosophila melanogaster III. The effect of temperature on scute-5.*

Claxton, J.H. (1967) *Patterns of abdominal tergite bristles in wild type and scute Drosophila melanogaster.* Genetics, *55*, 525-545.

Dubinin, N.P. (1933) *Step-allelo morphism in Drosophila melanogaster.* J. Genetics, *27*, 443-464.

Falk, R. (1963) *A search for a gene control system in Drosophila.* Amer. Nat. *97*, 129-132.

Fraser, A. (1967) *Variation of scutellar bristles in Drosophila XV. System of modifiers.* Genetics, *57*, 919-934.

Garcia-Bellido, A. (1977) *Inductive mechanisms in the process of wing rein formation in Drosophila.* W. Roxw's Arch. *182*, 93-106.

Garcia-Bellido, A. (1979) *Genetic analysis of the achaeta-scute system of Drosophila melanogaster.* Genetics, *91*, 491-520.

Garcia-Bellido, A. and Merriam, J. (1971a) *Parameters of the wing marginal disc development of Drosophila melanogaster.* Develop. Biol. *24*, 61-87.

Garcia-Bellido, A. and Merriam, J. (1971b) *Clonal parameters of tergite development in Drosophila.* Develop. Biol. *26*, 264-276.

Garcia-Bellido, A. and Merriam, J. (1971c) *Genetic analysis of cell heredity in imaginal discs of Drosophila melanogaster.* Proc. Natl. Acad. Sci. USA. *65*, 2222-2226.

Garcia-Bellido, A. and Santamaria, P. (1978) *Developmental analysis of the achaeta-scute system of Drosophila melanogaster.* Genetics, *88*, 469-486.

Ghysen, A. (1980) *Choice of the right pathway in Drosophila central nervous system.* Devel. Biol. *78*, 521-541.

Ghysen, A. and Richelle, J. (1979) *Determination of sensory bristles and pattern formation in Drosophila II. The achaete-scute locus.* Devel. Biol. *70*, 438-452.

Gottlieb, F.J. (1964) *Genetic control of pattern determination in Drosophila, the action of Hairy wing.* Genetics, *49*, 739-760.

Jimenez, F. and Campos-Ortega, J. (1979) *A region of the Drosophila genome necessary for central nervous system development.* Nature, *282*, 310-312.

Latter, B.D.H. (1973) *Selection for a threshold character in Drosophila. IV chromosomal analysis of plateaued populations.* Genetics, *73*, 497-512.

Lawrence, P.A. (1966) *Development and determination of hairs and bristles in the milkweed bug. Oncopeltus fasciatus (Lygaeidae, Hemiptera).* J. Cell Sci. *1*, 475-498.

Lawrence, P.A. (1973) *The development of spatial patterns in the integument of insects. In, Developmental Systems: Inspects.* (S.J. Counce and C.A. Waddington, eds.) vol. 2, pp 105-209). Academic Press, New York.

Lawrence, P.A., Struhl, G. and Morata, G. (1979) *Bristle patterns and compartment boundaries in the tarsi of Drosophila.* J. Embryol. Expt. Morph. *51* 195-208.

Lees, A.D. and Waddington, C.H. (1942) *The development of bristles in normal and some mutant types of Drosophila melanogaster.* Proc. Roy. Soc. (London) B, *131*, 87-110.

Lindsley, D.L. and Grell, E.H. (19680 *Genetic variations of Drosphila melanogaster.* Carnegie Inst. Wash. Publ. *627.*

Meinhardt, H. and Gierer, A. (1974) *Biological pattern formation involving lateral inhibition.* Lectures on Mathematics in Life Sciences, *7*, 163- 183.

Muller, H.J. (1955) *On the relation between chromosomes changes and gene mutations.* J. Heredity, *26*, 469-478.

Murphy, C. and Tokunga, C. (1970) *Cell lineage in the dorsal mesothoracic disc of Drosophila.* J. Exptl. Zool. *175*, 197-220.

Neel, J.V. (1941) *Studies on the interaction of mutations affecting the chaete of Drosophila melanogaster. I. The interaction of hairy, polychaetoid, and hairy wing.* Genetics, *26*, 52-68.

Poodry, C.A., Hall, L. and Suzuki, D.T. (1973) *Developmental properties of Shibiri : a pleiotropic mutation affecting larval and adult locomotion and development.* Devel. Biol. *32*, 373-386.

Rendel, J.M. (1976) *Is there a gene regulating the scute locus on the third chromosome of Drosophila melanogaster.* Genetics, *83*, 573-600.

Rendel, J.M. and Evans, M.J. (1978) *Canalization of the action of sc 1 in Drosophila melanogaster.* Heredity, *41*, 105-107.

Roberts, P. (1961) *Bristle formation controlled by the achaete locus in genetic mosaics of Drosophila melano gaster.* Genetics, *46*, 1241-1243.

Santamaria, P. and Garcia-Bellido, A. (1972) *Localisation and growth pattern of the tergite Anlage of Drosophila.* J. Embryol. Expt. Morph. *28*, 397-417.

Sondhi, K.C. (1962) *The evolution of a pattern.* Evolution, *16*, 186-191.

Stern, C. (1936) *Somatic crossing over and segregation in Drosophila melanogaster.* Genetics, *21*, 625-730.

Stern, C. (1938) *The innervation of setae in Drosophila.* Genetics, *23*, 325-346.

Stern, C. (1954) *Two or three bristles.* Am. Scientist, *42*, 213-247.

Sturtevant, A.H. (1929) *The claret mutant type of Drosophila simulans: a study of chromosome elimination and cell lineage.* Z. Wiss. Zool. *135*, 323- 356.

Sturtevant, A.H. (1932) *The use of mosaics in the study of developmental effects of genes.* Proc. 6th Intern. Congr. Genet. *1*, 304-307.

Sturtevant, A.H. (1970) *Studies on the bristle pattern of Drosophila.* Devel. Biol. *21*, 48-61.

Thoday, (1958) *Homeostasis in a selection experiment.* heredity *12*, 401-415.

Tokunaga, C. (1962) *Cell lineage and differentiation in the male foreleg of Drosophila melanogaster.* Devel. Biol. *4*, 489-516.

White, K. (1980) *Defective neural development in Drosophila embryos deficient for the tip of the X-chromosome.* Develop. Biol.

## Questions

*RM Brown Jr*
When the chaeta cell develops this extension is it modulating chitin synthesis in some specific way perhaps?

*Garcia-Bellido*
The classical differentiation is dead - namely, when we start seeing different proteins in that amount it does not mean that we have differentiation. The thing is, we start seeing a different habit much later than that. Chitin formation is in the puparium and these things are telling you what happened 48 hours - five cell divisions - before that. And I think it is a nice message; it also tells us that if we are waiting to see the proteins which are characteristic of the cell type, we may be very far away from the actual genetic operation that tells the cell to go one way or another - that is a big waste of time - to go from gene activation to expression in mensurable terms.

*Eisen*
If you make mosaics and you put in a cell you have cloned that has nothing to do with scute or hairy etc., then you would predict on your model that if you kill off cells in one region it would alter the pattern in the surrounding region. Is that what happens?

*Garcia-Bellido*
This actually goes back to the question namely: what happens if we generate a mosaic in which the cells, in the homozygous, are they chaete minus (because in that particular experiment, chaete minus was looked at). The results are that the neighbouring cells can respond to the position. To put it in other words - the definition of the site is not a geometrically unique point; it is spreading a little and has been called a little morphogenetic field. So, if one cell cannot respond then the other wild-type cell will do it. But the rest, namely those that are two or three cell diameters away, are completely normal. So the computation is a computation between neighbours again and this question is a nice one because it is an old one and can be answered in this way: it tells you that the decision is not computed in the entire anlage but is computed between neighbours. And this is another indication that the cells do talk and they say, 'If you do not answer, then I will answer; it is not a case of you die because I do not know what you are doing; no, they are keeping an eye and saying, 'are you dying alone?', because otherwise I will do it. (Laughter).

*Pardee*
I wonder if there are temperature-sensitive mutants in, say, the H-locus so that the dosage changes as if it were a labile protein.

*Garcia-Bellido*
Yes, there are temperature-sensitive mutations, so you can ask yourself two things: what does temperature do at that particular mutation and this was asked, again by Childs in 1936, that if you have a particular mutant (say, scute 1) and you rear these flies at different temperatures, you change the pattern. So, the pattern of chaetae moves, so that pattern is changed depending on the temperature in which the cells were grown, for a particular division. Secondly, when is the time that it changes the pattern and the answer is, the same time as the logic of the removal. Does this answer your question?

*Pardee*
Yes. I was thinking in particular of the case where you had four copies of the Hc locus and you were barely able to hold it down with the heterozygous H+ that should be especially temperature-sensitive, I would think, if you were destroying.

*Garcia-Bellido*
This has not been tried. But in this experiment you are dealing not with mutants but with the number of wild-type doses. It is very different because a

mutant could just leak to a constitution -to a product - which is working about half-way. The thing we cannot deal with in *Drosophila* (because we know how dangerous it is by experience) is half genes. The thing we cannot check is just a leak. And this is the reason why whenever we ask a question we want to go all the way to remove that gene because otherwise the phenotype is going to be a left-over phenotype ..so we have to crack out the genes and it is only then that we understand the function. So temperature, with respect, I do not think is going to help - it will add more noise to the system.

*Wolpert*
Antonio, just to defend a position. It does seem to me that you do not really have...

*Garcia-Bellido*
...I have to say I keep interupting because you are right (Laughter).

*Wolpert*
...just to say, it is possible to think of a way how the cells could use positional information.

*Garcia-Bellido*
The only thing is that you have now to reduce the system for positional information to discontinuities which are one or two cell diameters - if this is enough, that is fine but if the discontinuities are just one cell diameter that is as much as saying that is no positional information. Right? (Silence)

*Hartley*
So, you are right.

*Garcia-Bellido*
I will wait until you die to say 'you see, up to now I did not admit' (Laughter).

*Coffino*
This is an experimentally naive question.

*Garcia-Bellido*
No, there are only naive answers.

*Coffino*
But, it seems to me that the information does not have to be in the cells that you are making differentiate. In one of your early slides you showed that you could order a series of mutations in the scute locus, so that the mutations are an ordered set and it seems to me that all you need is to make different amounts of something that causes different numbers of cells to differentiate and then perhaps some sets of sites that have nothing to do with the cells except cells like them - like them in some hierachical sort of way - you make one, it goes to the highest affinity site, you make to it goes to that one.

*Garcia-Bellido*
I cannot just give you the background of insect genetics... this answer involves thinking that there is some place, like in a plant, that is producing cells and when those cells are committed they go, they move and they lock-in. I have to say to this no, they do not move; the cells differentiate according to where they are in the project. So there is no migration that can account for that. So this problem is not a problem of migration, it is a problem of responding to the position or to the 'talking' (whatever is the actual basic mechanism) without migrating.

*Sager*
I want to ask you also about a kind of positional information but at a different level and this has to do with position in DNA. There are translations which involve scute... if a particular allele which has a particular expression in one location what is the story about what happens to that expression if it is modified by cells in the genome because this is another way at getting at this question of what is determining the phenotype. In other words, if you can take a gene and move it into a heterochromatic region in which you are presumably altering the level of gene expression (say, decreasing the level of gene expression) is there some kind of a 1:1 way that you can explain those cha-

nges in terms of changes in the phenotype in scute?

*Garcia-Bellido*

Until we have the DNA mapped, we cannot make sense of this phenotype because there are huge distances with no complementation ...we cannot understand that in terms of classical transcription and classical translation.

# 8
# Summary and Discussion

# Chairman's Summary
*David A Rees*

In introducing this summarising discussion, may I first go back to the feelings
we had about the programme while it was still in the planning stage to check
how the outcome has compared against expectations. Some of the feelings of
myself and fellow-organisers have been similar to those of an expectant father:
In this situation, you wonder anxiously what sort of creature is going to
emerge, you know that it will make an awful lot of noise and you are not sure
whether you will like it! There is, however, some comfort in the fact that once
past the first point of commitment, the product depends not on your own
labours, but those of others.

More rationally, we also worried whether it would be possible to have
intelligent communication across such a very wide spread of topics - and from
this point of view we are greatly reassured that the meeting has been a success.
The chief evidence has been the intensity of the discussion and the wide range
of people who have become involved in it, both in the formal sessions and
outside the lecture hall. I would like to thank not only the speakers who have
stimulated all this, but also the discussants who haven't hesitated to jump in
and stir the debate. If I were to offer any prizes, perhaps I might offer one to
Ruth Sager who, with a cunningly planned loss leader on the function of
mitochondrial DNA yesterday afternoon, won that important concession from
Piet Borst on male inferiority.

We also wondered to what extent we could succeed in making the topics hang
together, and whether they would be so disparate that they had to lead to a
disconnected series of conversations; perhaps this question is really what our
discussion time should be about now. So I will quickly run over the subject
material to the best of my ability, in an account which must be rather patchy
because there are few who are equipped to cover this wide area of biology in
detail. I won't follow the chronological order, but instead try to relate to the
main aspects of differentiation that we seem to have been considering during
the course of these three days. I suggest these have been:

1) The way the cell takes readings from its environment in the control of differentiation;
2) The changes in organisation and biochemistry of the cytoplasm either as the result of differentiation or to bring differentiation about;
3) Changes in gene expression;
4) Important issues which we have only touched upon briefly, namely the nature and the role of communication between the cell surface and the cytoplasm and between the cytoplasm and the nucleus and;
5) How all this relates to pattern development in tissues.

From a personal vantage point, it seemed from this Meeting that the best understood of these areas is that which has to do with changes in the organisation and biochemistry in the cytoplasm. In Klaus Weber's lecture, we saw some interesting principles beginning to emerge as to how the actomyosin system (and all that implies for cell and tissue morphology) is controlled through calcium levels which affect the cross-linking of actin and the stimulation of myosin ATPase in non-muscle cells. In turn, Philip Cohen's lecture showed that we are clearly deriving quite a comprehensive picture of how phosphorylation of calcium-binding proteins affects the activity of other proteins in a coordinate manner and of how this results from hormone activity or the action potential at the cell surface. As for how the cell processes signal molecules received at the cell surface, Mark Willingham showed structural evidence for down-regulation of hormone receptors and how this can actually occur at the surfaces of tissue culture cells. All of this adds up to the beginnings of a very useful general understanding, even though the game isn't over yet by any means and there are important gaps. For example, although we know where the calcium is stored in skeletal muscle and how it is released to stimulate contraction, we don't know for non-muscle cells where the relevant calcium is stored - nor how its level is actually regulated. Again, although Mark Willingham showed how surface receptors may function in down-regulation, this still leaves the question alluded to by Philip Cohen of how the receptor actually passes the message across the cell surface - how in fact communication occurs between cell surface and the cytoplasm. It was most impressive for me as an outsider to this part of the area, to see how the new technologies have led to enormous increase in the mapping of gene structure - mitochondrial as well as nuclear DNA - and also (as Dr Wasylyk outlined) the roles of special sequences in DNA transcription. But I didn't hear as much as I expected of how gene expression is actually controlled and to what extent it really is the dominant and overriding factor in differentiation as opposed to say control at the level of RNA processing or even at the level of protein activity, or how translation is controlled. It was gratifying, therefore, that in his very significant lecture Harvey Eisen described a major protein which appears in chromatin following an extracellular signal such as the action potential in the visual system or a hormone which turns on terminal differentiation. Another exciting possibility for controlling gene activity was mentioned by Ruth Sager in discussion - of how methylation of DNA may serve to turn off genes during differentiation.

So far we have heard parts of a story concerning the dialogue between genes and environment but it seems that we shall have to wait until more is known about these and other relay devices before the subtleties of this conversation can be fully appreciated. We might then understand what controls the direction of communication and how forcefully the environment can talk back to genes.

A good example of how the environment affects the maintenance of a particular phenotype was provided by Antti Vaheri who, in telling us of the rapid advances in molecular characterisation of the extracellular matrix, described how the expression of certain tissue-type characteristics in culture (such as the production of particular types of collagen) was strongly influenced by the nature of the extracellular matrix with which the cells were in contact. It is still controversial, though, whether contacts with the extracellular matrix do trigger cytoplasmic events or merely follow them. This is an important point which we need to clear up over the next couple of years but the answer will surely help us understand the patterns of movement and the involvement of the extracellular matrix in vertebrate embryogenesis.

The quality of the matrix may also be important in growth control. For instance, a questioner after Klaus Weber's lecture asked whether signalling from extracellular contacts could provide the explanation of the phenomenon of anchorage dependence of growth for normal cells in culture. Certainly there are strong hints that interaction between the extracellular matrix and the cytoskeleton is involved in growth control as well as in crawling movements and cell adhesion. There are, of course, other levels of growth control and Dr Coffino's description of a histone protein synthesised in $G_1$ phase but not actually incorporated into the nucleus until later in the cell cycle may be relevant here and Dr Pardee and Dr Sager's evidence and speculations on the changes that follow DNA damage and implications for growth control and the development of cancer also began to raise important issues in this area. But in this general area we do indeed see through a glass darkly, and the relative complexity of the cytoplasm of eukaryotes compared with prokaryotes would suggest that it will be difficult in the future to extrapolate from what we know about the control of gene expression in prokaryotes to the eukaryotic system, so there is a great deal more work ahead.

When we get to higher levels of organisation still, such as those described by Sydney Brenner and Don Metcalf, by Dr Teich, by Professor Gardner and Dr Garcia-Bellido this morning, some overall principles are beginning to become visible like fragments of a jigsaw. The observation, described in different systems by Sydney Brenner and Don Metcalf, that the induction of differentiation occurs only after a preliminary cell division and then a complete cell cycle, showed a fascinating parallel. In terms of the stimulation of cell division, or individual events which are part of the expression of differentiation, some of the component biochemical steps can be described and generalised as Phil Coffino and others have discussed - but we are nowhere near an understanding of how the whole process can be coordinated overall. Finally, coming to the last two lectures, we are still confronted with the problem of positional information and how it relates to cell contacts or molecular messengers and it is to this higher level of questions that cell and molecular biologists must address themselves if we are ever to understand how cells build tissues and organs. At this point I suggest we open the general discussion.

# Open Discussion:
# What is Differentiation?

*Hunt*

I would like to ask a question, what is differentiation? I have a feeling that we are all thinking about different things in using that word. Some of us are thinking about differential gene activity, some of us about bristles in a pattern, some of us about cytoplasmic regulation of already existing elements. What are we really talking about?

*Hartley (Session Chairman)*

I am not prepared to answer this question. (Laughter)

*Lodish*

I will make a stab at it. I think that what has been missing is a separation of the terms 'commitment' from actual 'expression'. We all have a naive idea of what differentiation means : it's cells doing something a little bit different. Much of what people are studying that passes for differentiation is differential activation of genes in cells which are already committed. Going back to stem cells, for instance, such as those that Dr Metcalf talked about, commitment occurs very, very early on and I think that should be made explicit. You then have a sub-set of cells which are programmed to become erythrocytes or - rather - they have something in them that says they can only become erythrocytes, they may or may not according to the environment. The real mystery here is what commitment is. It's much easier to think of gene expression. We are all familiar with promoters and hormone receptors which can switch genes on or off but the critical question is why certain genes are switched on or off in a regulated fashion in a particular sub-set of cells. So, in answer to your question, I think differentiation can be thought of as two parts : commitment and the actual expression of that commitment into a recognisable phenotype. The difficulty is, on can not generally identify a committed cell.

*Housman*

Harvey, can I get back to that? I would agree with part of that in the sense that I

I think it's very important to identify where the commitment in a particular pathway occurs but what I think you have to do is to recognise that there are many commitments that occur along a differentiation programme. We have no models at all for this. I think that that is what we might want to discuss - is what might be going on the molecular level that sets a programme in motion instead of what keeps it operating?

*Wolpert*

I think it would be helpful if we could have a discussion along those lines if we have a chance to, but really it is a question of how cells remember. Even though we do not know how a committed cell gets turned on, there is, in a committed cell, some memory of its past and I would have thought that a key question was whether this memory is a structural modification at the level of DNA or is it some sort of Monod-type operator/feed-back loop. I know that Antonio Garcia-Bellido has some information which relates to what I regard as an absolutely central problem: that is, whether memory involves structural modification or does it involve something more tenuous such as a loop.

*Garcia-Bellido*

I will come to Lewis' (Wolpert) question later but I would like to go back a bit first. We have to get the idea of what we mean by differentiation clear, so that we know what we want to explain. By differentiation we may not want to mean the infinite graduation of qualitative, quantitative and spatial differences. This would have to be first described and would take years. What I think is critical to differentiation are the not-graded differences: alternative pathways. The choice of these alternatives could happen by a continuous series of interactions and cascade events or by 2. the singling out of few, specific genes, appearing through evolution to precisely permit discontinuous decisions, alternatives. I think the question is: does differentiation come about by very complex and sophisticated mechanisms, as those we have seen in phosphorylation reactions, for example, or is differentiation more simple and involve fewer variables, only few genes? Metabolic regulations are invariant in all organisms and all cells and yet organisms have different parts, shapes and functions. Does regulation in cell differentiation depend on the same complex interactions? My feeling (and at this part of the story we have to talk about feelings) is that it is more simple. To me the questions are: are there genes that take alternative decisions? and how are they regulated? In *Drosophila* there are genes that seem to act this way.

I come now to Lewis' question. I do not think there is a different situation between commitment and expression, it is probably the same operation. The only thing that looks different, let's say with respect to gene regulation in *E coli*, is that once the 'on' or 'off' decision has been taken it is maintained throughout subsequent cell divisions. The question of memory could be stated: is such maintenance due to the activity in the cells of the same elements involved in the decision or is something new left there, so that you remove the signalling elements and the effect is retained? In *Drosophila* we can manipulate gene activity during ontogenesis, because we can change the genetic constitution of the cells (by mitotic recombination), and so we can ask what is the effect of such a change, at different times of development upon differentiation. Well, the experience we have with *Drosophila*, in one single case, is that probably the system is maintained active or inactive because of a feed-back loop of gene interactions. Let me now be more specific. That system is called *bithorax*. The genes in this system specify the different thoracic and abdominal segments (Lewis, 1978. Nature *276*: 565). This specification occurs in the blastoderm stage and is implemented already in the individual cells. We cannot yet see the effect of the implementation in the appearance of proteins but differences in cell recognition and other characteristics do exist. These cells maintain this decision throughout cell proliferation as long as the *bithorax* wildtype genes are present in the cells. We can remove the *bithorax* wildtype genes during development (by mitotic recombination) and the differentiation of the cells collapses to segment O (the maximal repression state). Now we come to the first step; the initiation step, in which the *bithorax* genes are signalised to be 'on' or 'off'. In this step there are at least two other genetic elements involved: one of them is similar to the regulator gene in the lac operon. The products of this gene, if they are above the concentration of an inducer (related to the other gene), will repress *bithorax* and switch it 'off' (segment O); if below the inducer's concentration the *bithorax* genes switch 'on' (segments 1-8). Now the question is: what happens if we change the genetic constitution of the cells, during subsequent proliferation, for the regulator gene. If the *bithorax* system is maintained by *cis*-changes in the DNA or tertiary or quaternary structure in the chromatin, the removal of the regulator wildtype gene would go without effect. What we find is that this change in genetic constitution (again by mitotic recombination) leads to a depression of the *bithorax* gene: the transformation of the cells of all the segments to the differentiation of abdominal 8th characteristics. This change could come about in many possible ways, but it is easier to understand if the maintenance mechanism is based on a feedback loop between the regulator gene and the structural gene: the 'on' original condition is maintained by production by the active *bithorax* genes, of an hypothetical antirepressor, and the 'off' original condition by the continuous repression of the inactive *bithorax* genes.

In this scheme initiation and maintenance use the same regulatory elements acting by *trans*-interactions rather than by *cis*-modifications.

In this one case we have the apparent paradox that a cell is differentiated and yet this differentiation is reversible - manipulating the activity of certain genes in the genome. I do not think irreversibility is an inherent property of differentiation.

*Hartley*

That is a fantastic addition to the situation in very complex organisms. I wonder if I might make a simple observation. One of the things that contributed greatly to my perception of the differentiation process was to see that poster outside on the clonal oil palm which shows little plants growing out of callus tissue. I see Professor Steward is here. I wonder if he will remind us that some of these cosmic rules that we deal with in animals may not necessarily be the same in plants.

*Steward*

As one of the few botanists here I am glad of this opportunity to speak. The organisers of this symposium chose to build it about organisms other than higher plants. But as one who has worked exclusively with plants, mostly angiosperms, I make my comments from this point of view. Plants are not animals and their problems of differentiation and development are distinctive. This became clear at the outset. Sydney Brenner's nematodes as he so clearly explained, after a few divisions produce a few cells that give rise to developments that are fixed, defined, determined and irreversible. Angiosperm growing points, of shoot and root, developed from the egg in the embryo, are not so. They make organs, with great diversity of biochemistry and function repetitively by even potentially unlimited growth. But they do this, as Haberlandt prophesied long ago, without loss of the totipotency of their cells. We know now that we can take cells at the end of this process of development - provided they contain nuclei and cytoplasm - from different organs (as in the case of carrot) and make new embryos out of single cells. For me, therefore, one of the big questions is how the genome is affected as a whole, knowing that it is in all the cells in all organs, to tell it to do such very different things, not only in different organs but in adjacent cells in a tissue. In plants one of the main sources of control over all this development is the environment - telling the shoot growing point how to evoke its great potentialities for diversity. Plants emerge as stable physical systems somehow. Environmental characteristics 'mould' the growing point - lengths of day, interactions between day and night temperatures etc. All of this impinges on the outcome of what was born in an egg to start with and goes through all the business of forming leaves and roots, shoots and stems and hairs and yet can start all over again, without resorting to sexual reproduction. In carrot, or other plants, one can take cells from roots or tubers, or leaves or particularly somatic cells from floral organs and do it all over again. I appeal, therefore, that in a future symposium we give to angiosperms - so important for food and fibre and in climatology - the position they merit.

*Raff*

I would like to make a point about memory - a question that Lewis Wolpert was asking. I think it is already clear that there is not one answer. For example, one answer, that may well turn out to be unique, concerns B lymphocyte differentiation, where differentiation involves DNA deletion and is therefore irreversible. And so what Garcia-Bellido was saying is clearly not true for B lymphocytes. Moreover, it seems likely that there are other molecular mechanisms of commitment and differentiation for which there are no precedents now and will only be discovered in the future.

*Eisen*
Since we are considering organisms which have been forgotten in this symposium, I would like to mention phage lambda. This is perhaps the only organism which 'differentiates' both temporally and functionally, for which we have an understanding at the molecular level. The regulation of repressor synthesis during the various phases of phage infection is a good example. Here a single cistron has multiple promoters which are subject to different regulatory proteins. All of the proteins which regulate repressor synthesis have been purified and the regulation can be done in simple *in vitro* systems. Such phenomena are beginning to appear in higher organisms except that the lack of genetic systems makes their analysis complicated.

*Southern*
Could I add another organism to this list? In connection with the previous statement by Garcia-Bellido about memory in terms of what the genome can remember and by implication, what the DNA can remember. I think there have been hints from Ruth Sager that methylation is one of these systems of remembering. Against all of that, there is all the early nuclear transplantation experiments of Gurdon which suggest that if you have a memory that you can wipe it out and start again.

*Garcia-Bellido*
The fact that you can start all over again in such experiments, is still compatible with de-methylation or de- whatever is supposed to be a general cause for memory. The same is true for regeneration from highly differentiated cells. You can say the fact that they do it does not mean that the memory is forever but only 'as long as...'. But still, we do not know the mechanism. There are hints in higher organisms ...and *Drosophila* is higher because at least it flies... that we can also change subtle things in the genome. This is the classical phenomenon of trans-determination and we do not know the mechanism. By the pure description of a chromosome that happens to have methyl groups or non-methyl groups that happen to be correlated with a tissue which is differentiating or not differentiating we are not going to see if this is the mechanism because it could very well be that the mechanism is more subtle than that - it is really an open system like in lambda only it is implemented later

on in terms of a particular kind of folding of the chromatin or phosphorylation of the protein etc etc. The question is, to know - genetically speaking - what is the signal that goes to one cell, coming to one chromosome, to one locus and says, work or not work. From the pure description from the outside we do not have a functional experiment which allows us to deduce the normal mechanism and so we are going to go around and around about 'correlation'.

*Southern*

Can I come back to that? Speaking as a DNA chemist, I think it is really quite important to know whether we should be looking for something which is absolutely irreversible or for something which is reversible. That is the question that has not been answered for me. Is commitment absolute in the systems people are talking about.

*Sager*

Thank you very much. That is what I wanted to hear. I am very grateful to Lewis Wolpert because everytime I have a discussion with him it confirms my feeling that the only thing to do that's real is to work on DNA.. '(Wolpert. 'It certainly was not my intention. Laughter....because what it seems to me that the solid mechanisms and the solid answers are coming are the ones from DNA. Secondly, in the DNA field there are a lot of new ideas and a lot of new techniques which have not yet been applied to this problem. So I was very sympathetic with Dr Rees when he said, 'Why didn't somebody talk about it?'(ie. DNA)

People who think about differentiation are traditionally people who do not think about DNA but I think that what has happened with immunoglobulins points very strongly in the direction, that at least some kinds of differentiation mechanisms are going to be of the sort where we can now look for DNA splicing and that one kind of terminal and irreversible differentiation is the kind where you throw some of the DNA away. Once it has gone - that is the end. What is fascinating about plants is that apparently they never throw any of their DNA away because as long as differentiation is reversible it means maybe it has been re-arranged but it is still all there and even the re-arrangements, apparently, may be reversible. Right now, that there are many obvious things that need to be looked at if you are willing to start thinking about differentiation as a process at the DNA level - as a process at the chromatin level. Nucleosome changes probably have a great deal to do with the control of the expression, but those may all be reversible. In the adipocyte system, for instance, which Howard Green has described so beautifully, you can keep cells in a pre-adipocyte condition indefinitely as long as they are kept dividing and it is only those last terminal stages that I'll bet involve not only the accumulation of fat but the throwing away of some of the key DNA. So, I would propose that differentiation becomes irreversible where there have been irreversible changes in DNA.

*Lodish*
I wish to disagree emphatically. There is a certain tenor to the discussion that bothers me; namely, I get the feeling that people think there is one kind of differentiation or one thing which is meant by commitment. I would like to go back to one of the first examples I ever learned in developmental biology: there are two types of embryos; there are regulated embryos and mosaic embryos. You can take the first few cells that arise by the division of an egg and you can separate them. In some cases each cell will go on to produce a normal organism - in many cases the right size and shape etc. - in many cases it will not. This can have many meanings: it could be in the DNA; alternatively many people feel it is in the cytoplasm and there is no question that immunoglobulin differentiation is mediated at least in past by gene re-arrangements. I do not know of anyone who is willing to say that the only thing that determines a cell to becoming a B cell is moving a V gene locus to a J gene, I think that is absolutely not going to be the case and; as far as I know, re-arranged genes or no re-arranged genes, immunoglobulins are never trans cribed in any other cell. So, things are really very, very complex and as the field matures, people are going to become aware of how all these different levels interdigitate and I think one has to keep a very open mind.

*Raff*
I think that Harvey's point underlines the semantic nature of this problem and makes one wonder whether it is really worth discussing. A B cell's commitment to making a particular V region of an antibody molecule seems to me to be a *bona fide* example of differentiation. I do not agree with Ruth Sager that DNA deletion is likely to be a common mechanism of irreversible differentiation, although the nuclear transplantation experiments and plant cloning experiments cannot exclude that some DNA deletion accompanies differentiation. For example, one can imagine that a nucleus from a B lymphocyte transplanted into an enucleated egg might give rise to a normal mouse with only some minor impairment in its antibody repertoire.

*Sager*
Plants still.....

*Raff*
....don't have an immune system. We know they have not thrown away their DNA.

*Gardner*
I think there is a real problem of equating the stability of the process to the possibility of some change at the level of DNA. In the early mouse embryo at 4 days there are two populations of cells within the inner cell mass. All manipulations to alter them fail but it is nevertheless true that you can take an

embryo from the uterus beyond that stage of development and by the act of
ectopically grafting it you can get a teratocarcinoma from which you can pull
out a totipotent population of cells that are now capable of doing all things that
line (since it came from the ectoderm) should have forgotten how to do. So the
stability in the one situation may be somewhat analogous to the process that
occurs in *Drosophila* in trans-determination which you can break down. Then
there is the other situation of X chromosome inactivation - which occurs in
development at a fairly early stage - particularly shown by Barbara Migeon's
work. Once you've switched off an X - let us say X for wild-type allele for
HGPRT - you can then take those cells from a heterozygote and grow them to
high density you can then challenge them by withdrawing support; either they
must activate the wildtype allele, or die. They commit suicide and the
frequency with which you get reversion is of the same order as of mutation. The
story was nice and simple at one time because the only cell line you have got to
worry about activating the second X or having two X's active is in the female
germ line and the dogma was that the germ-line segregates before the rest of the
embryo undergoes X-inactivation. Very strong evidence is now accumulating
that this is not true. The germ-line also X-inactivates but normally and
efficiently reverses.

*Sager*

......of course, there are many levels of reversibility and irreversibility. The
question is, how stable is whatever it is that Harvey Eisen's protein is doing, I
would like to hear something about that and how firmly does that histone bind
and what is the relationship of its presence or its coming off to the stability of
the phenotype.

*Eisen*

*In vivo*, I do not think we can say very much except for experiments in which
one withdraws the maintenance hormone, where we see it will disappear with a
half-life of approximately a day. That seems to be due in part to normal turnover of the protein. In cells which are not dividing, it is clearly being turned-
over somewhat. Evidence for its turn-over comes from the fact that we can
detect its messenger in tissues which have little or no cellular turnover. It must
mean that either the message is not being translated *in vivo* or that it is being
turned over. In tissue culture we can study it somewhat better and in that
situation we can induce it in essentially any cell with butyric or propionic acid.
Butyric acid is complicated since it has so many effects, so aside from inducing
this protein it blocks cells in the $G_1$ phase etc. But once the protein is induced
(14-15 hours for maximal level) it remains there with little turn-over so long as
the cells are maintained in butyric acid. If butyric acid is removed, it
disappears with a half life of 12-24 hours. Propionic acid is a little more
interesting because it doesn't block the cells in $G_1$ - the cells continue to divide.

Again one sees the accumulation, also identically with butyric acid, but after a while the protein starts to go down and reaches a steady-state level which is much lower than the peak which could be 40% of the lysine-rich histone. So in that situation it looks like something is regulating its expression - both at the time when it was induced and at the steady-state level where it is being made at a much lower rate.

*Sager*
It is still maintaining the phenotype?

*Eisen*
Yes, but what the phenotype is, is another question because what you see is not so much the appearance of new things but the loss of old things. You see a certain class of spots on a 2-D gel which disappear without others being altered at all. You rarely see new things showing up except when you look specifically for haemoglobin or other specific differentiation-linked proteins.

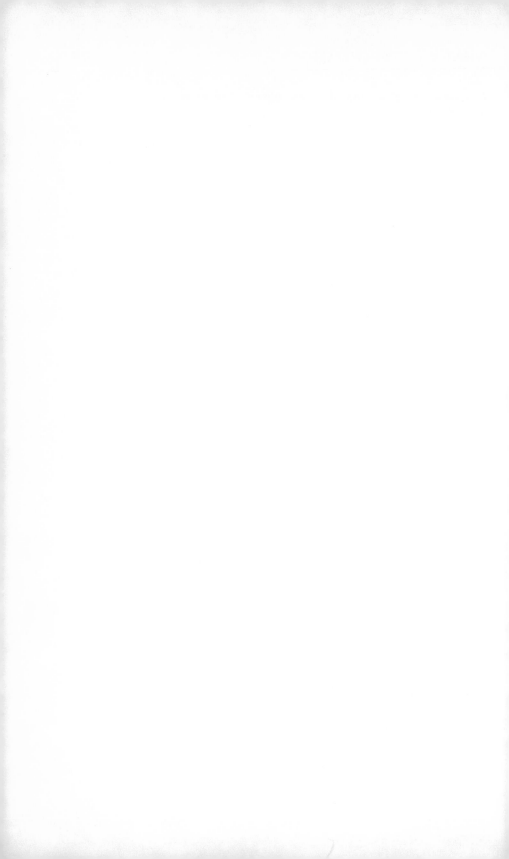

# List of Participants

Dr PJ Anderson, Head of Laboratory, Unilever Research Port Sunlight Laboratory, Bebington, UK.

Dr RA Badley, Biochemistry, Unilever Research Colworth Laboratory, Sharnbrook, UK.

Dr S Bayley-Gibson, Cell Biology, Unilever Research Colworth Laboratory, Sharnbrook, UK.

Mr RK Beerthuis, Background Research Coordination, Unilever Research Vlaardingen Laboratory, Netherlands.

Prof Dr DW van Bekkum, TNO, Rijswijk, Netherlands.

Dr DC Bennett, Imperial Cancer Research Fund, London, UK.

Dr M Bernfield, Stanford University, Stanford, USA.

Dr J van den Biggelaar, Zoological Laboratory, Utrecht, Netherlands.

Prof Dr IL Bonta, Erasmus Universiteit, Rotterdam, Netherlands.

Prof Dr D Bootsma, Erasmus Universiteit, Rotterdam, Netherlands.

Prof BB Boycott, Kings College, London, UK.

Prof G Boyd, Edinburgh University, Edinburgh, UK.

Dr EM Bradbury, School of Medicine, Davis, U.S.A.

Dr R Bravo, Div. of Biostructure, Arhus, Denmark.

Dr RF Brooks, Imperial Cancer Research Fund, London, UK.

Mr. JN Brouwer, Taste Perception, URL, Vlaardingen, Netherlands.

Mr P Brown, Academic Press, London, UK.

Prof R Brown, Dalhousie University, Halifax, Canada.

Prof RM Brown, University of North Carolina, Chapel Hill, USA.

Dr JE Celis, Div. of Biochemistry, Arhus, Denmark.

Dr EJ Christ, Biochemistry, Unilever Research Vlaardingen Laboratory, Netherlands.

Dr JR Couchman Cell Biology, Unilever Research Colworth Laboratory, Sharnbrook, UK.

Dr D Critchley, University of Leicester, UK.

Dr BA Cross, Institute of Animal Physiology, Babraham, Cambridge, UK.

Dr MJ Crumpton, Imperial Cancer Research Fund, London, UK.
Dr G Dunn, Strangeways Research Laboratory, Cambridge, UK.
Dr L Edens, DNA Recombinant Research, Unilever Research Vlaardingen Laboratory, Netherlands.
Dr PS Ellington, Business Member Research Division Executive, Unilever Limited, London, UK.
Dr DJ Frost, Secretary Research Division Executive, Unilever Limited, London, UK.
Dr U Gehring, Institute of Biological Chemistry, Heidelberg, Germany.
Dr DL Georgala, Head of Laboratory, Unilever Research Colworth Laboratory, Sharnbrook, UK.
Dr WT Gibson, Cell Biology, Unilever Research Colworth Laboratory, Sharnbrook, UK.
Dr GW Gould, Bacteriology, Unilever Research Colworth Laboratory, Sharnbrook, UK.
Dr R Grand, University of Birmingham, Birmingham, UK.
Mr EHM Greuell, Biosciences, Unilever Research Vlaardingen Laboratory, Netherlands.
Prof Dr K Halbrock, University, Freiburg, Germany.
Dr T Hardingham, Kennedy Institute of Rheumatology, London, UK.
Dr J Heath, Strangeways Research Laboratory, Cambridge, UK.
Dr S Higgins, University of Leeds, Leeds, UK.
Dr WPM Hoekstra, Vakgroep Moleculaire Celbiologie, Utrecht, Netherlands.
Dr B Hogan, Imperial Cancer Research Fund, London, UK.
Dr M Hook, University of Alabama, Birmingham, USA.
Dr F ten Hoor, Pathophysiology, Unilever Research Vlaardingen Laboratory, Netherlands.
Prof CRHopkins, University of Liverpool, Liverpool, UK.
Dr D Housman, Massachusetts Institute of Technology, Boston, USA.
Mr JM Hubert, Administrative Member Research Division Executive, Unilever Limited, London, UK.
Dr RC Hughes, MRC National Institute for Medical Research, London, UK.
Dr SG Hughes, Molecular Genetics, Unilever Research Colworth Laboratory, Sharnbrook, UK.
Dr T Hunt, University of Cambridge, Cambridge, UK.
Dr WP James, Dunn Nutrition Unit, Cambridge, UK.
Prof Dr H Jansz, Laboratory for Physiological Chemistry, Utrecht, Netherlands.
Dr LH Jones, Botany, Unilever Research Colworth Laboratory, Sharnbrook, UK.
Mr R Kenworthy, Veterinary Medicine, Unilever Research Colworth Laboratory, Sharnbrook, UK.

Mr R Keuning, Member Management Committee, Unilever Research Vlaardingen Laboratory, Netherlands.
Dr AD Krikorian, State University, New York, USA.
Dr M Kurkinen, University of Helsinki, Helsinki, Finland.
Dr A Ledeboer, DNA Recombinant Research, Unilever Research Vlaardingen Laboratory, Netherlands.
Dr CW Lloyd, Cell Biology, Unilever Research Colworth Laboratory, Sharnbrook, UK.
Prof HF Lodish, Massachusetts Institute of Technology, Boston, USA.
Dr J Maat, DNA, Recombinant Research, Unilever Research Vlaardingen Laboratory, Netherlands.
Mr T McCallum, Public Relations Dept., Unilever Limited, London, UK.
Prof Dr M van Montagu, State University Gent, Gent, Belgium.
Dr A Mottura-Rollier, Istituto di Biologia Generale, Milan, Italy.
Dr H Muir, Kennedy Institute of Rheumatology, London. UK.
Dr P Newmark, Nature, London. UK.
Prof D HJJ Nijkamp, Vrije Universiteit, Amsterdam, Netherlands.
Dr DH Nugteren, Lipid Biochemistry, Unilever Research Vlaardingen Laboratory, Netherlands.
Dr B Obrink, University of Uppsala, Uppsala, Sweden.
Dr FJG van der Ouderaa, Protein Chemistry, Unilever Research Vlaardingen Laboratory, Netherlands.
Dr M Parker, Imperial Cancer Research Fund, London, UK.
Dr DC Peters, Biotechnology, Unilever Research Port Sunlight Laboratory, Bebington, UK.
Dr P Porter, Immunology, Unilever Research Colworth Laboratory, Sharnbrook, UK.
Dr C Prottey, Skin Research, Unilever Research Port Sunlight Laboratory, Bebington, UK.
Dr RS Quatrano, Oregon State University, Corvallis, USA.
Prof M Raff, University College of London, London, UK.
Prof J Schell, State University Gent, Gent, Belgium.
Dr J Scholes, MRC Cell Biophysics Unit, London, UK.
Dr R Shields, Cell Biology, Unilever Research Colworth Laboratory, Sharnbrook, UK.
Dr AR Slabas, Lipid Biochemistry, Unilever Research Colworth Laboratory, Sharnbrook, UK.
Dr C Smart, Member Management Committee, Unilever Research Port Sunlight Laboratory, Bebington, UK.
Dr EM Southern, MRC Mammalian Genome Unit, Edinburgh, UK.
Dr L Sperling, Centre de Genetique, Gif-sur-Yvette, France.
Dr RA Steinberg, University of Connecticut, Storrs, USA.
Prof FC Steward, Charlottesville, USA.

Dr P Thorogood, University of Southampton, Southampton, UK.
Dr BP Toole, Dept. of Medicine, Harvard Medical School, Boston, USA.
Dr J Tooze, EMBO, Heidelberg, Germany.
Dr P Uster, University of California, Davis, USA.
Mr KH, Veldhuis, Research Director, Unilever NV, Rotterdam.
Dr AJ Vergroesen, Nutrition, Unilever Research Vlaardingen Laboratory, Netherlands.
Dr CT Verrips, DNA Recombinant Research, Unilever Research Vlaardingen Laboratory, Netherlands.
Mr H Vonkeman, Skin Research, Unilever Research Port Sunlight Laboratory, Bebington, UK.
Prof Dr O Vos. Erasmus Universiteit, Rotterdam, Netherlands.
Prof Dr A de Waard, Sylvius Laboratories, Leiden, Netherlands.
Dr MC Weiss, Centre de Genetique, Gif-sur-Yvette, France.
Mr H van der Wel, Taste Perception, URL, Vlaardingen, Netherlands.
Dr EJ Welsh, Skin Research, Unilever Research Colworth Laboratory, Sharnbrook, UK.
Dr J Williams, Imperial Cancer Research Fund, London, UK.
Dr G Wilson, Biochemistry, Unilever Research Colworth Laboratory, Sharnbrook, UK.
Prof L Wolpert, Middlesex Hospital Medical School, London, UK.
Prof M Yeoman, Edinburgh University, Edinburgh, UK.

**Advisory Scientific Committee**
Prof Dr J Boldingh, Gravenzande, Netherlands.
Prof BS Hartley, Imperial College, London, UK.
Prof DA Rees, Unilever Research Colworth Laboratory, Sharnbrook, UK.
Prof Dr A Rorsch, TNO, Den Haag, Netherlands.
Prof Dr EC Slater, BCP Jansen Institute, Amsterdam, Netherlands.

**Unilever Planning and Coordination**
Prof Dr WJ Beek, Head of Laboratory, Unilever Research Vlaardingen Laboratory, Netherlands.
Mr RK Beerthuis, Background Research Coordination, Unilever Research Vlaardingen Laboratory, Netherlands.
Dr EJ Christ, Unilever Research Vlaardingen Laboratory, Netherlands.
Mr G van Hattem, Unilever NV, Rotterdam, Netherlands.
Dr HJ Heinrich, Unilever NV, Rotterdam, Netherlands.
Prof DA Rees, Unilever Research Colworth Laboratory, Sharnbrook, UK.
Mrs DL Wedderburn, International Affairs Department, Unilever UK. Central Resources Limited, London. UK.